Oral Pathology for the
DENTAL HYGIENIST

Oral Pathology for the DENTAL HYGIENIST

Olga A.C. Ibsen, RDH, MS

Adjunct Professor, University of New Haven
West Haven, Connecticut
Adjunct Professor, Department of Oral Pathology
New York University College of Dentistry
New York, New York

Joan Andersen Phelan, DDS

Professor and Chair, Department of Oral Pathology
New York University College of Dentistry
New York, New York

FOURTH EDITION

SAUNDERS
An Imprint of Elsevier

SAUNDERS
An Imprint of Elsevier

11830 Westline Industrial Drive
St. Louis, Missouri 63146

ORAL PATHOLOGY FOR THE DENTAL HYGIENIST,
  FOURTH EDITION

NOTICE

Dental hygiene is an ever-changing field. Standard safety precautions must be followed, but as new
research and clinical experience broaden our knowledge, changes in treatment and drug therapy may
become necessary or appropriate. Readers are advised to check the most current product information provided by the manufacturer of each drug to be administered to verify the recommended dose,
the method and duration of administration, and contraindications. It is the responsibility of the li-
censed prescriber, relying on experience and knowledge of the patient, to determine dosages and the
best treatment for each individual patient. Neither the publisher nor the author assumes any liabil-
ity for any injury and/or damage to persons or property arising from this publication.

Previous editions copyrighted 2000, 1996, 1992

Acquisitions Editor: **Penny Rudolph**
Developmental Editor: **Shirley Kuhn**
Publishing Services Manager: **Linda McKinley**
Project Manager: **Ellen Kunkelmann**
Design Manager: **Gail Morey Hudson**
Cover Design: **M-W Design, Inc.**

ISBN-13: 978-0-7216-9946-2

ISBN-10: 0-7216-9946-4

Printed in the United States of America

Last digit is the print number: 9 8 7 6 5

Dedication

To
Shirley Kuhn
Our editor and friend at Elsevier
for her dedication, sincere interest, and guidance
through all four editions of
Oral Pathology for the Dental Hygienist.

We thank her for her support,
expertise, and encouragement.

We are indeed most grateful to Shirley for her support
through the years.

Contributors

Anthony J. Casino, DDS
Clinical Associate Professor
Department of Oral and Maxillofacial Surgery
School of Dental Medicine
State University of New York at Stony Brook
Chief, Division of Oral and Maxillofacial Surgery
Department of Dentistry
University Medical Center at Stony Brook
Chief, Section of Oral and Maxillofacial Surgery
Department of Veterans Affairs Medical Center
Northport, New York
Diseases Affecting the Temporomandibular Joint

Margaret J. Fehrenbach, RDH, MS
Adjunct Faculty, Dental Hygiene Program
Marquette University Dental School
Milwaukee, Wisconsin
Inflammation and Repair; Immunity

Kenneth E. Fleisher, DDS
Assistant Professor
Oral and Maxillofacial Surgery
New York University College of Dentistry
New York, New York
Assistant Professor
Oral and Maxillofacial Surgery
Bellevue Hospital Center
New York, New York
Diseases Affecting the Temporomandibular Joint

Paul D. Freedman, DDS
Director, Section of Oral Pathology
The New York Hospital Medical Center of Queens
Director, Oral Pathology Laboratory
Flushing, New York
Neoplasia

Joen Iannucci Haring, DDS, MS
Professor of Clinical Dentistry
Section of Primary Care
Director, Sterilization Monitoring Service
The Ohio State University College of Dentistry
Columbus, Ohio
Developmental Disorders

Olga A.C. Ibsen, RDH, MS
Adjunct Professor, University of New Haven
West Haven, Connecticut
Adjunct Professor, Department of Oral Pathology
New York University College of Dentistry
New York, New York
*Introduction to Preliminary Diagnosis of Oral
Lesions; Developmental Disorders; Nonneoplastic
Diseases of Bone; Oral Manifestations of Systemic
Diseases*

Anne Cale Jones, DDS
Professor, The University of Texas Health Science
Center at San Antonio
San Antonio, Texas
Neoplasia; Nonneoplastic Diseases of Bone

Joan Andersen Phelan, DDS
Professor and Chair, Department of Oral Pathology
New York University College of Dentistry
New York, New York
*Inflammation and Repair; Immunity; Infectious
Diseases; Neoplasia; Nonneoplastic Diseases of
Bone; Oral Manifestations of Systemic Diseases*

Heddie O. Sedano, DDS, Dr. Odont.
Professor Emeritus, University of Minnesota
Lecturer, Pediatric Dentistry and Oral Diagnosis
School of Dentistry
University of California, Los Angeles
Los Angeles, California
Genetics

Anthony T. Vernillo, DDS, PhD
Professor of Oral Pathology
Associate Coordinator
Teaching Program for Oral Medicine and Pathology
New York University College of Dentistry
New York, New York
Oral Manifestations of Systemic Diseases

Contributors to the New CD-ROM

Sandra D'Amato-Palumbo, RDH, MPS
Assistant Professor and Director
Department of Dental Hygiene
University of New Haven
West Haven, Connecticut

Olga A.C. Ibsen, RDH, MS
Adjunct Professor, University of New Haven
West Haven, Connecticut
Adjunct Professor, Department of Oral Pathology
New York University College of Dentistry
New York, New York

Joan Andersen Phelan, DDS
Professor and Chair, Department of Oral Pathology
New York University College of Dentistry
New York, New York

We are delighted to have made some exciting changes in this edition, which we hope will contribute significantly to the teaching and learning process of oral pathology. This edition includes 10 chapters. We reorganized the information already in the text to make the material easier to teach and learn. In previous editions, Chapter 3, "Immunology," was a very long chapter. This edition breaks the information into two chapters: Chapter 3, "Immunity," and Chapter 4, "Infectious Diseases." A chapter on nonneoplastic bone diseases (Chapter 8) was also added. The bone diseases included in this chapter were formerly scattered throughout the text. We believe the new reorganization of material into these chapters provides for an easy flow of text information that is appropriately organized and less overwhelming.

We received enthusiastic responses from faculty and students on the full-color clinical illustrations throughout the text in the third edition. Our goal has always been to facilitate teaching and learning. The third edition was meant to serve two purposes—to become an oral pathology resource text as well as a color atlas. In this fourth edition, we are delighted to present the entire text in *full color!* All photomicrographs are now in color, in addition to the clinical illustrations and appropriate anatomic drawings. Without a doubt, the color photomicrographs will make the microscopic appearance of the lesions easier to understand.

Each chapter has been updated with vocabulary, terminology, and references. All questions at the end of each chapter now offer five selections for answers. We hope that this format will assist the student in preparing for National Board Examinations. Additionally, the CD of case studies included in the text presents the text material in another format to assist the learning process. Summaries at the end of chapters briefly outline the most critical information pertinent to each lesion, disease, or condition, thus providing a quick reference that can be used in the clinical setting.

We hope that this *full-color* oral pathology text, specifically written for dental hygienists, will continue to provide dental hygienists with the highest-standard oral pathology text and that instructors will use it in other courses, such as radiology, oral histology, and all clinical courses. Dental hygienists have earned a reputation for excellence in identifying abnormal oral findings. The integration of oral pathology throughout the dental hygiene curriculum ensures more comprehensive patient care by the student and the dental hygiene practitioner.

Olga A.C. Ibsen, RDH, MS
Joan Andersen Phelan, DDS

Acknowledgments

Through the years, many individuals have contributed to the success of *Oral Pathology for the Dental Hygienist.*

Shirley Kuhn, our Editor at Elsevier, has nagged, supported, and cajoled us through all four editions. We sincerely appreciate her guidance and encouragement and are delighted to dedicate this fourth edition to her. Congratulations and thank you, Shirley!

Helaine Tobin, our Developmental Editor, worked with us on the third and fourth editions. We thank her for "pulling it all together"! We are also grateful to Penny Rudolph, our newly "acquired" Editor, for taking care of all the details. Ellen Kunkelmann, Project Manager at Elsevier, guided us through the final stages in the production process.

We acknowledge Dr. William Forbes from Dover-Foxcroft, Maine, and Dr. Elias Kopti from Fargo, North Dakota, who provided detailed critiques of the first and second editions. It was Dr. Kopti who recommended that we include the valuable summaries at the end of each chapter.

We will always be grateful to our Oral Pathology teachers: Drs. Melvin Blake, Ernest Baden, Leon Eisenbud, Paul Freedman, Stanley Kerpel, Harry Lumerman, Michael Marder, James Sciubba, Philip Silverstein, Marshal Solomon, David Zegarelli, and Edward V. Zegarelli. Olga A.C. Ibsen is especially grateful to two individuals who influenced her personal and professional life: her dad, the late Dr. Joseph A. Cuttita, and her godfather, the late Dr. Edward V. Zegarelli. All of these individuals strongly influenced our passion for pathology!

In addition to being a mentor, role model, and outstanding educator, Dr. Edward V. Zegarelli shared his expertise and extensive library of color illustrations. He truly influenced our quest to develop an oral pathology text for dental hygienists. We dedicated the last edition to him. He was indeed a legend. His legacy in oral pathology will live on. We truly miss him.

Gloria Turner of the Diagnostic Pathology Laboratory at NYU College of Dentistry prepared most of the slides used for the color photomicrographs that enhance the fourth edition of *Oral Pathology for the Dental Hygienist.* We extend our sincere appreciation for her outstanding work. Additionally, color photomicrographs were also provided by the Oral Pathology Laboratory, Inc., Flushing, New York.

Sandra D'Amato-Palumbo, RDH, MPS, Director of Dental Hygiene, University of New Haven, contributed significantly to the preparation of the CD of case studies in this edition. Thank you, Sandra, for your expertise and significant contribution to this teaching and learning tool.

Finally, we thank our husbands, Lawrence and Jerry, who have assisted us in innumerable ways. We extend special thanks, appreciation, and love for their support.

We are proud to present the fourth edition of *Oral Pathology for the Dental Hygienist.*

Olga A.C. Ibsen, RDH, MS
Joan Andersen Phelan, DDS

About This Edition

The fourth edition of *Oral Pathology for the Dental Hygienist* enjoys all the same features as earlier editions, along with some new components that further enhance this text as a very effective learning and teaching tool.

See what is new in the fourth edition:

- *All* clinical illustrations, photomicrographs, and line drawings are now in full color. Color photomicrographs are sure to make identifying the microscopic appearance of lesions easier and more meaningful for students.
- Case studies are presented on a CD-ROM to help students master much-needed critical thinking skills that they will need when working in the clinical setting.
- A chapter on nonneoplastic bone diseases has been added.
- Information previously covered in the "Immunology" chapter has been separated into two chapters. Chapter 3 covers immunology and immunologic diseases, and Chapter 4 discusses infectious diseases.
- An electronic image collection of more than 400 full-color clinical oral pathology photos and photomicrographs, plus 50 case studies, is also available.

Other outstanding features include:

- Each chapter begins with a list of objectives that provides an overview of what is covered in the chapter. These objectives clearly define what the student is expected to learn and guide the faculty in test question preparation.
- New vocabulary words along with definitions and pronunciations are presented at the beginning of each chapter to help students learn essential new dental terminology to help them perform effectively in the classroom as well as in the clinical setting.
- Each chapter concludes with a very useful synopsis that briefly outlines the most critical information pertinent to each lesion, disease, or condition discussed in the chapter. This handy feature enables students to review all the disorders discussed in the chapter at a glance. This also serves as a quick reference for practicing hygienists in the clinical setting.
- Review questions at the end of each chapter help students test their knowledge of the chapter material and serve as good practice for taking the national board exam. All questions now have five selections for answers, consistent with the national exam.
- Answers to the review questions are provided at the end of the book to provide immediate feedback.
- An extended list of references appears at the end of each chapter. References have been updated in this edition to reflect new research.
- A comprehensive glossary at the end of the text provides easy access to the definitions of all the vocabulary words.

Contents

CHAPTER 3:

Immunity

Margaret J. Fehrenbach
Joan A. Phelan

Introduction to Preliminary Diagnosis of Oral Lesions

Olga A.C. Ibsen

Objectives

After studying this chapter, the student will be able to:

1. Define each of the terms in the vocabulary list for this chapter.
2. List and define the eight diagnostic categories that contribute to the diagnostic process.
3. Name a diagnostic category and give an example of a lesion, anomaly, or condition for which this category greatly contributes to the diagnosis.
4. Describe the clinical appearance of Fordyce granules (spots), torus palatinus, mandibular tori, and lingual varicosities, and identify them in the clinical setting or on a clinical photograph.
5. Describe the radiographic appearance and historical data (including the age, sex, and race of the patient) that are relevant to periapical cemento-osseous dysplasia (cementoma).
6. Define "variant of normal" and give three examples of such lesions involving the tongue.
7. List and describe the clinical characteristics and identify a clinical picture of fissured tongue, median rhomboid glossitis, geographic tongue, ectopic geographic tongue, and hairy tongue.
8. Describe the clinical and histologic differences between leukoedema and linea alba.

Vocabulary

Clinical Appearance of Soft Tissue Lesions

Bulla (adjective, bullous; plural, bullae) A circumscribed, elevated lesion that is more than 5 mm in diameter, usually contains serous fluid, and looks like a blister.

Lobule (adjective, lobulated) A segment or lobe that is a part of the whole; these lobes sometimes appear fused together **(Figure 1-1).**

Macule An area that is usually distinguished by a color different from that of the surrounding tissue; it is flat and does not protrude above the surface of the normal tissue. A freckle is an example of a macule.

Papule A small, circumscribed lesion usually less than 1 cm in diameter that is elevated or protrudes above the surface of normal surrounding tissue.

Pedunculated Attached by a stemlike or stalk base similar to that of a mushroom **(Figure 1-2).**

Pustules Variously sized circumscribed elevations containing pus.

Sessile Describing the base of a lesion that is flat or broad instead of stemlike **(Figure 1-3).**

Vesicle A small, elevated lesion less than 1 cm in diameter that contains serous fluid.

Figure 1-1 Lobulated torus palatinus.

Figure 1-2 Fibroma with a pedunculated base. Arrow points to the stemlike base.

Soft Tissue Consistency

Nodule A palpable solid lesion up to 1 cm in diameter found in soft tissue; it can occur above, level with, or beneath the skin surface.

Palpation The evaluation of a lesion by feeling it with the fingers to determine the texture of the area; the descriptive terms for palpation are *soft, firm, semifirm,* and *fluid filled;* these terms also describe the consistency of a lesion.

Color of Lesion

Colors Red, pink, salmon, white, blue-black, gray, brown, and black are the colors used most frequently to describe oral lesions; they can be used to identify specific lesions and may also be incorporated into general descriptions.

Erythema An abnormal redness of the mucosa or gingiva.

Pallor Paleness of the skin or mucosal tissues.

Size of Lesion

Centimeter (cm) One hundredth of a meter; equivalent to a little less than one-half inch (0.393 of an inch) **(Figure 1-4).**

Millimeter (mm) One thousandth of a meter (a meter is equivalent to 39.3 inches); the periodontal probe is of great assistance in documenting the size or diameter of a lesion that can be measured in millimeters (general terms such as small, medium, or large are sometimes used, but these terms are not as specific) **(Figure 1-5).**

Surface Texture

Corrugated Wrinkled.

Fissure A cleft or groove, normal or otherwise, showing prominent depth.

Papillary Resembling small, nipple-shaped projections or elevations found in clusters.

Smooth, rough, folded Terms used to describe the surface texture of a lesion.

Radiographic Terms Used to Describe Lesions in Bone

Coalescence The process by which parts of a whole join together, or fuse, to make one.

Diffuse Describes a lesion with borders that are not well defined, making it impossible to detect the exact parameters of the lesion; this may make treatment more difficult and, depending on the biopsy results, more radical **(Figure 1-6).**

Multilocular Describes a lesion that extends beyond the confines of one distinct area and is defined as many lobes or parts that are somewhat fused together, making up the entire lesion; a multilocular radiolucency is sometimes described as resembling soap bubbles; an odontogenic keratocyst often presents as a multilocular, radiolucent lesion **(Figure 1-7).**

Radiolucent Describes the black or dark areas on a radiograph; radiant energy can pass through these structures; less dense tissue, such as the pulp, is seen as a radiolucent structure **(Figure 1-8).**

Figure 1-3 Fibroma with a sessile base.

Figure 1-4 A ruler measuring centimeters is used to measure all specimens submitted for microscopic examination.

Figure 1-5 **A,** Probe measuring the diameter of a fibroma with a sessile base. **B,** Gutta-percha point used to explore a radiographic defect. **C,** Periodontal probe placed before a radiograph.

Radiolucent and radiopaque Terms used to describe a mixture of light and dark areas within a lesion usually denoting a stage in the lesion's development; for example, in a stage I periapical cemento-osseous dysplasia (cementoma) **(Figure 1-9, *A*),** the lesion is radiolucent; in stage II it is radiolucent and radiopaque **(Figure 1-9, *B*).**

Radiopaque Describes the light or white area on a radiograph that results from the inability of radiant energy to pass through the structure; the more dense the structure, the more light or white it appears on the radiograph; this is illustrated in **Figure 1-10.**

Root resorption Observed radiographically when the apex of the tooth appears shortened or blunted and ir-

Figure 1-6 Squamous cell carcinoma of the hard palate showing diffuse borders. (Courtesy Drs. Paul Freedman and Stanley Kerpel.)

Figure 1-7 Odontogenic keratocyst *(arrow),* illustrating a multilocular lesion. (Courtesy Dr. Victor M. Sternberg.)

regularly shaped; it occurs as a response to stimuli, which can include a cyst, tumor, or trauma; **Figure 1-11** illustrates resorption of the roots as a result of a rapid orthodontic procedure (see Figure 1-27); external resorption arises from tissues outside the tooth, such as the periodontal ligament, whereas internal resorption is triggered by pulpal tissue reaction from within the tooth; in the latter the pulpal area can be seen as a diffuse radiolucency beyond the confines of the normal pulp area.

Scalloping around the root A radiolucent lesion that extends between the roots, as seen in a traumatic bone cyst; this lesion appears to extend up the periodontal ligament **(Figure 1-12).**

Unilocular Having one compartment or unit that is well defined or outlined as in a simple radicular cyst **(Figure 1-13).**

Well circumscribed Term used to describe a lesion with borders that are specifically defined and in which one can clearly see the exact margins and extent **(Figure 1-14).**

Figure 1-8 Prominent pulp chambers, horns, and canals in mandibular molars.

Figure 1-9 **A,** Stage I periapical cemento-osseous dysplasia (cementoma). **B,** Stage II periapical cementoosseous dysplasia (cementoma).

Figure 1-10 Amalgam restorations on the occlusal surfaces of the maxillary and mandibular molars.

Figure 1-11 Resorption of the roots on maxillary anteriors as a result of rapid orthodontic movement.

Figure 1-12 Traumatic bone cyst around the roots. (Courtesy Drs. Paul Freedman and Stanley Kerpel.)

Figure 1-14 Well-circumscribed median palatal cyst.

Figure 1-13 Radicular cyst at the apex of the maxillary lateral incisor illustrating a unilocular lesion.

To understand the material in this text, it is imperative that the reader approaches the material in a systematic manner. Significant time is spent in the dental hygiene curriculum identifying and describing normal structures. Before one can identify the abnormal condition, it is necessary to have a solid understanding of the basic and dental sciences, such as human anatomy and physiology, histology, and dental anatomy. Once one has a solid understanding of normal structures and those that are variants of normal, findings that deviate from normal and pathologic conditions are more easily recognized. The preliminary evaluation and description of these lesions are within the scope of dental hygiene practice and are truly among the most challenging experiences in clinical practice.

In the first part of this chapter, the definitions of commonly used terms that describe the clinical and radiographic features of a lesion, including terms used for normal, variants of normal, and pathologic conditions discussed throughout this text, are presented. The reader is encouraged to use these terms in the clinical setting so that they become part of an everyday professional vocabulary, thereby facilitating communication between the hygienist and other dental practitioners in the clinical setting.

The second part of this chapter focuses on the eight diagnostic categories that provide a systematic approach to the preliminary evaluation of oral lesions. Each area is described, and the strength of that area in the diagnostic process is illustrated using specific examples of lesions.

The final part of the chapter includes conditions that are considered variants of normal and those that are benign conditions of unknown cause. Most are diagnosed from their distinct clinical appearance and history.

The Diagnostic Process

MAKING A DIAGNOSIS

How is a diagnosis made? What are the essential components? The answers to these questions begin with data collection. The process of diagnosis requires gathering information that is relevant to the patient and the lesion being evaluated; this information comes from various sources.

Certain distinct diagnostic categories should be thought of as pieces in a puzzle—each piece playing a significant role in the final diagnosis. The eight categories that contribute segments of information leading to the definitive or final diagnosis are (1) clinical, (2) radiographic, (3) historical, (4) laboratory, (5) microscopic, (6) surgical, (7) therapeutic, and (8) differential findings. It is important to note that usually one area alone does not provide sufficient information to make a diagnosis; the strength of the diagnosis is often derived from one or two areas. As the reader becomes more aware of the diseases and conditions discussed in this text, it will be most helpful to use the diagnostic categories as a guide to the evaluation of a lesion.

Clinical Diagnosis

Clinical diagnosis suggests that the strength of the diagnosis comes from the clinical appearance of the lesion. By observing the area in a well-illuminated clinical setting and palpating the area if necessary, the clinician can establish a diagnosis for some lesions based on color, shape, location, and history of the lesion. Because a diagnosis can be made based on these unique clinical features, biopsy or surgical intervention is not necessary. Examples of lesions that can be clinically diagnosed are Fordyce granules **(Figure 1-15)**, torus palatinus **(Figure 1-16)**, mand-

Figure 1-15 Fordyce granules.

Figure 1-16 Lobulated torus palatinus. (Courtesy Dr. Edward V. Zegarelli.)

ibular tori **(Figure 1-17)**, melanin pigmentation **(Figure 1-18)**, retrocuspid papillae **(Figure 1-19)**, and lingual varicosities. These lesions are described later in this chapter.

Other benign conditions of unknown cause that are recognized by their distinct clinical appearance include fissured tongue **(Figure 1-20)**, median rhomboid glossitis **(Figure 1-21)**, geographic

Figure 1-17 Arrows point to mandibular tori.

Figure 1-18 Melanin pigmentation.

Figure 1-19 Arrows point to the retrocuspid papillae on the gingival margin of the lingual aspect of the mandibular cuspids.

Figure 1-20 Fissured tongue.

Figure 1-21 Median rhomboid glossitis *(top arrow)* and geographic tongue *(bottom arrows)*.

Figure 1-22 Geographic tongue. Arrows point to areas of depapillation.

tongue **(Figure 1-22)**, and hairy tongue **(Figure 1-23,** *A* to *C*)**.** These conditions are also discussed later in this chapter.

Sometimes the diagnostic process requires historical information in addition to the clinical findings. For example, an amalgam tattoo can be observed as a blue-to-gray patch on the gingiva or mucosa where an amalgam restoration is or has been located **(Figure 1-24).** Although this condition is usually easily observed and a clinical diagnosis made, any history involving the area can still be very helpful in confirming the clinical impression. The patient in Figure 1-24 had root canal therapy and a retrograde amalgam on a deciduous tooth. The amalgam tattoo is observed in the apical area of the permanent cen-

Figure 1-23 A, White hairy tongue. **B,** White hairy tongue showing a circumvallate papilla *(arrow).* **C,** Black hairy tongue.

tral incisor; no evidence of an amalgam restoration exists in the entire anterior area. The history helped confirm the clinical diagnosis.

Radiographic Diagnosis

In a radiographic diagnosis, the radiograph provides sufficient information to establish the diagnosis. Although additional clinical and historical information may contribute, the diagnosis is obtained from the radiograph. Conditions for which the radiograph provides the most significant information include periapical pathosis (PAP) (**Figure 1-25**, *A* and *B*), internal resorption (**Figure 1-26**), external resorption (**Figure 1-27**), heavy interproximal calculus (**Figure 1-28**), dental caries (**Figure 1-29**, *A* to *C*), compound odontoma (**Figure 1-30**), complex odontoma (**Figure 1-31**, *A* and *B*), supernumerary teeth (**Figure 1-32**, *A* and *B*), impacted or unerupted teeth (**Figure 1-33**, *A* and *B*), and calcified pulp (**Figure 1-34**). Normal anatomic landmarks are also easily observed radiographically. In some cases the radiograph may show very distinct and well-defined structures, such as the nutrient canals seen in **Figure 1-35**, *A* and *B*, and the mixed dentition seen in Figure 1-35, *C*. Unusual radiographic findings are illustrated in **Figure 1-36**, *A* to *K*.

Text continued on p. 19

Figure 1-24 Arrow points to an amalgam tattoo at the apical area of the patient's maxillary right central incisor. This patient had a root canal procedure on a deciduous tooth. No other amalgam restoration is in the area; therefore it was helpful to know the patient's past dental history to confirm this diagnosis.

A **B**

Figure 1-25 A, Periapical pathosis (PAP); a radiolucency is seen at the apex of the mandibular second premolar. **B,** In another patient a fistula is seen on the maxillary lateral incisor. A fistula is usually an indication of PAP. When a fistula is observed clinically, a radiograph is necessary for diagnostic and treatment purposes.

Figure 1-26 Arrow points to the area of internal resorption on the maxillary first molar.

Figure 1-28 Heavy interproximal calculus.

Figure 1-27 External resorption on a mandibular central incisor. (Courtesy Dr. Gerald P. Curatola.)

A

Figure 1-29 A, Dental caries. The reader should observe the interproximal radiolucencies. Clinical examination is necessary to confirm the involvement of some of the areas. **B,** Periapical radiograph taken September 1989. A subtle carious area can be seen on the distal aspect of the mandibular second premolar. **C,** The patient in **B** was seen in June 1990. During the scaling procedure, a defect on the distal aspect of the mandibular second premolar was detected. This vertical bite-wing radiograph was taken. The reader should note the definite radiolucent, carious area on the distal aspect of the mandibular second premolar. This example emphasizes the need for careful clinical and radiographic evaluation. (**B** and **C,** Courtesy Dr. Victor M. Sternberg.)

B

C

Figure 1-30   Arrow points to compound odontoma.

Figure 1-31 **A,** Complex odontoma rather easily diagnosed from the radiograph alone. **B,** Complex odontoma not diagnosed from the radiograph alone. (**B,** Courtesy Drs. Paul Freedman and Stanley Kerpel.)

Figure 1-32 **A,** Mesiodens. A supernumerary tooth is located between the maxillary central incisors. **B,** A radiograph showing a supernumerary mandibular premolar *(arrow)* surrounded by a radiolucent area diagnosed as a dentigerous cyst. Clinically this area was thought to be a mandibular torus (until the radiograph was taken).

Figure 1-33 A, Impacted mandibular cuspid. **B,** Impacted maxillary cuspid.

Figure 1-34 Calcified pulp in the mandibular first molar.

Figure 1-35 A, Nutrient canals in the anterior maxillary arch. **B,** Nutrient canals in the mandibular anterior area. **C,** The mixed dentition of a 5-year-old child is observed in this radiograph.

Figure 1-36 A, Arrow points to a 7-carat cubic zirconia (a round stone) that was glued to this patient's maxillary left central incisor. **B,** The radiopaque area on the distal aspect of the mandibular second premolar *(arrow)* is an amalgam fragment. There was a subtle clinical amalgam tattoo in the interproximal papilla that was not detected or charted on initial examination, which included a full-mouth series of radiographs and incomplete scaling. When the radiographs were viewed after the patient was dismissed, the radiopaque area was thought to be the tip of a broken instrument. Further evaluation of the instruments used at that appointment ruled out the possibility of a broken instrument. When the patient returned for an additional appointment 2 weeks later, another radiograph, using the same long cone and precision Rinn instruments, was taken of the area. The radiopaque fragment remained in the exact same place. Clinically a very close look at the interproximal papilla in the area then revealed a subtle bluish-black area. The dentist surgically slit the papilla on the buccal aspect and revealed the amalgam particle. **C,** This patient wore wide-framed eyeglasses during the radiographic procedure. The arrow points to a **U**-shaped radiopacity from the eyeglass frame. **D,** This radiograph reveals an obvious radiopaque overhang from the amalgam restoration on the distal aspect of the mandibular first molar.

Continued

Figure 1-36, cont'd E, Instruments from a root canal procedure were broken in these two maxillary lateral incisors *(arrows)*. **F,** The broken tip of a curet *(arrow)* is observed as a radiopaque area on the distal aspect of the maxillary first premolar. **G,** The arrow points to a retained deciduous tooth with an amalgam restoration. **H,** The arrow points to a radiopaque area that identifies a retained shotgun pellet on the distal aspect of the mandibular third molar. **I,** The arrow points to a radiopaque circular area that is a nose ring.

Figure 1-36, cont'd J, Periapical radiograph showing a radiopaque area at the apex of the mesial root of the mandibular second molar. This object was a retained piece of shrapnel. **K,** A panoramic radiograph of the same patient showing the same object. This radiograph gives a more accurate view of the location of the object. It was found to be in the soft tissue in the area and not within bone.

Figure 1-37 A, One of the clinical appearances of amelogenesis imperfecta. **B,** The radiographic aspect of amelogenesis imperfecta. (Courtesy Dr. Edward V. Zegarelli.)

Historical Diagnosis

Historical data constitute an important component in every diagnosis; occasionally when historical data are combined with observation of a lesion's clinical appearance, the historical information constitutes the most important contribution to the diagnostic process. Personal history, family history, past and present medical and dental histories, history of drug ingestion, and history of the presenting disease or lesion can provide information necessary for the final diagnosis. Thorough medical and dental histories must be a part of every patient's permanent record. The clinician should carefully review these docu-

ments and update them with the patient at each visit. Pathologic conditions in which the family history contributes a significant role in the diagnosis include amelogenesis imperfecta (**Figure 1-37,** *A* and *B*), dentinogenesis imperfecta (**Figure 1-38,** *A* and *B*), and many other genetic disorders. Additionally, clinical findings and radiographs also provide significant assistance to the diagnostic process of these conditions.

A patient's medical or dental status, including drug history, can also contribute significant information to a diagnosis. For example, a history of ulcerative colitis may contribute to the diagnosis of oral ulcers (**Figure 1-39,** *A*), which could be related to this

Figure 1-38 **A,** The clinical appearance of dentinogenesis imperfecta. **B,** The radiographic appearance of dentinogenesis imperfecta. (Courtesy Dr. Edward V. Zegarelli.)

Figure 1-39 **A,** Oral ulcers on the soft palate associated with ulcerative colitis. (Courtesy Dr. Edward V. Zegarelli.) **B,** Gingival enlargement seen in a patient taking nifedipine, a calcium channel blocker.

medical condition. Another example of the value of this type of information is the patient in Figure 1-39, *B,* who experienced gingival enlargement; drug history revealed that the patient was taking a calcium channel blocker.

A history of a skin graft from the hip to the ridge and mucobuccal fold area in the anterior mandible in a patient can provide significant information relevant to the diagnosis of a white- or brown-pigmented area on the mandibular anterior ridge and vestibule (**Figure 1-40,** *A* and *B*).

Periapical cemento-osseous dysplasia (cementoma) is another lesion in which the patient's personal history contributes significantly. It is found most frequently in black women in the third decade of life. Other characteristics of the lesion reveal that it is asymptomatic and that the teeth involved are vital (see Figure 1-19).

Figure 1-40 Skin grafts performed to enhance the mandibular ridge in a white **(A)** and a black patient **(B).** Without the patients' past medical and dental histories, it would be difficult to diagnose this anomaly of melanosis accurately.

Laboratory Diagnosis

Clinical laboratory tests, including blood chemistries and urinalysis, can provide information that contributes to a diagnosis. An elevated serum alkaline phosphatase level is significant in the diagnosis of Paget disease. This feature, in addition to a distinctive radiographic appearance that includes a "cotton-wool effect" **(Figure 1-41)** and hypercementosis, provides conclusive information for a definitive diagnosis. Laboratory cultures are also helpful in determining the diagnosis of oral infections.

Microscopic Diagnosis

Microscopic examination is of particular importance in the diagnostic process and therefore is discussed separately from laboratory diagnosis. The microscopic examination of the biopsy specimen taken from the lesion in question contributes significant information. This procedure is often the main component of the definitive diagnosis. However, the skill of the practitioner performing the biopsy is of equal importance. It is most important that an adequate tissue sample be removed for microscopic evaluation. If other diagnostic information, such as clinical features or history of the lesion, indicates the strong possibility of malignancy and the biopsy report does not concur, a second biopsy should be performed.

Figure 1-41 The radiographic appearance of Paget disease, showing the traditional irregular radiopacities ("cotton-wool effect") in bone, characteristic of this disease.

A new technique called a *brush biopsy* can be used to obtain information from oral mucosal epithelium. This technique uses a circular brush to obtain cells from the full thickness of the epithelium, including cells from the keratin layer through the basal layer. Microscopic examination of the individual cells is used to assess whether normal, abnormal, or dysplastic cells are present. The results of this test may help determine if a scalpal biopsy is needed to establish a definitive diagnosis.

A white lesion (**Figure 1-42,** *A*) cannot be diagnosed based on its clinical appearance alone. The microscopic appearance of this type of white lesion can vary from a thickening of the epithelium or surface keratin layer to epithelial dysplasia, which can be premalignant (**Figure 1-42,** *B*).

Surgical Diagnosis

The strength of a surgical diagnosis comes from surgical intervention. Diagnosis is made using the information gained during the surgical procedure for the traumatic bone cyst (**Figure 1-43**) and lingual mandibular bone concavity, also referred to as a static bone cyst or Stafne bone cyst (**Figure 1-44**). A traumatic or simple bone cyst may appear as a radiolucency that scallops around the roots. Surgical intervention provides conclusive evidence when the lesion is opened and an empty void within the bone is found. The void usually fills with bone and heals after the surgical procedure. Lingual mandibular bone concavity is a developmental anomaly and is

A

B

Figure 1-42 A, A white lesion is seen on the anterior floor and ventral surface of the tongue. **B,** Microscopic examination of the white lesion showed a thickened keratin layer called hyperkeratosis and some atypical changes in the basal layer of the epithelium (mild epithelial dysplasia).

Figure 1-43 Traumatic bone cyst. (Courtesy Dr. Edward V. Zegarelli.)

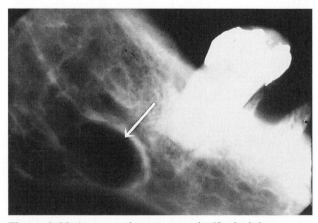

Figure 1-44 Arrow points to a static (Stafne) bone cyst. (Courtesy Dr. Edward V. Zegarelli.)

often bilateral. Surgical examination of the well-circumscribed radiolucent area reveals salivary gland tissue entrapped during development; no treatment is indicated.

Therapeutic Diagnosis

Nutritional deficiencies are common conditions to be diagnosed by therapeutic means. Although angular cheilitis **(Figure 1-45)** may be associated with a deficiency of the B-complex vitamins, it is most commonly a fungal condition and responds to topical application of an antifungal cream or ointment such as nystatin. A thorough patient history should be obtained to rule out contributory nutritional deficiency.

Necrotizing ulcerative gingivitis (NUG) has distinct clinical features (**Figure 1-46,** *A* and *B*) and constitutional signs. It responds to hydrogen peroxide rinses because the anaerobic bacteria that cause NUG cannot survive in an oxygenated environment. Prescribing hydrogen peroxide rinses and observing the results without culturing the bacteria applies the principle of therapeutic diagnosis because it is based solely on clinical and historical information. Antibiotic therapy is also used in the management of NUG.

Differential Diagnosis

The differential diagnosis is that point in the diagnostic process when the practitioner decides which test or procedure is required to rule out the conditions originally suspected and establish the definitive or final diagnosis. All the previously discussed components are applied to the differential diagnosis. The final diagnosis emerges from a thorough evaluation of the suspected lesions.

CASE STUDY

The following case illustrates how the diagnostic processes work together and how the differential diagnosis is used.

An 11-year-old white girl came to the dental office with her mother. The mother was concerned about the interdental papilla on the child's labial aspect between the maxillary right central and lateral incisors **(Figure 1-47).** Nothing in the medical history explained the condition; the child had been wearing orthodontic appliances for about 1 year. Clinically the interdental papilla was enlarged and had a papillary surface that bled easily when probed. The sessile lesion measured 5 mm cervicoincisally by 3 mm mesiodistally. No pain was felt in the area. Information pertinent to the history of the lesion was secured from the mother. The lesion had been there for about 1 year and was first noticed around the time the child began wearing braces. At times, tags of the lesion or pieces of it "fell off" during

Figure 1-45 Angular cheilitis.

Figure 1-46 **A,** Necrotizing ulcerative gingivitis (NUG). **B,** NUG. The reader should note the gingival contours and punched-out, blunted papillae.

brushing. The orthodontist "pulled most of it off" at one point, but it was never surgically removed or submitted for microscopic examination and seemed to grow back. Additional questioning revealed that the child had a wart on her foot within the last year. A biopsy was performed, and the tissue sample was placed in formalin and sent to an oral pathology laboratory with the following differential diagnosis:

- Pyogenic granuloma: The spongy inflammatory tissue was possibly caused by the mechanical irritation from the orthodontic bands, thereby causing pyogenic granuloma.
- Papilloma: Based on the papillary surface texture of the lesion, it was thought to be a papilloma.
- Verruca vulgaris: Because the child had a wart and could have spread the virus, verruca vulgaris was suggested. In addition, histologically a wart has lateral lipping, and it was thought that this could explain why pieces of the lesion fell off periodically during brushing. However, the surface of a verruca vulgaris is usually keratinized and therefore whiter than the lesion illustrated in Figure 1-47.

The microscopic examination revealed stratified squamous epithelium covering a core of loose and edematous fibrous connective tissue. The stroma contained numerous endothelium-lined, blood-filled capillaries and a dense infiltrate of lymphocytes, plasma cells, and neutrophils.

The definitive or final diagnosis was pyogenic granuloma.

Figure 1-47 Arrow points to a pyogenic granuloma between the patient's right maxillary central and lateral incisors. (Courtesy Dr. Victor M. Sternberg.)

To arrive at a diagnosis, the data collection included the patient's medical and dental health histories, the history of the lesion in question, a clinical description and evaluation, and biopsy and microscopy reports. This case illustrates the fact that arriving at a diagnosis involves a process. As stated previously, it can be thought of as a puzzle, because the information from each diagnostic category becomes part of the entire diagnostic process. In this case the microscopic examination contributed most significantly to the definitive or final diagnosis. The differential diagnosis included three possible diagnoses; the biopsy and microscopic examinations provided conclusive information in the diagnostic process.

The hygienist can be effective in the preliminary evaluation of the lesion by calling it to the attention of the dentist and then gathering and preparing all the data for the clinician who will perform the biopsy. In addition, it is both challenging and stimulating to discuss diagnostic impressions with other professionals based on the data available at the time.

Variants of Normal

FORDYCE GRANULES

Clusters of ectopic sebaceous glands are called **Fordyce granules.** They are most commonly observed on the lips and buccal mucosa. Clinically they appear as yellow lobules in clusters and are usually distributed over the buccal mucosa or vermilion border of the involved lips. The surrounding tissue is normal. Because more than 80% of adults over 20 years of age have Fordyce granules, they are considered a variant of normal. Microscopically, Fordyce granules appear as normal sebaceous glands. They are asymptomatic and require no treatment **(Figure 1-48).**

TORUS PALATINUS

Torus palatinus or palatal torus is an exophytic growth of normal compact bone. Palatal tori are inherited and occur more frequently in women. They are asymptomatic, develop gradually, and are observed clinically in the midline of the hard palate. Palatal tori may take on various shapes and sizes, may be lobulated, and are covered by normal soft tissue. It is not unusual for the palatal torus to be traumatized, which can cause discomfort and possible ulceration on the surface of the torus. When the lesion is large, it may be seen as a radiopaque mass on the radiograph. No treatment is indicated unless the torus interferes with speech, swallowing, or a prosthetic appliance (**Figure 1-49**, *A* and *B*).

MANDIBULAR TORI

Outgrowths of normal dense bone found on the lingual aspect of the mandible in the area of the premolars above the mylohyoid ridge are **mandibular tori.** They are usually bilateral, often lobulated or nodular, can appear fused together, and have no predilection for either sex. Mandibular tori do not usually require treatment unless the patient needs a prosthodontic appliance (denture) and the tori interfere with proper fabrication and placement (**Figure 1-50**, *A* and *B*).

MELANIN PIGMENTATION

Melanin is the pigment that gives color to the skin, eyes, hair, mucosa, and gingiva. **Melanin pigmentation** of the oral mucosa or gingiva is most commonly observed in dark-skinned individuals (**Figure 1-51**; see Figure 1-18).

RETROCUSPID PAPILLA

A **retrocuspid papilla** is a sessile nodule on the gingival margin of the lingual aspect of the mandibular cuspids (see Figure 1-19).

LINGUAL VARICOSITIES

Prominent lingual veins, called *lingual varicosities,* are usually observed on the ventral and lateral surfaces of the tongue. Clinically, red-to-purple enlarged vessels or clusters are seen. They are not associated with other systemic diseases; however, a relationship

A

B

Figure 1-49 A, The radiopaque appearance of torus palatinus. **B,** The clinical appearance of a torus palatinus.

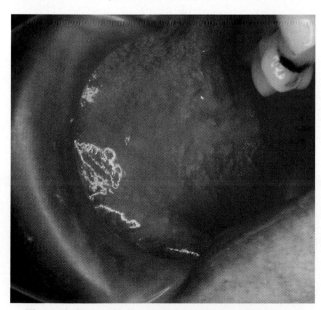

Figure 1-48 Fordyce granules on the buccal mucosa.

Figure 1-50 **A,** The clinical appearance of lobulated mandibular tori. **B,** The radiopaque appearance of mandibular tori in same patient. (Courtesy Dr. Edward V. Zegarelli.)

Figure 1-51 Melanin pigmentation of the mandibular gingiva.

Figure 1-52 Lingual varices. (Courtesy Dr. David Zegarelli.)

between varicosities in the legs and prominent lingual veins has been reported. Lingual varices are most commonly observed in individuals older than 60 years of age and are therefore thought to be related to the aging process **(Figure 1-52).**

LINEA ALBA

Linea alba is a "white line" that extends anteroposteriorly on the buccal mucosa along the occlusal plane. It may be bilateral and can be more prominent in patients who have a clenching or bruxing habit **(Figure 1-53).**

LEUKOEDEMA

A generalized opalescence is imparted to the buccal mucosa by **leukoedema.** It is most commonly observed in black adults (up to 85%), suggesting an ethnic predisposition. Leukoedema can also be seen in whites. Clinically a gray-white film is diffused throughout the buccal mucosa, giving the mucosa an opaque quality. If the mucosa is stretched, the opalescence becomes less prominent. The condition becomes more pronounced in smokers. The opalescence is an integral part of the buccal tissue and

Figure 1-53 Arrow points to linea alba on the buccal mucosa.

Figure 1-55 Median rhomboid glossitis. (Courtesy Dr. Edward V. Zegarelli.)

Figure 1-54 Leukoedema of the buccal mucosa showing an opalescent, velvety texture.

cannot be removed. Histologically, significant intracellular edema in the spinous cells and acanthosis of the epithelium is seen. It is a benign anomaly that requires no treatment **(Figure 1-54).**

Benign Conditions of Unknown Cause

LINGUAL THYROID NODULE

The thyroid gland begins to develop during the first month of fetal life and is initially located in the area of the foramen cecum on the posterior tongue. In normal development the thyroid gland descends to its normal location in the neck. When thyroid tissue either does not descend or remnants become entrapped

in the tissue that makes up the tongue, a developmental anomaly called a **lingual thyroid nodule** results. Research has indicated a high predilection in females, and studies have linked the emergency of the lingual thyroid nodule with hormonal changes because its onset appears to be associated with puberty, pregnancy, and menopause. Clinically a lingual thyroid nodule is observed as a mass in the midline of the dorsal surface of the tongue posterior to the circumvallate papillae in the area of the foramen cecum. The lesion usually has a sessile base and is 2 to 3 cm in width. On histologic examination, normal thyroid tissue is found. Treatment requires careful evaluation of the patient to determine whether the thyroid gland is present in its normal location. Surgical intervention is not always required.

MEDIAN RHOMBOID GLOSSITIS

The cause of **median rhomboid glossitis** is not clear. Research has suggested that it may be associated with a chronic fungal infection from *Candida albicans*. Clinically, median rhomboid glossitis appears as a flat or slightly raised oval or rectangular erythematous area in the midline of the dorsal surface of the tongue, beginning at the junction of the anterior and middle thirds and extending posterior to the circumvallate papillae. It is devoid of filiform papillae, and therefore its texture is smooth. If the remaining surface of the tongue is coated, the rectangular area appears more prominent. No specific treatment exists; however, sometimes an antifungal agent is applied and the lesion resolves, but this is not always the case. Occasionally the condition resolves with no specific treatment at all **(Figure 1-55).**

GEOGRAPHIC TONGUE

The cause of **geographic tongue** (erythema migrans, benign migratory glossitis) is not clear. The familial occurrence of geographic tongue suggests that genetic factors play a role. Some investigators suggest that it is exacerbated by stress, and studies exist that associate the histologic findings with those found in psoriasis. The clinical appearance involves the dorsal and lateral borders of the tongue. Diffuse areas devoid of filiform papillae can be observed. These areas appear as erythematous patches that are surrounded by a white or yellow perimeter. The fungiform papillae appear distinct within the erythematous patch. The condition does not remain static; there appears to be remission and changes in the depapillated areas. Occasionally a patient complains of a burning discomfort associated with geographic tongue. Usually no treatment is indicated (**Figure 1-56,** *A*).

Ectopic geographic tongue is the term used to describe the condition when it is found on mucosal surfaces other than the tongue. In **Figure 1-56,** *B,* it is seen in the mandibular anterior mucobuccal fold.

FISSURED TONGUE

The cause of **fissured tongue** is unknown. It is seen in about 5% of the population. Familial patterns of occurrence suggest that genetic factors are probably involved. Clinically the dorsal surface of the tongue appears to have deep fissures or grooves that may become irritated if food debris collects in them. No treatment is indicated for the condition. However, a patient with a fissured tongue may be advised to brush the tongue gently with a soft toothbrush to keep the fissures clean of debris and irritants (**Figure 1-57;** see Figure 1-20).

HAIRY TONGUE

Hairy tongue is a condition in which the patient has an increased accumulation of keratin on the filiform papillae that results in a white, "hairy" appearance. This may be the result of either an increase in keratin production or a decrease in normal desquamation. Unless otherwise pigmented, the elongated filiform papillae are white (**Figure 1-58**). In the condition known as black hairy tongue, the papillae are a brown-to-black color because of chromogenic bacteria (**Figure 1-59**). Tobacco and certain foods may also discolor the papillae. Although the cause is unknown, hydrogen peroxide, alcohol, or chemical rinses have been suggested to stimulate the elongation of the filiform papillae that results in the appearance of hairy tongue.

Treatment involves directing the patient to brush the tongue gently with a toothbrush (wet with water only) to remove debris. The condition usually clears completely but may recur.

A   **B**

Figure 1-56 A, Geographic tongue. **B,** Ectopic geographic tongue observed in the mandibular anterior mucosa.

Figure 1-57 Fissured tongue and attrition.

Figure 1-58 White hairy tongue.

Figure 1-59 Black hairy tongue.

Selected References

Books

Darby ML: *Mosby's comprehensive review of dental hygiene,* ed 5, St Louis, 2002, Mosby.

Neville BW et al: *Color atlas of clinical oral pathology,* Philadelphia, 1991, Lea & Febiger.

Neville BW et al: *Oral and maxillofacial pathology,* ed 2, Philadelphia, 2002, WB Saunders.

Regezi JA, Sciubba JJ: *Oral pathology: clinical pathologic correlations,* ed 4, Philadelphia, 2003, WB Saunders.

Sonis ST, Fazio RC, Fang L: *Principles and practice of oral medicine,* ed 2, Philadelphia, 1995, WB Saunders.

Journal Articles

Bouquot JE, Gundlach KKH: Odd tongues: the prevalence of common tongue lesions in 23,616 white Americans over 35 years of age, *Quintessence Int* 17:719, 1986.

Chapnick L: External root resorption: an experimental radiographic evaluation, *Oral Surg Oral Med Oral Pathol* 67:578, 1989.

Comfort M, Wu PC: The reliability of personal and family medical histories in the identification of hepatitis B carriers, *Oral Surg Oral Med Oral Pathol* 67:531, 1989.

Daley TD. Pathology of intraoral sebaceous glands, *J Oral Pathol Med* 22:241, 1993.

Kalan A, Tarig M: Lingual thyroid gland: clinical evaluation and comprehensive management, *Ear Nose Throat J* 78:340, 1999.

Kaugars GE, Miller ME, Abbey LM: Odontomas, *Oral Surg Oral Med Oral Pathol* 67:2172, 1989.

Lydiatt DD, Hollins RR, Peterson GP: Multiple idiopathic root resorption: diagnostic considerations, *Oral Surg Oral Med Oral Pathol* 67:208, 1989.

McCann AL, Wesley RK: A method for describing soft tissue lesions of the oral cavity, *J Dent Hyg* 304, 1986.

Neupert EA, Wright JM: Regional odontodysplasia presenting as a soft tissue swelling, *Oral Surg Oral Med Oral Pathol* 67:193, 1989.

Pogrel MA, Cram D: Intraoral findings in patients with psoriasis with a special reference to ectopic geographic tongue (erythema circinata), *Oral Surg Oral Med Oral Pathol* 66:184, 1988.

Rosen DJ et al: Traumatic bone cyst resembling apical periodontitis, *J Periodontal* 68:1019, 1997.

Suzuki M, Sakae T: A familial study of torus palatinus and torus mandibularis, *Am J Phys Anthropol* 18:263, 1960.

Review Questions

1. After arriving at a differential diagnosis, information from which one of the following categories will best establish a final or definitive diagnosis?
   A. Clinical
   B. Historical
   C. Microscopic
   D. Radiographic
   E. Clinical laboratory test

2. The descriptive term that would best be used for a freckle is a:
   A. Bulla
   B. Vesicle
   C. Lobule
   D. Macule
   E. Papule

3. Which one of the following terms describes the base of a lesion that is stalklike?
   A. Sessile
   B. Lobulated
   C. Bullous
   D. Macule
   E. Pedunculated

4. Clinical diagnosis can be used to determine the final or definitive diagnosis of all of the following *except*:
   A. Fordyce granules
   B. Unerupted supernumerary teeth
   C. Mandibular tori
   D. Geographic tongue
   E. White hairy tongue

5. Radiographic diagnosis would most likely be sufficient to determine the final or definitive diagnosis of:
   A. Internal resorption
   B. Periapical cemento-osseous dysplasia
   C. Odontomas
   D. Dental caries
   E. All of the above

6. To determine the presence of blood dyscrasias, which one of the following would provide the most definitive information?
   A. Laboratory blood tests
   B. Bleeding during probing
   C. Pallor of the gingiva and mucosa
   D. Patient complaint of weakness
   E. Medication history

7. When response to the application of an antifungal ointment or cream to angular cheilitis is used as a diagnostic procedure, which of the following diagnostic categories is being used?
   A. Clinical
   B. Historical
   C. Laboratory
   D. Differential
   E. Therapeutic

8. Yellow clusters of ectopic sebaceous glands commonly observed on the buccal mucosa and evaluated through clinical diagnosis are most likely:
   A. Lipomas
   B. Fibromas
   C. Cheek bites
   D. Linea alba
   E. Fordyce granules

9. A slow-growing, bony, hard exophytic growth in the midline of the hard palate is developmental and hereditary in origin. The diagnosis is determined through clinical evaluation. The hygienist suspects:
   A. Torus palatinus
   B. Mixed tumor
   C. Palatal cyst
   D. Nasopalatine cyst
   E. Ranula

10. The "white line" observed clinically on the buccal mucosa that extends from anterior to posterior along the occlusal plane is:
    A. Leukoedema
    B. Leukoplakia
    C. Linea alba
    D. Lichen planus
    E. Cheek biting

11. Which one of the following occurs as an erythematous area that is devoid of filiform papillae, somewhat rectangular in shape, and on the midline of the dorsal surface of the tongue?
    A. Median rhomboid glossitis
    B. Geographic tongue
    C. Fissured tongue
    D. Lingual thyroid
    E. White hairy tongue

12. Which one of the following diagnostic categories would the hygienist most easily apply to the preliminary evaluation of oral lesions?
    A. Microscopic
    B. Clinical

C. Therapeutic
D. Differential
E. Laboratory

13. These examples of exostoses are found on the lingual aspect of the mandible in the area of the premolars. They are benign, bony, hard, and require no treatment. Radiographically they appear as radiopaque areas and are often bilateral. The hygienist suspects:
    A. Retrocuspid papilla
    B. Lingual mandibular bone concavity
    C. Genial tubercles
    D. Mandibular fossa
    E. Mandibular tori

14. Which one of the following terms is most often used when describing mandibular tori?
    A. Bullous
    B. Lobulated
    C. Sessile
    D. Pedunculated
    E. Macule

15. Which of the following is the condition that is considered a variant of normal; has a diffuse gray-to-white, opalescent, filmy appearance on the buccal mucosa; and is most commonly seen in black individuals?
    A. Leukoplakia
    B. Linea alba
    C. Ectopic geographic tongue
    D. Lichen planus
    E. Leukoedema

16. A patient has the clinical signs of NUG. Other constitutional signs are also evident. The hygienist has the patient begin hydrogen peroxide rinses without culturing the bacterial flora. This action applies which one of the following diagnostic categories?
    A. Therapeutic
    B. Microscopic
    C. Clinical
    D. Final or definitive
    E. Clinical

17. A small circumscribed lesion usually less than 1 cm in diameter that is elevated and protrudes above the surface of normal surrounding tissue is called a:
    A. Bulla
    B. Macule
    C. Vesicle

D. Papule
E. Freckle

18. The base of a sessile lesion is:
    A. Broad and flat
    B. Stemlike
    C. Corrugated
    D. Lobulated
    E. Nodular

19. The identification of which one of the following is not determined by clinical diagnosis?
    A. Fordyce granules
    B. Tori
    C. Compound odontoma
    D. Retrocuspid papilla
    E. Hairy tongue

20. Another term for geographic tongue is:
    A. Allergic tongue
    B. Median rhomboid glossitis
    C. Scalloped tongue
    D. White hairy tongue
    E. Migratory glossitis

21. The cause of supernumerary teeth is most likely:
    A. Genetic
    B. Traumatic
    C. Cystic
    D. Systemic
    E. Syndrome related only

22. Historical diagnosis can include:
    A. Age and sex
    B. Sex and family history
    C. Race and medical history
    D. Duration of a lesion
    E. All of the above

23. Which condition is most often seen on the buccal mucosa?
    A. Melanin pigmentation
    B. Fordyce granules
    C. Nicotine stomatitis
    D. Retrocuspid papilla
    E. Ectopic geographic tongue

24. Which one of the following is not considered a variant of normal?
    A. Migratory glossitis
    B. White hairy tongue
    C. Fissured tongue
    D. Geographic tongue
    E. Hairy leukoplakia

Chapter 1 Synopsis

Condition/Disease	Cause	Age/Race/Sex	Location
Fordyce Granules	Variant of normal	Age—adults	Most common on the buccal mucosa & lips
Torus Palatinus	Genetic	F>M Develops after age 13 Increased prevalence in Native Americans	Midline of palate
Mandibular Tori	Genetic	Develops after age 13	Lingual mandibular premolar area
Melanin Pigmentation	Variant of normal	Increased prevalance with increased skin pigmentation	Gingiva & oral mucosa Most prominent in dark-skinned individuals
Retrocuspid Papillae	Developmental	†	Lingual gingival margin of the mandibular cuspids
Lingual Varicosities	Aging process	>Age	Most common on ventral and lateral surfaces of the tongue
Linea Alba	Clenching/bruxing habit		Buccal mucosa at occlusal plane
Leukoedema	Unknown	Black	Buccal mucosa
Lingual Thyroid Nodule	Developmental Thyroid tissue entrapped in tongue	F>M	Midline of tongue posterior to circumvallate papillae in area
Median Rhomboid Glossitis	Unknown, associated with candida	Adults Rare in children	Midline of dorsal tongue
Geographic Tongue	Genetic Associated with stress Some cases associated with psoriasis	†	Dorsal and lateral borders of tongue
Hairy Tongue	Unknown Associated with smoking, peroxide rinses, alcohol	†	Dorsal midposterior tongue

†Not included in text.

Clinical Features	Radiographic Features	Microscopic Features	Treatment	Diagnostic Process
Tiny, yellow lobules in clusters	N/A	Normal sebaceous gland lobules	None	Clinical
Bony hard exophytic structure	Radiopaque	Compact bone	None	Clinical
Bony hard exophytic structures	Radiopaque	Compact bone	None	Clinical
Most prominent in dark-skinned individuals Brown to gray-black pigmented mucosa	N/A	Melanin pigment in the basal cell layer of the epithelium and subjacent connective tissue	None	Clinical
Red, sessile nodule	N/A	FIbrous connective tissue with large stellate-shaped cells	None	Clinical
Red to purple enlarged blood vessels	N/A	Thick walled blood vessels	None	Clinical
Anterior-posterior white line	N/A	Epithelial hyperplasia and hyperkeratosis	None	Clinical
Gray-white film that gives the mucosa an opalescent quality	N/A	Intracellular edema & acanthosis of the epithelium	None	Clinical
Exophytic mass	N/A	Normal thyroid tissue	None	Clinical
Flat or slightly raised erythematous, rectangular area anterior to the circumvallate papillae	N/A	Epithelial hyperplasia	None	Clinical
Erythematous, depapillated areas with white borders Occasional c/o burning discomfort	N/A	Epithelial hyperplasia with tiny collections of neutrophils near the surface	None Avoid spicy foods	Clinical
Elongated filiform papillae (black, white, yellow, etc.)	N/A	N/A	Gently brush tongue without toothpaste	Clinical

Inflammation and Repair

Margaret J. Fehrenbach
Joan A. Phelan

Objectives

After studying this chapter, the student will be able to:

1. Define each of the words in the vocabulary list for this chapter.
2. List the five classic signs of inflammation that occur locally at the site of inflammation.
3. List three systemic signs of inflammation.
4. Describe the microscopic events associated with each of the classic signs of inflammation.
5. List and describe the microscopic events of the inflammatory process.
6. List the types of white blood cells that participate in inflammation and describe how each is involved.
7. Describe the differences between acute and chronic inflammation.
8. Define and contrast hyperplasia, hypertrophy, and atrophy.
9. Describe the microscopic events that occur during the repair of a mucosal wound.
10. Describe and contrast healing by primary intention, healing by secondary intention, and healing by tertiary intention.
11. Describe local and systemic factors that can impair healing.
12. Describe and contrast attrition, abrasion, and erosion.
13. Describe the pattern of erosion seen in bulimia.
14. Describe the relationship between bruxism and abrasion.
15. Describe the cause, clinical features, and treatment of each of the following: aspirin and phenol burns, electric burn, traumatic ulcer, frictional keratosis, linea alba, and nicotine stomatitis.
16. Describe the clinical features, cause (when known), treatment, and histologic appearance of each of the following: traumatic neuroma, postinflammatory melanosis, solar cheilitis, mucocele ranula, necrotizing sialometaplasia, pyogenic granuloma, giant cell granuloma, chronic hyperplastic pulpitis, and irritation fibroma.
17. Describe the difference between a mucocele and a ranula.
18. Define sialolithiasis.
19. Describe the difference between acute and chronic sialadenitis.
20. Describe the clinical features, radiographic appearance, and histologic appearance of a periapical abscess, a periapical granuloma, and a periapical (radicular) cyst.
21. Describe and contrast internal and external tooth resorption.

Vocabulary

Acute (ah-kūt) Of short duration or of short and relatively severe course.

Atrophy (at′-ro-fe) Atrophy is the decrease in size and function of a cell, tissue, organ, or whole body.

Central (sen-′tral) Within bone.

Chemotaxis (ke″mo-tak′sis) The directed movement of white blood cells to the area of injury by chemical mediators.

Chronic (kron′ik) Persisting over a long time.

Emigration (em″ə gra′shun) The passage of white blood cells through the endothelium and wall of the microcirculation into the injured tissue.

Erythema (er″ə-the′mah) Redness of the skin or mucosa.

Exudate (eks′u-dat) Inflammatory fluid formed as a reaction to injury of tissues and blood vessels.

Fever (fe′ver) An elevation of body temperature to greater than the normal of 98.6° F (37° C).

Hyperemia (hi″per-e′me-ah) An excess of blood in a part of the body.

Hyperplasia (hi″per-pla′ze-ah) An enlargement of a tissue or organ resulting from an increase in the number of normal cells.

Hypertrophy (hi-per′tro-fe) An enlargement of a tissue or organ resulting from an increase in size but not in number of cells.

Leukocytosis (loo″ko-si-to′sis) A temporary increase in the number of white blood cells circulating in blood.

Local (lo′kal) Confined to a limited part, not general or systemic.

Lymphadenopathy (lim-fad″ĕ-nop′-ah-thē) A condition associated with various disease processes that affect lymph nodes, such that they become enlarged and palpable.

Margination (mar″jĭ-nā-′shun) A process during inflammation in which white blood cells tend to move to the periphery of the blood vessel wall.

Microcirculation (mi′kro-sur-kūl-a′shin) Small blood vessels, including arterioles, capillaries, and venules, all of which can be affected by local changes as the result of inflammation.

Necrosis (nĕ-kro′sis) The pathologic death of one or more cells or a portion of tissue or organ resulting from irreversible damage.

Pavementing (pāv′ment-ing) Adherence of white blood cells to the walls of a blood vessel during inflammation.

Peripheral (pĕ-rif′er-al) Located away from the center; indicates that the location of a lesion is in the soft tissue surrounding a bone.

Phagocytosis (fag″o-si-tol′ĭ-sis) A process of ingestion and digestion by cells.

Purulent (pu′roo-lent) Containing or forming pus.

Regeneration (re-gen-er-a′-shun) The process by which injured tissue is replaced with tissue identical to that present before the injury.

Repair (re-pār′) The restoration of damaged or diseased tissues.

Serous (se′rus) Having a watery consistency relating to serum.

Systemic (sis-tem′ik) Pertaining to or affecting the body as a whole.

Wheal (hwēl) A localized swelling of tissue because of edema during inflammation, often accompanied by severe itching.

Inflammation and **repair** are the body's responses to injury. Inflammation allows the human body to eliminate injurious agents, contain injuries, and heal defects. The specific lesions included in this chapter occur in response to injury. Many of these lesions are quite common and are likely to be encountered when the dental hygienist examines the hard and soft tissues of the oral cavity. Lesions that occur as a result of destruction through activity of the immune system are included in Chapter 3. Lesions that occur as a result of infection are included in Chapter 4.

Injury

Injury is an alteration in the environment that causes tissue damage. Injury to oral tissues can be caused by many different factors. Physical injury can affect teeth, soft tissue, and bone. Chemical injury can occur from the application of caustic materials to oral tissues. Microorganisms can cause injury by invading oral tissues. Nutritional deficiencies can render oral tissues more susceptible to injury from other sources.

Natural Defenses Against Injury

The body has a number of mechanisms to protect against injury. Intact skin or mucosa acts as a physical barrier to injury. Enzymes in saliva, such as lysozyme, have antibacterial activity, and the flushing action of tears, saliva, urine, and diarrhea removes foreign substances.

Inflammation

Inflammation is a nonspecific response to injury and occurs in the same manner regardless of the nature of the injury. The extent and duration of the injury determine the extent and duration of the inflammatory response. The inflammatory response may be local and limited to the area of injury, or it may become systemic if the injury is extensive. The inflammatory response may be acute or chronic. If the injury is minimal and brief and its source is removed from the tissue, only **acute inflammation** occurs.

The duration of acute inflammation is short, lasting only a few days. The tissue may return to its original state (regeneration), or repair of the tissue may begin immediately. If the inflammatory response is longer lasting, it is referred to as **chronic inflammation.** Chronic inflammation may last weeks, months, or even indefinitely. Chronic inflammation occurs if injury to the tissue continues. The inflammatory response is a dynamic process, changing continually. Thus transitional stages exist during which the response is changing from one type of inflammation to the next; in addition, an acute inflammatory response may be superimposed over a chronic inflammatory response. Occasionally an overwhelming inflammatory response may lead to further injury. Repair of the tissue occurs only if the persistent source of injury is removed. Inflammation of a specific tissue is denoted by the suffix **"itis"** combined with the name of the tissue, such as in *tonsillitis, pulpitis,* and *gingivitis.*

MICROSCOPIC EVENTS AND CLINICAL SIGNS OF INFLAMMATION

Microscopic events occur within the injured tissues during both acute and chronic inflammation. These events cause changes that can be seen clinically. Local clinical changes at the site of injury are called the **classic signs of inflammation;** these local changes include redness, heat, swelling, pain, and loss of normal tissue function **(Table 2-1).** Systemic signs of inflammation may be present when the response is more extensive; these include an increase in body temperature **(fever),** an increase in the number of white blood cells **(leukocytosis),** and enlargement of lymph nodes **(lymphadenopathy) (Figure 2-1).** The microscopic events of inflammation involve the **microcirculation** (arterioles, capillaries, and venules) in the area of injury, certain white blood cells, and chemicals called chemical mediators. Normally, blood flows through the microcirculation, and exchange of oxygen and nutrients occurs as fluid passes between the endothelial cells lining the vessel walls. Most of the fluid reenters the circulation through the venules. The lymphatic vessels carry away fluid that cannot reenter the blood vessels.

In inflammation the underlying microscopic events proceed faster than the visible clinical changes. A summary of the sequence of microscopic events that occur during the inflammatory response is as follows:

1. Injury to tissue
2. Constriction of the microcirculation
3. Dilation of the microcirculation
4. Increase in permeability of the microcirculation
5. Exudate leaves the microcirculation
6. Increased blood viscosity
7. Decreased blood flow through the microcirculation
8. Margination and pavementing of white blood cells
9. White blood cells escape the microcirculation and enter tissue
10. White blood cells ingest foreign substances

The first microscopic event of the inflammatory response is a brief, immediate reflex constriction of the microcirculation in the area of the injury. This is followed by a dilation of the same small blood vessels. Dilation is an increase in the diameter of the vessels and is caused by chemical mediators that are released at the time of the injury. Dilation of the microcirculation results in increased blood flow through the vessels. The increased blood flow that fills the capillary beds in the injured tissue is called

Table 2-1 Local and Systemic Clinical Signs of Inflammation and Associated Microscopic Events

Clinical Feature	Associated Microscopic Events
Localized Signs of Inflammation	
Redness (erythema) and heat	Hyperemia resulting from dilation of microcirculation
Swelling	Permeability of microcirculation leads to exudate formation in the tissues
Pain	Pressure on nerves by exudate formation
	Release of chemical mediators
Loss of normal tissue function	Events associated with swelling and pain
	Repair
Systemic Signs of Inflammation	
Fever	Production of pyrogens affects the hypothalamus, which influences body temperature
Leukocytosis	Increased circulating white blood cells from increased formation and release from bone marrow
Lymphadenopathy	Hyperplasia and hypertrophy of lymphocytes

hyperemia. Hyperemia is responsible for two clinical signs of inflammation: (1) redness **(erythema)** and (2) heat. Erythema is easily visible in most oral tissues. Local temperature changes may be more difficult to recognize.

While hyperemia is occurring, the permeability of the microcirculation also increases. This increased permeability is caused by blood vessel injury, chemical mediators, or an opening of the junctions of the endothelial cells that line the vessels. As a result, blood plasma and proteins flow into the injured tissues as a fluid that is called **exudate.** The presence of exudate in the injured tissue helps to dilute injurious agents that may be present. This results in excess fluid in the tissues. This excess fluid in the tissue is called edema. Two main types of exudate are (1) serous and (2) purulent. **Serous exudate** is composed mainly of plasma fluids and proteins with a few white blood cells. **Purulent exudate** (suppuration) contains tissue debris and many white blood cells in addition to plasma fluids and proteins.

Swelling of the injured area develops as the exudate escapes into the tissue **(Figure 2-2)**. If the swollen tissue area is further injured, the exudate flows out of the tissue as either a thin, clear fluid (serous exudate) or a thick, white-to-yellow pus (purulent exudate).

The formation of exudate may be so excessive that it interferes with repair of the tissue. The injured tissue may allow the excess exudate to drain by formation of a drainage passage that bores through the tissue, allowing drainage to the outside. This channel through the tissue is called a **fistula (Figure 2-3)**; it is formed at the expense of healthy, functioning tissue in the area, which is lost as the tissue becomes necrotic. Sometimes excessive exudate in damaged tissue has to be mechanically drained by making an incision in the surface of the swollen area, often placing a drainage tube in the site of the incision. This procedure is called incision and drainage and is usually accompanied by the administration of an antibiotic to treat infection and medication to reduce inflammation **(Figure 2-4)**. Exudate formation results in pain as the exudate presses on sensory nerves in the area. In addition, some chemical mediators in inflamed tissue can also cause pain. The swelling and

Figure 2-1 Enlarged cervical lymph node.

Figure 2-2 Swelling caused by increased local edema associated with a dental infection. The patient was hospitalized for treatment of the swelling. (Courtesy Dr. Sidney Eisig.)

Figure 2-3 Fistulas formed from periapical abscesses. **A,** A fistula formed from an abscess associated with a mandibular first molar. **B,** The opening of a fistulous tract from a mandibular incisor is seen here on the skin of the chin. **C,** A periapical radiolucency at the area of abscess causing the fistula to the skin in **B.**

pain in tissue resulting from the inflammatory process may cause a loss of normal tissue function, another clinical sign of inflammation.

In addition to exudate formation, blood vessel permeability also leads to increased blood viscosity because of the loss of plasma fluids. The blood becomes thicker and cannot flow as easily. This eventually results in decreased flow through the microcirculation. As the blood flow slows down, the red blood cells begin to pile up in the center of the blood vessels and the white blood cells are displaced to the periphery of the blood vessels. This movement of the white blood cells to the periphery of the vessel is called **margination.** The white blood cells are now in position to adhere themselves to the injured and "sticky" inner walls of the blood vessel because of specific cell factors. This lining of the walls by white blood cells is called **pavementing (Figure 2-5).**

Figure 2-4 An intraoral abscess has been incised and a drain *(arrow)* placed to allow the escape of purulent exudate from the tissue. (Courtesy Dr. Sidney Eisig.)

Figure 2-5 Margination and pavementing during inflammation. Neutrophils *(N)* are seen at the periphery of a small blood vessel (high magnification).

After pavementing the vessel walls, the white blood cells begin to escape from the blood vessels along with the plasma fluids and enter the injured tissue. This process by which the white blood cells escape from the blood vessels through the gaps between the endothelial cells lining the blood vessels is called **emigration.** Emigration occurs as a result of a combination of events: increased blood flow in the microcirculation causing increased pressure, opening of the junctions of the endothelial cells that line the blood vessels, increased mobility of the white blood cells involved, and chemical mediators in the injured tissue that cause directed movement of the white blood cells in the injured tissue.

This directed movement of white blood cells toward the site of the injury is called **chemotaxis,** and substances that enhance this directed movement are called chemotactic factors. Emigration and chemotaxis of the white blood cells to the area of injury allows these cells to be mobilized in the body's defense against the injury. At first these cells try to wall off the site of the injury from the surrounding healthy tissue. In the injured tissue the white blood cells remove foreign substances from the site by ingesting and then digesting them. This is called **phagocytosis (Figure 2-6).** The ingested substances may include pathogenic microorganisms or tissue debris. The presence of these substances interferes with the repair process; therefore they must be removed for the inflammation to resolve and any necessary tissue repair to proceed.

Figure 2-6 Phagocytosis of a foreign substance (bacterium) by a white blood cell. The foreign substance will later be destroyed by digestion within the cell by lysosomal enzymes that are contained within lysosomes.

CELLS INVOLVED IN THE ACUTE INFLAMMATORY RESPONSE

Emigration and chemotaxis of white blood cells **(leukocytes)** from the blood vessels into the site of injury is an important part of the process of inflammation. Six different kinds of white blood cells exist: (1) neutrophils, (2) monocytes, (3) lymphocytes, (4) plasma cells, (5) eosinophils, and (6) mast cells. The **neutrophil (polymorphonuclear [PMN] leukocyte)** is the first cell to arrive at the site of injury and is the primary cell involved in acute inflammation. The **monocyte** or **macrophage** is the second cell to participate in the inflammatory response. The **lymphocyte** and **plasma cell** are involved in both chronic inflammation and the immune response, and the **eosinophil** and **mast cell** participate in both inflammatory and immune responses.

As inflammation begins and as it continues, changes take place in the types of white blood cells present in the tissue **(Figure 2-7).** Initially the

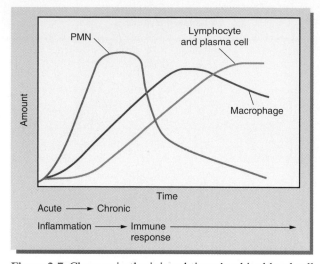

Figure 2-7 Changes in the injured tissue's white blood cell population over time, starting with acute inflammation, continuing to chronic inflammation, and extending to the beginning of the immune response. *PMN,* Polymorphonuclear neutrophils.

Figure 2-9 Microscopic view of chronic inflammation and the beginning of the immune response, mainly showing macrophages, lymphocytes, and plasma cells (medium magnification).

Figure 2-8 Microscopic view of acute inflammation showing an increase in the number of neutrophils. Macrophages are also present (medium magnification).

neutrophil is the most common inflammatory cell present **(Figure 2-8)** during acute inflammation. The monocyte circulating in blood becomes a macrophage as it enters the tissue and is the second type of white blood cell at the site of injury. As inflammation continues, the number of neutrophils decreases. If the injury persists and chronic inflammation occurs, macrophages, lymphocytes, and plasma cells become the predominant cells in the tissue instead of neutrophils **(Figure 2-9)**.

Neutrophils

Neutrophils constitute 60% to 70% of the entire white blood cell population. Like all white blood cells, the neutrophil is derived from a precursor cell called a stem cell, which is located in the bone marrow **(Figure 2-10)**. Neutrophils possess a multilobed nucleus, which is the reason they are also called PMNs, and a granular cytoplasm, which contains enzymes called lysosomal enzymes **(Figure 2-11)**. Neutrophils are produced throughout life and are mobile cells.

The main function of the neutrophil is phagocytosis of substances such as pathogenic microorganisms and tissue debris. The cells are recruited into the area of injury in response to chemotactic factors. Lysosomal enzymes contained within vacuoles in the cytoplasm destroy substances after the cell has engulfed them. The removal of these substances from the site of injury is necessary to allow the process of healing to occur.

The neutrophil dies shortly after phagocytosis, during which lysosomal enzymes and other damaging cellular substances that were meant only for intracellular destruction of foreign substances leak from the cells. This leakage can cause further tissue damage.

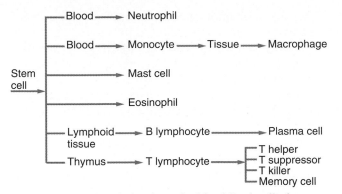

Figure 2-10 The derivation of white blood cells from a stem cell in the bone marrow.

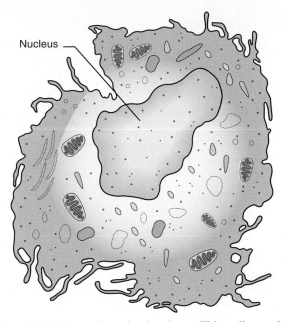

Figure 2-12 Macrophage in the tissue. This cell was formerly a monocyte when circulating in blood.

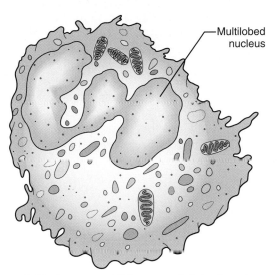

Figure 2-11 A neutrophil has a multilobed nucleus and granular cytoplasm.

Monocytes

As mentioned previously, the monocyte is the second white blood cell to emigrate from the blood vessels into the injured tissue, where it becomes a macrophage. Like the neutrophil, the monocyte is derived from the stem cell in the bone marrow (see Figure 2-10); later as a macrophage, it responds to chemotactic factors, is capable of phagocytosis, is mobile, and has lysosomal enzymes in its cytoplasm that assist in the destruction of foreign substances. The macrophage has a single round nucleus and a nongranular cytoplasm **(Figure 2-12)**. It constitutes 3% to 8% of the entire white blood cell population.

The macrophage has a somewhat longer life span than the PMN. In addition to its role in phagocytosis, the macrophage is an important cell in the immune response.

CHEMICAL MEDIATORS OF INFLAMMATION

Chemical agents called chemical mediators cause many of the events involved in the inflammatory response. Chemical mediators are essential to the inflammatory response and can start or amplify the response. During the response, basic mediators of inflammation can recruit other mediators and immune mechanisms, thus increasing the overall process. Some are derived from blood, some come from endothelial cells, some from white blood cells and platelets; others are produced by certain pathogenic microorganisms as they injure the tissue.

Three systems in the blood may be activated during inflammation: (1) the kinin system, (2) the clotting mechanism, and (3) the complement system. These systems are interrelated, and much interaction takes place during their activation, among their products, and within their various actions.

Kinin System

The kinin system mediates inflammation by causing increased dilation of the blood vessels at the site of injury and increasing the permeability of local blood vessels. This system is rapidly activated both by substances present in plasma and by substances present in injured tissues. Its role is limited to the early phases of inflammation. Components of the kinin system also induce pain.

Clotting Mechanism

The clotting mechanism functions primarily in the clotting of blood. It also mediates inflammation, because certain of its products that are activated when tissue is injured cause local vascular dilation and permeability by activating the kinin system. The clotting mechanism is also important in the repair process.

Complement System

This system involves the production of a sequential cascade of plasma proteins that are present in blood in an inactivated form. When the first of the complement substances is triggered—usually by antibody interlocked with an antigen—it sets in motion ripple effect. As each component is activated, it acts upon the next in a precise sequence of carefully regulated steps. Many of these plasma proteins function in both inflammation and immunity. Components of the complement system cause the white blood cells called mast cells to release the granules in their cytoplasm that contain the chemical histamine. Histamine causes an increase in vascular permeability and vasodilation. Other components of the complement system cause cell death (cytolysis) by creating holes in the cell's membrane. They also form chemotactic factors for white blood cells and enhance phagocytosis.

Other Chemical Mediators of Inflammation

In addition to the chemical mediators already mentioned, others are formed in the body during inflammation. Prostaglandins are involved in the inflammatory response by causing increased vascular dilation and permeability, tissue pain and redness, and changes in connective tissues. Lysosomal enzymes are released from the granules in white blood cells.

They act as chemotactic factors and can cause damage to connective tissues and to the clot.

Endotoxin and lysosomal enzymes that are released by pathogenic microorganisms may also serve as chemical mediators. Endotoxin is produced from the cell walls of gram-negative bacteria and can serve as a chemotactic factor, can activate complement, and can function as an antigen and damage bone tissue. During infection the lysosomal enzymes released from pathogenic microorganisms have a similar chemical composition and action to those released by the white blood cells.

Antiinflammatory Drugs

Antiinflammatory drugs block or suppress the inflammatory response, preventing or reducing the clinical signs of inflammation and adverse reactions to the injury. Diseases and conditions such as asthma, arthritis, organ transplants, and surgical trauma are treated with nonsteroidal or steroidal antiinflammatory agents. Examples of nonsteroidal antiinflammatory agents include aspirin, ibuprofen, and celecoxib. Prednisone is a steroidal antiinflammatory drug. Aspirin and some other antiinflammatory drugs exert their analgesic effects by inhibiting prostaglandin synthesis.

SYSTEMIC MANIFESTATIONS OF INFLAMMATION

In addition to the local features of inflammation, systemic signs may also occur. These include fever, an increase in the number of white blood cells (leukocytosis), and involvement of lymph nodes (lymphadenopathy) (see Table 2-1).

Fever

Body temperature is controlled by a regulatory center in the brain called the hypothalamic thermoregulatory center. Fever is an elevated body temperature higher than 98.6° F (37° C) and is associated with a systemic inflammatory response. White blood cells and pathogenic microorganisms produce fever-producing substances known as pyrogens. Pyrogens exert their effects by action on the hypothalamus, the regulatory center in the brain that increases the temperature of the body by way of prostaglandins, producing fever. The function of this increased body temperature is not clear. A moderately high fever may be helpful in combating some infections, because increased temperature slows down the growth of many pathogenic microorganisms. The body cannot tolerate excessively high fever for very long, however, and such fever could prove fatal. Drugs can be given to reduce high fever. Measuring body temperature with a thermometer is helpful in assessing whether a systemic inflammatory response is present.

Leukocytosis

The number of white blood cells circulating in the blood can be measured by a laboratory test, the white blood cell count. The normal number of white blood cells is 4000 to 10,000/mm^3 of blood. A systemic inflammatory response, particularly a response to infection, may result in an increase in the number of white blood cells circulating in blood from 10,000 to 30,000/mm^3. This increase is called **leukocytosis** and usually primarily involves the neutrophil. The body increases the number of circulating white blood cells by increasing their formation and releasing immature forms from the bone marrow into the blood. This increase in the number of circulating white blood cells is an attempt by the body to provide more cells for phagocytosis.

Lymphadenopathy

Involvement of superficial lymph nodes is clinically identified by enlarged and palpable lymph nodes **(lymphadenopathy)**. The enlarged lymph node or nodes can be felt (palpated) as a mass or masses in the area of inflammation and possibly along the associated lymphatic drainage route **(Figure 2-13)**. When palpated, the involved node feels firm and larger than normal and may be tender. Deeper lymph nodes may also be enlarged, but these cannot be palpated.

An enlarged lymph node results from changes in its lymphocytes. Lymphocytes are white blood cells that mature in lymphoid tissue and also travel from the node to the tissue, where they are involved in the immune response. The changes in the lymphocytes cause the change in size of the lymph nodes. These changes include an increase in the number of cells **(hyperplasia)**, resulting from increased cell division, and an enlargement of individual cells **(hypertrophy)**, resulting from cellular maturation. The lymphoid tissue in the Waldeyer's ring, which includes the pharyngeal and lingual tonsillar tissue, may also undergo these changes.

Figure 2-13 Location of lymph nodes in the neck. (From Jarvis C: *Physical examination and health assessment,* Philadelphia, 1996, WB Saunders.)

These changes in the lymphocyte population occur during prolonged or chronic inflammation. Lymphocytes are also the primary cells of the immune response.

CHRONIC INFLAMMATION

Chronic inflammation results from injuries that persist, often for weeks or months, possibly indefinitely. In addition to neutrophils and monocytes, other white blood cells are involved, as is the proliferation of fibroblasts. The cells involved in chronic inflammation include macrophages, lymphocytes, and plasma cells. Repair takes place at the same time that the chronic inflammation proceeds, but it cannot be completed until the source of the injury is removed.

A distinctive form of chronic inflammation is called granulomatous inflammation. It is characterized by the formation of granulomas, which are microscopic groupings of macrophages surrounded by lymphocytes and occasional plasma cells. They usually contain large macrophages that have multiple nuclei called multinucleated giant cells. Foreign material in tissue and certain infections, such as tuberculosis, tend to stimulate the formation of granulomas.

HYPERPLASIA, HYPERTROPHY, AND ATROPHY

A cell or its associated tissue or organ may respond to injury by undergoing an adaptive response such as hyperplasia, hypertrophy, or atrophy. *Hyperplasia* is defined as an increase in the number of cells in a tissue or organ whereby the size of the tissue or organ is increased in response to conditions that cause cellular stress. Pathologic hyperplasia frequently occurs in oral tissues. In the oral cavity, an increase in the number of epithelial cells and the increased thickness of the epithelium commonly occurs in response to chronic irritation or abrasion. As surface epithelial cells are lost, division of basal epithelial cells increases to replace the lost cells. The production of new cells is in excess of the original number of cells, so the epithelium becomes thickened and the tissue appears paler or whiter **(Figure 2-14)**. When the irritation subsides, the proliferation ceases; with time the epithelium usually returns to its normal size, and the color of the tissue returns to normal. Sometimes, however, the hyperplastic tissue persists even after the irritation is discontinued. Hyperplasia of fibrous connective tissue may also occur in response to

Figure 2-14 Microscopic appearance of epithelial hyperplasia (low magnification). The epithelium *(E)* is thickened because of an increase in the number of cells. *CT,* underlying connective tissue.

chronic injury and is common in the oral cavity. Oral lesions caused by epithelial and fibrous hyperplasia are described later in this chapter.

Hypertrophy is different from hyperplasia. **Hypertrophy** is a response to cellular stress that is defined as an increase in the size of a tissue or organ because of an increase in the size, not the number, of cells. For example, hypertrophy occurs in the smooth muscles of the uterus and the mammary glands in response to pregnancy, in cardiac muscle in response to long-standing high blood pressure, and in skeletal muscle in response to increased exercise. Hypertrophy and hyperplasia are often seen together.

Atrophy is the decrease in size and function of a cell, tissue, organ, or whole body in response to certain conditions of cellular stress. Atrophied cells are capable of increasing to their normal size after removing the stress. Atrophy can be seen in the muscular wasting that sometimes occurs in chronic disease states that do not allow mobility and thus function of the body ("use it or lose it"). It can also happen with changes in cellular growth, malnutrition, pressure, ischemia, or hormonal changes.

Regeneration and Repair

With resolution of the inflammatory response, the injured tissue undergoes either regeneration or repair. When tissue damage has been slight, the inflamed area may return completely to its normal structure and function. This is called **regeneration.** Regeneration is the most favorable end to acute inflammation and involves complete removal of all cells, by-products, and inflammatory exudate that enter the tissue during inflammation and return of the microcirculation to its preinflammatory state.

The process of **repair** takes place when complete return of the tissue to normal is not possible because the damage has been too great. Some tissues, such as epithelium, fibrous connective tissue, and bone, have the ability to undergo repair. Other tissues, such as enamel, do not.

Repair is the body's final defense mechanism in its attempt to restore injured tissue to its original state. During the repair process, destroyed cells and tissue are replaced with live cells and new tissue components, but the repair process cannot be completed until the source of injury is removed or the injurious agents are destroyed. Repair is not always a perfect process. Functioning cells and tissue components are often replaced by nonfunctioning scar tissue. Many studies are currently investigating ways to enhance the repair process.

MICROSCOPIC EVENTS THAT OCCUR DURING REPAIR

After an injury, microscopic events occur in both the epithelium and connective tissue **(Figure 2-15)**. These events are different for each of these tissues but occur almost simultaneously and are dependent on each other for optimal healing. If the source of the injury is removed, the repair process for both tissues is usually completed in 2 weeks. The repair process is slightly different in mucosa than in skin, because mucosal tissues are wet and a scab does not form.

Day of Injury

A clot forms as the blood flows into the injured tissue. The clot or meshwork of fibrin is produced in the area of injury as a result of activation of the clotting mechanism. The clot consists of locally produced fibrin, clumped (aggregated) red blood cells, and platelets. Platelets, also called thrombocytes, are found in blood and are extremely important in the formation of a clot. Hereditary factors, drugs, extensive injury, or certain diseases may affect the formation of the clot and prevent or delay tissue repair.

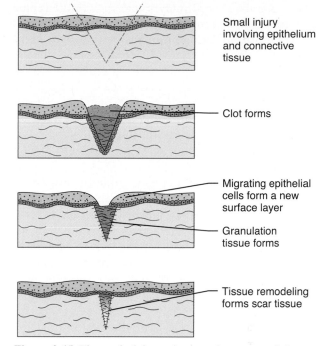

Small injury involving epithelium and connective tissue

Clot forms

Migrating epithelial cells form a new surface layer

Granulation tissue forms

Tissue remodeling forms scar tissue

Figure 2-15 The underlying microscopic events of the repair process from the day of injury to 2 weeks later.

One Day after Injury

Acute inflammation is taking place in the area of repair. The neutrophils emigrate from the microcirculation into the injured tissue, and phagocytosis of foreign substances and necrotic tissue occurs as part of the inflammatory response.

Two Days after Injury

The monocytes emigrate from the microcirculation into the injured area as macrophages. Macrophages continue phagocytosis in a manner similar to that of the neutrophils. Neutrophils are reduced in number as the chronic inflammatory process proceeds. Fibroblasts increase in number within the injured connective tissue. They begin to produce new collagen fibers, using the fibrin meshwork as a scaffold.

The initial tissue formed in the connective tissue portion of the injury is called granulation tissue. It is an immature tissue, with many more capillaries and fibroblasts than mature connective tissue. Sometimes the growth of this tissue is excessive (exuberant). Lesions resulting from exuberant granulation tissue are described later in this section. Exuberant granulation tissue is a vivid red. It may interfere with the repair process until it is removed surgically.

If the surface epithelium has been destroyed by the injury, the epithelial cells create a new surface tissue at the same time that granulation tissue forms in the injured connective tissue. The epithelial cells from the borders of the healing injured area lose their cell junctions and become mobile. They then divide and migrate across the injured tissue, using the fibrin meshwork as a guide to form a new surface layer.

In addition to serving as a guide for migrating epithelial cells and as a scaffold for forming connective tissue, the fibrin meshwork serves to protect the two newly formed tissues from further injury. Thus it is important for the clot to remain in place during this time to allow optimal repair in both tissues. Dressings placed over the clot may prove beneficial to the healing process in some injuries.

At the end of 2 days, lymphocytes and plasma cells begin to emigrate from the surrounding blood vessels into the injured area as chronic inflammation and an immune response begin. The macrophages already present in the area now assist the lymphocytes in the immune response occurring at the site of injury.

Seven Days after Injury

The fibrin is digested by tissue enzymes and sloughs off, and the initial repair of the tissues is completed. Clinically the surface of the repaired injury remains redder because of the thinness of the new epithelium and the increased vascularity of the new connective tissue. If the source of the injury has been completely removed, the inflammatory and immune responses in the tissue are nearly complete.

Two Weeks after Injury

The initial granulation tissue and its fibers have been remodeled, giving the tissue its full strength. The new tissue is now called scar tissue; it appears whiter or paler at the surface of the repaired injury because of the increased number of collagen fibers and decreased vascularity. The amount of scar tissue remaining after an injury depends on many factors, such as heredity, the strength and flexibility needed in the tissue, the type of repair that has occurred, and the tissue involved. The oral mucosa is less prone to scar formation than the skin.

TYPES OF REPAIR

Healing by Primary Intention

This refers to the healing of an injury in which little loss of tissue takes place, such as in a surgical incision. In this type of healing, the clean edges of the incision are joined with sutures to form only a small clot, and very little granulation tissue forms **(Figure 2-16)**. Thus less scar tissue forms, and the patient retains more normal tissue. The use of sutures in an accidental injury is an attempt to try to join the edges of the injury surgically so that healing by primary intention occurs and scarring is minimized.

Healing by Secondary Intention

This involves injury in which tissue is lost, so the edges of the injury cannot be joined during healing. A large clot slowly forms, resulting in increased formation of granulation tissue (e.g., extraction site) **(Figure 2-17)**. After healing, scar tissue increases and normal tissue function is greatly reduced. Scar tissue formation can be so excessive in the epithelium and

Sutured injury

Small clot   Decreased granulation tissue   Less scar tissue

Figure 2-16 The use of sutures in an unintentional injury to encourage healing by primary intention.

connective tissue that surgical correction is sometimes needed. Excessive scarring in skin is called a **keloid (Figure 2-18).**

Healing by Tertiary Intention

If infection occurs at the site of a surgical incision that is healing by primary intention, healing by secondary intention may ensue. This transformation occurs because of an enlargement of the injured area and an increase in the magnitude and duration of the inflammatory and immune responses triggered by the presence of pathogenic microorganisms. In some cases an infected injury is left open and the edges are not surgically joined until the infection is controlled. Waiting to perform surgical tissue repair until the infection is resolved is called healing by tertiary intention.

Large injury

Large clot   Increased granulation tissue   Increased scar tissue

Figure 2-17 Healing by secondary intention (without the use of sutures) in a large injury.

Figure 2-18 An example of keloid formation (excessive scar tissue formation) after an injury. (Courtesy Dr. Harold Baurmash.)

Factors That Impair Healing

Certain local factors impair healing; these include bacterial infection (primarily by *Streptococcus* species), tissue destruction and necrosis, hemorrhage into the tissue (hematoma), excessive movement of the injured tissue, and poor blood supply. Systemic factors, such as those resulting from malnutrition (especially when protein, zinc, calcium, and vitamin C are severely reduced in the diet), can also impair healing. If the body is undergoing immunosuppression because of steroid use or chemotherapy, healing will also be impaired. Certain genetic connective tissue disorders (osteogenesis imperfecta, Marfan syndrome) (see Chapter 6) and metabolic disorders resulting from age, renal failure, and diabetes mellitus (see Chapter 9) can reduce the effectiveness of the natural healing mechanism. Smoking has also been shown to impair healing.

BONE TISSUE REPAIR

Repair of a bone injury is similar to the process that takes place in fibrous connective tissue except that it involves the creation of bone tissue. Bone-forming cells called osteoblasts, which are found on the inner and outer surfaces of bone, produce this tissue. Nutrition, age, and tobacco use can influence the repair process. At the site of the injury, blood supply and growth factors can further modulate the process. Removal of osteoblast-producing tissues or increased movement of the bone can interrupt the healing of a bone injury; edema, infection in the tissue, and excessive or inadequate movement of the involved bone can also delay it.

Injuries to Teeth

ATTRITION

Attrition is the wearing away of tooth structure during mastication. It is a normal occurrence and happens as an individual ages. It involves the incisal, occlusal, and proximal surfaces of the teeth and is rarely seen on any other tooth surfaces unless teeth are abnormally placed in the arch **(Figure 2-19).** Attrition occurs in both deciduous and permanent dentitions; it is usually a slow process that starts as soon as the teeth are in contact and continues for the duration of the contact.

The first sign of attrition is the disappearance of the mamelons on incisal teeth and the flattening of

Figure 2-19 **A**, Attrition of adult dentition. **B,** Attrition of adult dentition (incisal view).

Figure 2-20   Attrition has caused the flattening of the cusps (wear facets) of both the maxillary and mandibular cuspid teeth.

Figure 2-21 Attrition of the mandibular anterior teeth resulting from bruxism.

the occlusal cusps **(Figure 2-20).** The rate of attrition is influenced by diet. A diet of more fibrous food causes greater attrition. Bruxism, the use of chewing tobacco, and certain occupations and environments in which abrasive dust particles enter the mouth accelerate attrition. Attrition increases as patients grow older, and the rate of attrition has been reported to be greater in men than in women.

Bruxism

Grinding and clenching the teeth together for nonfunctional purposes is called **bruxism.** The signs and symptoms resulting from bruxism and their extent are related to the intensity of the grinding and clenching. They are varied and include "wear facets" visible on enamel surfaces, an abnormal rate of attrition **(Figure 2-21),** hypertrophy of masticatory muscles (especially the masseter muscle), increased muscle tone, muscle tenderness, muscle fatigue, cheek biting, pain in the temporomandibular joint area (see Chapter 10), tooth mobility, and pulpal sensitivity to cold.

The incidence of bruxism varies greatly according to the population studied. In a university student population, 5% of individuals showed signs and symptoms of bruxism. In studies of patients with periodontal disease, 60% to 90% had evidence of bruxism. In children aged 2 to 5 years, the average prevalence reported was 20% to 30%, but the highest prevalence reported was 78%.

The cause of bruxism is unclear. Local factors such as occlusal interferences in combination with stress and tension are considered to be triggering factors. A relationship has been reported between bruxism and anxiety, hostility, and hyperactivity. Other studies have characterized the individual who engages in bruxism as emotionally fragile with meticulous character traits, more headaches and muscle pains, and more success in school. Certain conditions such as seizure disorders have been related to bruxism. The higher prevalence of bruxism reported in certain occupations is possibly related to the amount of stress associated with those occupations.

Management of the individual with bruxism includes eliminating the occlusal interferences through occlusal adjustments and protecting the teeth and supporting tissues from further destruction by fabricating an acrylic splint that can be worn as a protective device.

The dental hygienist may identify signs of bruxism while taking the patient's history and during the oral examination. Active wear facets, muscle tenderness, and excessive attrition are clues to the presence of bruxism.

ABRASION

Abrasion is the pathologic wearing away of tooth structure that results from a repetitive mechanical habit. It is most commonly seen in exposed root surfaces because the cementum and dentin are not as hard as enamel; however, abrasion also occurs on enamel surfaces. The process of abrasion is usually slow, and the dentin responds by laying down a protective layer of secondary dentin. Therefore pulpal exposure does not usually result.

Abrasion most frequently presents as a notching of the root surface in areas of gingival recession and may occur from an improper tooth-brushing technique, most commonly a back-and-forth scrubbing motion using excessive pressure. The use of an abrasive dentifrice or a hard toothbrush may also cause abrasion **(Figure 2-22)**. Today most dentifrices manufactured in the United States have a very low abrasive index, and toothbrushes with soft bristles are recommended. Other causes of abrasion include opening bobby pins with the teeth or holding needles or pins in the teeth. These practices result in a notching of the maxillary incisors. Musicians who play wind instruments may also exhibit forms of abrasion of the teeth in the area of the mouth where the instrument is placed, and pipe smokers may show evidence of abrasion in the area of pipe placement.

The diagnosis of abrasion can often be made by correlating the clinical appearance of the lesions with information gained from questioning the patient

Figure 2-22 Abrasion at the cervical area of mandibular bicuspids caused by toothbrushing.

about possible factors that may be causing the lesions. The patient should be informed of the cause of the abrasion, and corrective measures should be taken to prevent further destruction of tooth structure. Restorative dental treatment to repair the defect may be appropriate.

ABFRACTION

Abfraction typically appears as wedge-shaped lesions at the cervical areas of teeth. These lesions occur in adults, and the cause may be related to fatigue, flexure, fracture, and deformation of tooth structure as the result of biomechanical forces on the teeth. The weakened tooth structure is more susceptible to abrasion, particularly toothbrush abrasion. The lesions may be treated using composite or glass ionomer materials, but the forces on the teeth may result in dislodging of the restorations.

EROSION

Erosion is the loss of tooth structure resulting from chemical action. The loss may occur on the smooth facial or lingual surfaces of the teeth and on the proximal and occlusal surfaces **(Figure 2-23)**. The area of erosion appears smooth and polished and is usually extensive, involving several teeth. If erosion occurs in an area where restorations exist, the tooth structure is lost around the restoration, making it appear as if

Figure 2-23 Erosion of buccal and labial surfaces of teeth that occurred as a result of accidental exposure to sulfuric acid.

A

B

Figure 2-24 Erosion caused by bulimia. **A,** Decreased tooth size. **B,** Erosion of maxillary lingual surfaces.

the restoration is standing on its own. This phenomenon is not seen in abrasion or attrition because the restoration would be worn down along with the tooth surface.

Erosion may be seen in individuals who work in industries in which acid is used, such as battery manufacturing, plating companies, and soft-drink manufacturing. The erosion occurs because the workers breathe the acid in the air. Proteolytic enzymes in the workplace have also caused abrasion and erosion. Erosion of teeth associated with intraorally applied cocaine hydrochloride has been reported. Erosion of the facial surfaces of the teeth may also occur as a result of frequently sucking on lemons; erosion of the lingual surfaces of the teeth may occur as a result of chronic vomiting.

The location of erosion and abrasion cannot reliably identify the cause. The patient's history must be correlated with the location and cause.

Bulimia is an eating disorder characterized by food binges, usually of very high caloric intake, followed by self-induced vomiting. Because of the pattern of erosion of the lingual surfaces of the teeth caused by frequent vomiting **(Figure 2-24)**, the dental hygienist may be the first health care professional to identify a patient with bulimia and may assist in encouraging the patient to seek treatment. Bulimia differs from anorexia nervosa, another eating disorder, which is characterized by a distorted perception of body image, in addition to depression, intense fear of gaining weight, and self-imposed starvation. The patient with bulimia maintains a normal body weight but is secretive about eating habits. Vomiting after eating is a component of bulimia and not of anorexia nervosa. Electrolyte imbalance and signs of malnutrition may be present. Irritation of the oral mucosa and lips may occur, and there may be lesions on the back of the fingers caused by their continual use to induce vomiting. Generalized erosion of the lingual surfaces of teeth is common and results from frequent vomiting.

Dental management of patients who vomit frequently includes an effort to minimize the effects of acid on tooth enamel by encouraging the daily use of fluoride rinse and toothpaste containing fluoride. Rinsing the mouth with water and thoroughly cleaning the teeth immediately after vomiting episodes also lessens the effects of acid.

Injuries to Oral Soft Tissues

ASPIRIN BURN

An **aspirin burn** generally occurs when a patient with a toothache places an aspirin tablet directly on the painful tooth instead of swallowing it. Aspirin (acetylsalicylic acid) is an analgesic (pain reliever) and antiinflammatory agent that must be ingested to be effective. Topical application is a common misuse of aspirin. As a result of placing the aspirin on the soft tissue, the tissue becomes necrotic and white. The lesion is painful, and the necrotic tissue may separate from the underlying connective tissue and slough off, resulting in a large ulcer **(Figure 2-25)**. Questioning the patient should reveal the cause of the lesion, and the diagnosis is generally made without the need for biopsy of the tissue. An aspirin burn is painful and heals slowly because of the extent of destruction. However, the ulcer usually heals spontaneously in 7 to 21 days. The patient requires appropriate treatment of the painful tooth and medication for symptomatic relief of pain until the ulcer heals.

PHENOL BURN

Phenol is used in dentistry as a cavity-sterilizing agent and a cauterizing agent. When phenol comes into contact with the soft tissues, a whitening of the exposed area occurs as a result of tissue destruction. The surface tissue may slough off, exposing the underlying connective tissue. The resulting ulcer is painful, and the duration of healing depends on the extent of the destruction. The phenol should be removed immediately to minimize the destruction. If phenol is ingested, the patient should drink large amounts of water. Other agents used in dental treatment may also cause mucosal burns **(Figure 2-26,** *A*).

Phenol is also a component of some over-the-counter products that are advertised for relief of oral pain. Patients frequently misuse these preparations for oral ulcers, and the resulting destruction, in addition to being quite painful, may mask the diagnostic characteristics of the original ulcer.

ELECTRIC BURN

Electric burns in the oral area are usually seen in infants and young children who have bitten or chewed

Figure 2-25 **A** and **B,** Aspirin burns.

a live electric cord or have inserted something into an electric socket. The electric current can cause a great deal of destruction of the oral tissues. Any tissue in the area may be damaged, including the permanent tooth buds. Permanent disfigurement and scarring may result from this type of injury. Treatment may require a multidisciplinary approach that includes plastic surgery, oral surgery, and orthodontics.

OTHER BURNS

Mucosal burns from hot food are common. They occur most often on the palate and tongue **(Figure 2-26,** *B*). Over-the-counter products containing hydrogen peroxide or eugenol can also cause mucosal destruction.

Figure 2-26 Mucosal burns. **A,** Chemical burn caused by contact with caustic material during endodontic treatment. **B,** Thermal burn of palate caused by contact with hot soup. **C,** Ulcer of midline of palate caused by heat generated during the use of crack cocaine. (Reprinted by permission of ADA Publishing Co., Inc. from Mitchell-Lewis DA et al: Identifying oral lesions associated with crack-cocaine use, *J Am Dent Assoc* 125:1104, 1994. Copyright 1994, American Dental Association.)

LESIONS FROM SELF-INDUCED INJURIES

Habits of which the patient may or may not be aware can cause injury. Chronic lip, cheek, or tongue biting and trauma to the gingiva by a fingernail are examples of habits that may cause oral lesions. These lesions range from ulceration to epithelial hyperplasia and hyperkeratosis. Ulcers caused by continual self-induced injuries may be of long duration and may require biopsy and histologic examination to confirm the diagnosis. Treatment of self-induced lesions depends on the amount and type of destruction and may involve psychotherapy.

LESIONS ASSOCIATED WITH COCAINE USE

Lesions located at the midline of the hard palate that vary from ulcers to keratotic lesions to exophytic reactive lesions have been reported to result from the smoking of crack cocaine (**Figure 2-26,** *C*). When crack cocaine is smoked, the crack pipe directs extremely hot smoke to this part of the hard palate. Identification of these lesions is based on their location and the history of recent smoking of crack cocaine. Necrotic ulcers of the tongue and epiglottis related to smoking free-base cocaine have also been reported.

HEMATOMA

A **hematoma** is a lesion that results from the accumulation of blood within tissue as a result of trauma. In the oral cavity a hematoma appears as a red to purple to bluish-gray mass, most frequently seen on the labial or buccal mucosa. The size may vary from small to large, depending upon the extent of the trauma. No treatment is required because the lesion will spontaneously resolve.

TRAUMATIC ULCER

A **traumatic ulcer** occurs as a result of some form of trauma (**Figure 2-27,** *A* to *D*). Sources of trauma vary. Biting the cheek, lip, or tongue may result in a traumatic ulcer, as can irritation from a complete or partial denture or mucosal injury from sharp edges of food. The removal of a dry cotton roll from the oral tissue after a dental procedure can cause a traumatic ulcer, and it is not uncommon to see a patient present for a dental hygiene appointment with a traumatic injury to the gingival tissues or vestibular mucosa that results from overzealous brushing before the appointment. Persistent trauma may result in a hard (indurated), raised lesion called a **traumatic granuloma** (**Figure 2-27,** *D*).

Traumatic ulcers are usually diagnosed based on the relationship of the history to the lesion. Healing is usually uneventful and occurs in 7 to 14 days unless the trauma persists. If trauma persists, ulcers may last for weeks to months. The patient is followed until healing is ensured. If an ulcer does not heal in 7 to 14 days, a biopsy is usually indicated. Microscopically the inflammatory infiltrate associated with a trau-

matic ulcer includes many eosinophils in addition to neutrophils, lymphocytes, and plasma cells. Rapid healing after biopsy of persistent traumatic granulomas occurs frequently.

FRICTIONAL KERATOSIS

Chronic rubbing or friction against an oral mucosal surface may result in a thickening of the keratin on the surface, which is called hyperkeratosis. This results in an opaque, white appearance of the tissue and represents a protective response. It is analogous to a callus on the skin. An example of frictional keratosis is an increase in surface keratin that results from chronic cheek and tongue chewing and chewing on

Figure 2-27 **A,** Traumatic ulceration caused by irritation of gingiva by fingernails. **B,** Traumatic ulcer caused by denture. **C,** Traumatic ulcer on lateral tongue caused by chronic trauma to tongue by teeth. **D,** Traumatic ulcer (traumatic granuloma) of buccal mucosa.

edentulous alveolar ridges **(Figure 2-28)**. Frictional keratosis is not associated with malignancy.

The diagnosis of frictional keratosis is made by identification of the trauma causing the lesion, elimination of the cause, and observing the resolution of the lesion. The keratosis may take a while to disappear on keratinized surfaces such as the gingiva.

Frictional keratosis must be distinguished from other white lesions that arise spontaneously and are not caused by trauma because idiopathic leukoplakia may be a premalignant lesion. Biopsy is indicated for any questionable lesion.

LINEA ALBA

Linea alba is a white, raised line that forms most commonly on the buccal mucosa at the occlusal plane and is usually considered a variant of normal **(Figure 2-29)**. In some patients the line becomes prominent as a result of a teeth-clenching habit. The line follows the pattern of the teeth at the occlusal plane. Although it is most commonly seen on the buccal mucosa, linea alba may form on the labial mucosa as well. Histologically the white, raised line is caused by epithelial hyperplasia and hyperkeratosis. No treatment is indicated. However, the prominence of linea alba may be helpful in evaluating the severity of the clenching habit. (See Figure 1-53.)

NICOTINE STOMATITIS

Nicotine stomatitis is a benign lesion on the hard palate most typically associated with pipe and cigar smoking; however, it also occurs with cigarette

A

B

C

Figure 2-28 Frictional keratosis (indicated by *arrow*) caused by an opposing third molar **(A)**, and chronic tongue chewing **(B). C,** Microscopic appearance of hyperkeratosis (low magnification) showing an increase in surface keratin *(K).*

smoking. The development of the lesion indicates that the patient is smoking heavily. The intensity of smoking required to produce this lesion increases the patient's risk for development of malignancy elsewhere in the oral cavity and respiratory tract.

The initial response of the palatal mucosa to the heat from these substances is an erythematous appearance. Over time, keratinization occurs and results in increasing opacification. After the increase in keratinization, raised red dots are seen at the openings of the ducts of the minor salivary glands on the palatal surface **(Figure 2-30)**. The minor salivary glands be-

come inflamed as a result of obstruction by keratin at the mucosal opening of the ducts. The palate may develop a very similar clinical appearance as a result of the chronic intake of very hot liquids.

TOBACCO POUCH KERATOSIS

Individuals who chew tobacco may develop a white lesion in the area where the tobacco is habitually placed. The mucobuccal fold is the most common location. The epithelium usually has a granular or wrinkled appearance in early lesions. Long-standing lesions may be more opaquely white and have a corrugated surface **(Figure 2-31)**. The lesion often disappears when the tobacco is no longer placed in the area.

Long-term exposure to smokeless tobacco has been associated with an increased risk of squamous cell carcinoma. Lesions that do not resolve require

Figure 2-29 Linea alba.

A

Figure 2-30 Nicotine stomatitis.

B

Figure 2-31 Tobacco pouch keratosis. Note the rough texture of the surface. **A,** Labial mucosa. **B,** Anterior buccal mucosa.

biopsy and may show atypical epithelium. In addition the patient has an increased risk of caries, periodontal disease, attrition, and staining with this habit.

TRAUMATIC NEUROMA

A **traumatic neuroma** is a lesion caused by injury to a peripheral nerve. Nerve tissue is encased in a sheath composed of Schwann cells and their fibers. When this sheath is disrupted, the nerve loses its framework. When a nerve and its sheath are damaged, the proximal end of the damaged nerve proliferates into a mass of nerve and Schwann cells mixed with dense fibrous scar tissue. In the oral cavity, injury to a nerve may occur from injection of local anesthesia, surgery, or other sources of trauma.

Traumatic neuromas are often painful. The pain may range from pain on palpation to severe and constant pain. Most traumatic neuromas occur in adults, and the mental foramen is the most common location. However, a traumatic neuroma may occur in other locations as well. Although the clinical features, particularly the pain that is characteristic, may suggest that a lesion is a traumatic neuroma, the diagnosis is made based on a biopsy and microscopic examination. Traumatic neuromas are treated by surgical excision, and recurrence is rare.

AMALGAM TATTOO

An **amalgam tattoo** is a flat, bluish-gray lesion of the oral mucosa that results from the introduction of amalgam particles into the tissues (**Figure 2-32**, *A*). This may occur at the time of placement or removal of an amalgam restoration or at the time of tooth extraction if a piece of amalgam fractures off a restoration and remains in the tissue. The metallic particles disperse in the connective tissue and result in a permanent area of pigmentation. Over time the mercury-silver-tin amalgam changes, and it is mainly silver that remains in the tissue.

Amalgam tattoos may be seen in any location in the oral cavity but are most commonly found on the gingiva or edentulous alveolar ridge. The posterior region of the mandible is the most common location.

An amalgam tattoo is usually diagnosed based on the clinical appearance of the pigmented area. Often the particles of amalgam can be seen on a periapical radiograph (see **Figure 2 –32**, *B*). As amalgam particles diffuse in the tissue over time, the size of the amalgam tattoo may increase. Biopsy may be necessary to distinguish an amalgam tattoo from a me-

A

B

Figure 2-32 **A,** This blue-gray pigmentation of the gingiva is an amalgam tattoo. **B,** Periapical radiograph showing amalgam particles in the gingival tissue.

lanocytic lesion, particularly if it is located in an area other than the gingiva or alveolar ridge. Once the diagnosis of amalgam tattoo has been established, treatment is generally not indicated.

MELANOSIS

Normal physiologic pigmentation of the oral mucosa is common, particularly in dark-skinned individuals (see Figures 1-18 and 1-51). Melanin pigmentation may also occur after inflammation **(Figure 2-33).** The **oral melanotic macule** is a flat, well-circumscribed brown lesion of unknown cause. These are usually small (<1 cm in diameter) and may require biopsy and histologic examination for diagnosis. A similar lesion may occur on the vermilion of the lips. When occurring on the lips, the lesion may darken with exposure to sunlight.

Figure 2-33 Posttraumatic melanin pigmentation. Area of melanin pigmentation on the gingiva after healing of a traumatic injury.

Figure 2-34   Solar cheilitis.

Another type of melanosis is called **smoker's melanosis** or **smoking-associated melanosis.** In this type of melanosis, the melanin pigmentation is associated with smoking, and the intensity is related to the amount and duration of smoking. The pigmentation fades when smoking is discontinued. However, this may take months to years. The anterior labial gingiva is the most commonly affected site. Women are affected more frequently than men. A relationship to female hormones and birth control pills has been suggested. Oral mucosal melanin pigmentation may also be associated with genetic, bone, and systemic diseases (see Chapters 6, 8, and 9).

SOLAR CHEILITIS

Sun exposure, particularly in fair-skinned individuals, can result in degeneration of the tissue of the lips, called **solar cheilitis (Figure 2-34).** Solar cheilitis is also called **actinic cheilitis.** The development of this condition is related to the total cumulative exposure to sunlight and the amount of skin pigmentation; it may be seen in individuals of various ages. The lower lip is usually more severely involved than the upper lip. The epithelium is thinner than normal, and degenerative changes can be seen microscopically in the connective tissue.

The vermilion of the lips is affected. The color appears pale pinkish and mottled. The interface between the lips and the skin is indistinct, with fissures appearing at right angles to the skin and vermilion junction. The lips are dry and cracked.

No specific treatment is indicated. However, a strong relationship exists between these epithelial and connective tissue changes and the development of basal cell carcinoma of the skin or squamous cell carcinoma of the lips and skin. Smoking may increase this risk. Biopsy is indicated for persistent scaling or ulceration. Identification of patients at high risk and with early indications of sun damage can be helpful in preventing future lesions. Patients at risk should be advised to avoid sun exposure and use sun blocking agents for protection.

MUCOCELE

A **mucocele** is a lesion that forms when a salivary gland duct is severed and the mucous salivary gland secretion spills into the adjacent connective tissue. An inflammatory response occurs, granulation tissue forms, and the mucus is walled off to form a cystlike structure lined by compressed granulation tissue. This is not a true cyst because the cystic space is not lined by epithelium.

A mucocele presents as a swelling in the tissue that often increases and decreases in size over time. The lower lip is the most common site of occurrence **(Figure 2-35).** However, mucoceles may form in any area of the oral mucosa in which minor salivary glands are found. On the lower lip they are usually lateral to the midline. If a mucocele is near the surface, it may appear bluish. The color of the mucosa is normal if the mucocele is deeper in the tissue. A mucoepidermoid carcinoma may clinically resemble a mucocele and should be considered in the differential

Figure 2-36 Mucocele (mucous cyst) of the floor of the mouth.

Figure 2-35 Mucocele of the lower lip. **A,** Fluid-filled lesion is seen on the lower lip. **B,** Microscopic appearance of a mucocele showing a cystlike space lined by granulation tissue (low magnification).

diagnosis. Most mucoceles occur in children and adolescents. However, they may occur in adults as well. If they are chronic or persistent, treatment is by surgical excision and removal of the adjacent minor salivary glands.

Occasionally an epithelium-lined cystic structure occurs in association with a salivary gland duct. This is also called a **mucocele, mucous cyst,** or **mucous retention cyst (Figure 2-36)** and occurs much less frequently than the type described previously. Most of these are not true cysts but rather dilated salivary gland ducts that are believed to develop as a result of salivary duct obstruction. A ballooning of the duct

occurs, which appears microscopically as an epithelium-lined cyst. Mucous cysts usually occur in adults who are older than 50 years of age. They may occur anywhere in the oral cavity where minor salivary glands are found and are treated by removal of the affected minor salivary glands.

Ranula is a term used for a mucocele-like lesion that forms unilaterally on the floor of the mouth **(Figure 2-37).** It is associated with the ducts of the sublingual and submandibular glands. The name "ranula" is derived from *rana,* the Latin word for frog. The clinical appearance of the ranula resembles the outpouching that occurs under the jaw of the frog when croaking. Although obstruction of the duct is considered to be the most likely cause for its development, histologically a ranula may resemble either a mucocele or a mucous cyst. Ranulas are treated by surgery, and the cause of obstruction, often a salivary gland stone, must be removed.

NECROTIZING SIALOMETAPLASIA

Necrotizing sialometaplasia is a benign condition of the salivary glands characterized by moderately painful swelling and ulceration in the affected area **(Figure 2-38).** Histologically, necrosis of the salivary glands is seen. The salivary gland duct epithelium is replaced by squamous epithelium (metaplasia) and appears microscopically as islands of squamous epithelium deep in the connective tissue. If the duration of the ulcer is prolonged, a biopsy is needed to establish the diagnosis. However, the ulcer heals spontaneously by secondary intention, usually within a

Figure 2-37   Ranula.

Figure 2-38   Necrotizing sialometaplasia.

few weeks. The junction of the hard and soft palates is most often affected. Necrotizing sialometaplasia is thought to result from blockage of the blood supply to the area of the lesion.

SIALOLITH

A **sialolith** is a salivary gland stone. Sialoliths occur in both major and minor salivary glands and form by precipitation of calcium salts around a central core. They may cause obstruction of the involved salivary gland; when they occur in the floor of the mouth, they can often be seen as a radiopaque structure on an occlusal radiograph **(Figure 2-39)**.

Figure 2-39   Sialoliths. **A,** Occlusal radiograph showing a sialolith *(arrow)* in Wharton duct. **B,** Sialolith *(arrow)* in a minor salivary gland on the floor of the mouth. **C,** Microscopic appearance of a sialolith showing concentric rings. (**A** courtesy Dr. Barry Wolinsky.)

ACUTE AND CHRONIC SIALADENITIS

Both **acute** and **chronic sialadenitis** may occur as a result of obstruction of a salivary gland duct. They may also occur as a result of infection. In some cases the cause cannot be identified. Sialadenitis presents as a painful swelling of the involved salivary gland, usually one of the major glands. Diagnosis may require injection of a radiopaque dye into the gland, followed by taking a radiograph of the gland (sialography). Antibiotics may be necessary in cases of infection.

Reactive Connective Tissue Hyperplasia

Reactive connective tissue hyperplasia consists of proliferating, exuberant granulation tissue and dense fibrous connective tissue. These lesions result from overzealous repair. They may occur as a response to a single event or as a chronic low-grade injury. The reason for the exuberant overgrowth of reparative tissue is not known.

Periapical inflammation, radicular cyst, and **internal** and **external tooth resorption** are included in this classification because they are also examples of lesions associated with proliferating inflamed tissue.

PYOGENIC GRANULOMA

A **pyogenic granuloma** is a commonly occurring intraoral lesion that is characterized by a proliferation of connective tissue containing numerous blood vessels and inflammatory cells. It occurs as a response to injury. The term "pyogenic granuloma" is a misnomer. The lesion does not produce pus (pyogenic) and is not a true granuloma.

The pyogenic granuloma **(Figure 2-40)** is usually ulcerated, soft to palpation, and bleeds easily. It is deep red to purple because of the vascularity of the proliferating tissue. It is generally elevated and may be either sessile or pedunculated. When ulcerated, the fibrin membrane on the surface appears yellowish white. The gingiva is the most common location of occurrence, but the lesion also occurs in other areas, such as the lips, tongue, and buccal mucosa. Pyogenic granulomas may vary considerably in size, from a few millimeters to several centimeters. They usually develop rapidly and then remain static. Although they

are most common in teenagers and young adults, they may occur at any age. Some studies show a predominance in females.

Pyogenic granulomas often occur in pregnant women and have been called **pregnancy tumors (Figure 2-41).** The lesions are identical to those seen in men and in nonpregnant women and may be caused by changing hormonal levels and increased response to plaque. However, they often regress after delivery. Similar gingival lesions also occur during puberty.

Figure 2-40 Pyogenic granuloma.

Figure 2-41 Pyogenic granuloma of pregnancy (pregnancy tumor).

The pyogenic granuloma is treated by surgical excision if it does not resolve spontaneously. Occasionally the lesion may recur if the injurious agent (e.g., calculus) remains.

GIANT CELL GRANULOMA

A **giant cell granuloma** is a lesion that contains many multinucleated giant cells and well-vascularized connective tissue. Red blood cells and chronic inflammatory cells are also seen in this lesion. The cause of the giant cell granuloma is not clear. It occurs only in the jaws, seems to originate from the periodontal ligament or the periosteum, and is thought to be a response to injury. The giant cell granuloma occurs both on the gingiva (peripheral giant cell granuloma) and within bone (central giant cell granuloma). The term *peripheral* pertains to those lesions occurring outside the bone, generally on the gingiva or alveolar mucosa, and the term *central* refers to a lesion occurring within the maxilla and mandible.

Peripheral Giant Cell Granuloma

The **peripheral giant cell granuloma** always occurs on the gingiva or alveolar process, usually anterior to the molars. It is considered a reactive lesion usually occurring as a result of local irritating factors. It may resemble the pyogenic granuloma in clinical appearance **(Figure 2-42)**. Peripheral giant cell granulomas may vary in size from 0.5 to 1.5 cm in diameter and are usually dark red because of the numerous blood vessels present. The lesion may occur at any age but has been reported to be more frequent in people between 40 and 60 years of age and more common in women than men. Peripheral giant cell granulomas may cause superficial destruction of the alveolar bone; they are treated by surgical excision of the lesion and generally do not recur.

Central Giant Cell Granuloma

The central giant cell granuloma occurs within the bone of the maxilla or mandible, primarily in children and young adults. Studies have reported its occurrence more commonly in females than in males. These granulomas are common in the anterior segments of the maxilla and mandible and are uncommon in the ramus of the mandible. Patients

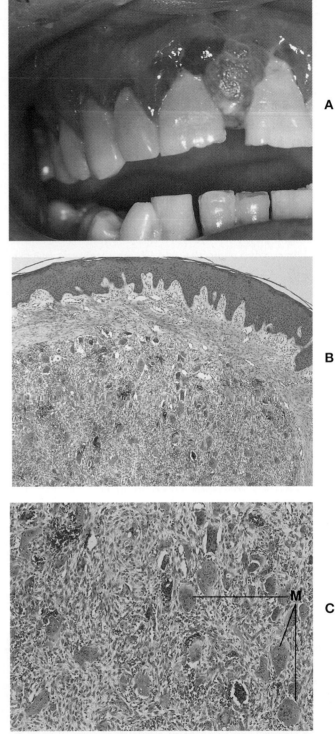

Figure 2-42 A, Peripheral giant cell granuloma. **B** and **C,** Microscopic appearance of a peripheral giant cell granuloma. Low magnification **(A)** shows the surface epithelium. Higher magnification **(B)** shows multinucleated giant cells *(M),* capillaries, and fibroblasts.

with central giant cell granulomas may complain of discomfort from the lesions, but pain is not a common feature. Most central giant cell granulomas are discovered on routine radiographs. The lesion is slow growing and destructive and produces a radiolucency in the bone. The borders of the radiolucency may be either sclerotic or ill defined, and they may be unilocular or multilocular **(Figure 2-43)**. Divergence of the roots of teeth adjacent to the lesion is a common feature of central giant cell granuloma. Lesions are treated by surgical removal but occasionally recur.

A lesion of bone identical to the central giant cell granuloma (often called **brown tumor**) occurs in patients with hyperparathyroidism (discussed in Chapter 9). They are not surgically removed because they resolve when the underlying disease is successfully treated.

IRRITATION FIBROMA

The **irritation fibroma** (also known as **fibroma** or **traumatic fibroma**) is a broad-based, persistent exophytic lesion that is composed of dense, scarlike connective tissue containing few blood vessels. It occurs as a result of chronic trauma or an episode of trauma such as habitual cheek chewing or cheek biting **(Figure 2-44)**. The irritation fibroma is usually a small lesion. Most are less than a centimeter in diameter, and fibromas greater than 2 cm in diameter are rare. The fibroma occurs most frequently on the buccal mucosa. It also occurs on the tongue, lips, and palate. It is the most common mass on the gingiva. The color of the irritation fibroma is usually lighter than that of the surrounding mucosa. The surface is covered by stratified squamous epithelium and may appear opaque and white if it has a thick keratin surface, or it may be ulcerated because of local secondary trauma.

An irritation fibroma is surgically removed. Many benign soft tissue tumors resemble the irritation fibroma in clinical appearance. Excision and microscopic examination of the tissue are important for diagnosis if the clinician is unsure about the nature of the lesion. Irritation fibromas usually do not recur at the same site, but additional lesions may occur as a response to additional trauma.

The **peripheral ossifying fibroma** is a common gingival lesion, the cause of which is not known. It is thought to originate in the periodontal ligament and is described in Chapter 7.

A

B

C

Figure 2-43 Radiographs of central giant cell granulomas showing multilocular radiolucencies in the mandible **(A)** and maxilla **(B)**. **C,** Microscopic appearance of a central giant cell granuloma showing the same features as a peripheral giant cell granuloma except for the absence of surface mucosa.

Figure 2-44 Irritation fibroma. **A,** The development of fibroma followed by the healing of a periodontal abscess. **B,** Irritation fibroma of the buccal mucosa. **C,** Microscopic appearance of a fibroma. (**A** courtesy Dr. Murray Schwartz.)

DENTURE-INDUCED FIBROUS HYPERPLASIA

Denture-induced fibrous hyperplasia is commonly called **epulis fissuratum** or **inflammatory hyperplasia.** This lesion is caused by an ill-fitting denture and is located in the vestibule along the denture border. It is composed of dense, fibrous connective tissue surfaced by stratified squamous epithelium, the same type of tissue seen in the irritation fibroma. The lesion is usually somewhat larger than the irritation fibroma. It is arranged in elongated folds of tissue into which the denture flange fits **(Figure 2-45).** The surface of the lesion is often ulcerated. Because this lesion does not resolve even with prolonged removal of the denture, treatment involves surgical removal of the excess tissue and construction of a new denture.

PAPILLARY HYPERPLASIA OF THE PALATE

Papillary hyperplasia of the palate, or **palatal papillomatosis,** is a form of denture stomatitis. It is almost always associated with a removable full or

Figure 2-45 Denture-induced fibrous hyperplasia (epulis fissuratum). **A,** With denture; **B,** without denture.

partial denture or an orthodontic appliance. The palatal mucosa, most commonly the vault area, is covered by multiple erythematous papillary projections that give the area a granular or "cobblestone" appearance **(Figure 2-46)**. Each of the papillary projections consists of fibrous connective tissue, usually chronically inflamed and surfaced by stratified squamous epithelium. The precise cause of this type of hyperplasia is not known. It is usually related to an ill-fitting upper denture or other removable prosthetic device that is worn continuously, 24 hours a day. Surgical removal of the hyperplastic papillary tissue before construction of a new denture is generally necessary.

GINGIVAL ENLARGEMENT

Gingival enlargement is characterized by an increase in the bulk of the free and attached gingiva, especially that involving the interdental papillae **(Figure 2-47)**. No stippling is seen, and the gingival margins are rounded. The tissue consistency may vary from soft to firm, and the appearance may vary from erythematous to a normal pink color, depending on the degree of inflammation. Gingival enlargement may be generalized or localized and may vary from mild focal enlargement of interdental papillae to severe generalized gingival enlargement that may cover the crowns of the teeth. The en-

Figure 2-46 Papillary hyperplasia of the palate. **A,** Full denture. **B,** Partial denture. (Courtesy Dr. Edward V. Zegarelli.)

Figure 2-47 Gingival enlargement. **A,** Fibrous; **B,** inflamed.

larged tissue may appear red, a normal mucosal color, or paler, depending on the amount of inflammation and degree of vascularity. Although generally called **gingival hyperplasia,** enlargement of the gingiva may also be the result of hypertrophy.

Most cases are the result of an unusual tissue response to chronic inflammation associated with local irritants such as plaque or calculus. Hormonal changes, such as those occurring in pregnancy and puberty, and certain drugs, such as phenytoin, calcium channel blockers, and cyclosporine, can increase the tissue response to local factors (see Chapter 9). Hereditary forms of gingival fibromatosis occur, beginning in early childhood (see Chapter 6). In some cases the cause of gingival hyperplasia cannot be identified.

If the tissue is inflamed and bleeds easily, biopsy and histologic examination of the tissue may be necessary to rule out the gingival enlargement that may occur in individuals with leukemia. (See Chapter 7.)

Gingivoplasty (reshaping the gingiva) or gingivectomy (removing gingival tissue) may be necessary to recontour the gingival tissue. Meticulous oral hygiene is helpful in reducing additional hyperplasia.

CHRONIC HYPERPLASTIC PULPITIS

Chronic hyperplastic pulpitis, or **pulp polyp,** is an excessive proliferation of chronically inflamed

Figure 2-48 Chronic hyperplastic pulpitis (pulp polyp) *(arrow).*

dental pulp tissue. In children and young adults, it occurs in teeth with large, open carious lesions; primary and permanent molars are often affected. Chronic hyperplastic pulpitis appears as a red or pink nodule of tissue that often fills the entire cavity in the tooth, with tissue protruding from the pulp chamber **(Figure 2-48).** It is usually asymptomatic; because the hyperplastic tissue contains so few nerves, it is usually insensitive to manipulation. The proliferation of pulp tissue rather than pulpal necrosis, which can also result from dental caries, may be related to the large root opening and blood supply of the tooth involved.

The hyperplastic tissue is granulation tissue. Inflammatory cells, primarily lymphocytes and plasma cells and sometimes neutrophils, are commonly present. The tissue is generally surfaced by stratified squamous epithelium. Because no epithelium exists in normal pulp tissue, this epithelium is thought to result from desquamation of the surface oral mucosa. Chronic hyperplastic pulpitis is treated by either extraction or endodontic treatment of the involved tooth.

Inflammatory Periapical Lesions

Dental caries or trauma to a tooth may result in a variety of responses: inflammation, infection, chronic hyperplastic pulpitis, and necrosis of the dental pulp. The inflammatory process begins in the dental pulp and then extends into the periapical area (the area surrounding the apical portion of the tooth root at the site of the apical foramen). This condition occurs because once the inflammatory process has been established in the dental pulp, the only route it can follow is through the root canal into the periapical area. The presence of accessory canals may lead to areas of inflammation located on the lateral portion of the tooth root.

PERIAPICAL ABSCESS

An acute **periapical abscess** is composed of a purulent exudate, or pus, surrounded by connective tissue containing neutrophils and lymphocytes **(Figure 2-49,** *A*). The patient complains of severe pain, which is the result of inflammation. The inflammatory exudate puts pressure on nerves, and chemical mediators can also cause pain. The periapical abscess may develop directly from the inflammation in the pulp, but it more commonly develops in an area of previously existing chronic inflammation. The pus that forms seeks a path of least resistance and finds either a channel or a fistula out of the tissue, or it spreads to contiguous areas through oral and facial tissue spaces (see Figure 2-3). The tooth associated with the abscess is usually quite painful and may be slightly extruded from its socket. If the acute abscess develops directly from pulpal inflammation, there may be no radiographic changes except for a slight thickening of the apical periodontal ligament space. If the abscess develops in a preexisting area of periapical chronic inflammation, a distinct radiolucent area is seen at the apex.

The clinician treats a periapical abscess by establishing drainage, either by opening the pulp chamber or by extracting the tooth. If the abscess has extended into adjacent tissue, an incision may be necessary to establish drainage. The patient may also be given antibiotic therapy.

DENTAL OR PERIAPICAL GRANULOMA

A **periapical granuloma** is a localized mass of chronically inflamed granula that forms at the opening of the pulp canal, generally at the apex of a nonvital tooth root **(Figure 2-49)**. This is a chronic process from the outset. Most cases are completely asymptomatic. Sometimes the tooth is sensitive to pressure and percussion because of the inflammation in the apical area. The tooth may also feel slightly extruded from its socket. The radiographic change may vary from a slight thickening of the periodontal ligament space in the area of inflammation to a diffuse radiolucency to a distinct, well-circumscribed radiolucency surrounding the root apex.

The periapical granuloma is composed of granulation tissue containing lymphocytes, plasma cells, and macrophages. Neutrophils may also be present, and areas of dense fibrous connective tissue are often seen. The periapical granuloma is different from the granuloma of granulomatous inflammation, which is a distinctive type of inflammation characteristic of certain diseases (e.g., tuberculosis). Epithelial rests of Malassez, which are remnants of tooth-forming tissue, are often present in the periapical granuloma. The periapical granuloma is treated by root canal therapy or extraction of the tooth.

Figure 2-49 A, Radiograph of a periapical granuloma. **B,** Microscopic appearance of a periapical granuloma showing a collection of inflammatory cells at the apex of a tooth (low magnification). (**A** courtesy Dr. Herbert Frommer.)

RADICULAR CYST (PERIAPICAL CYST)

A **radicular cyst**, or **periapical cyst**, is a true cyst consisting of a pathologic cavity lined by epithelium. It occurs in association with the root of a nonvital tooth **(Figure 2-50)**. It is the most commonly occurring cyst in the oral region. The epithelial lining of the cyst develops in a periapical granuloma as a result of proliferation of the epithelial rests of Malassez.

A periapical cyst develops when the epithelium within the inflamed connective tissue of the periapical granuloma proliferates, forming an epithelial mass that increases in size through division of the peripheral cells. The peripheral cells are the equivalent of the basal cell layer of the epithelium. As the cells

A

B

C

Figure 2-50 Radicular cyst. **A,** Diagram of a radicular cyst located around the root of an erupted tooth. **B,** Radiograph showing a well-circumscribed radiolucency around the root of a tooth. **C,** Microscopic features of a radicular cyst.

in the central portion of the mass become increasingly separated from the source of nutrition in the connective tissue, they degenerate centrally, forming a cavity (lumen) that is lined by epithelium and filled with fluid. Histologically the tissue surrounding this epithelial-lined cystic cavity is similar to that seen in the periapical granuloma.

Most periapical cysts are asymptomatic and are discovered on radiographic examination. The radiographic appearance of the radicular cyst is the same as that of the periapical granuloma. It appears as a radiolucency, usually well circumscribed, that is attached to a tooth root. It is not possible to differentiate reliably a periapical granuloma from a radicular cyst based on the radiographic appearance alone. A periapical cyst may form in association with any tooth. The cyst may occur lateral to the tooth root rather than at the apex, if it is associated with a lateral pulp canal. Other types of cysts can resemble a periapical cyst radiographically, and therefore removal of the cyst and microscopic examination of the tissue are necessary.

The radicular cyst is treated by root canal therapy, apicoectomy, or extraction and curettage of the periapical tissues. A **residual cyst** forms when the tooth is removed and all or part of a periapical cyst is left behind **(Figure 2-51)**. Radiographically a residual cyst is a well-circumscribed radiolucency located at the site of tooth extraction. It is treated by surgical removal of the cyst.

RESORPTION OF TEETH

Tooth structure can be resorbed in the same manner as bone. This occurs normally in the process of exfoliation of deciduous teeth and may also occur in other situations. Resorption of the tooth structure beginning at the outside of the tooth is called external resorption. This usually involves the root of a tooth but can occasionally involve the crown of an impacted tooth.

Like bone resorption, tooth resorption can occur when inflammatory tissue is present. Resorption of the root of a tooth sometimes occurs when a periapical granuloma is present. Bone resorption as a response to pressure allows orthodontic tooth movement to occur. Pressure can also cause resorption of tooth structure. This can occur from excessive occlusal or orthodontic forces and with benign and malignant tumors. When a tooth that has been avulsed is reimplanted, the root is resorbed and re-

A   B

C

D

Figure 2-51 A, Diagram of a residual cyst. **B,** Radiograph of a residual cyst showing a radiolucency at the site of a previously extracted tooth. (Courtesy Drs. Paul Freedman and Stanley Kerpel.)

placed by bone. Occasionally, resorption may involve the crown of an impacted tooth or the roots of teeth, and the cause cannot be identified. This is called **idiopathic tooth resorption.**

External root resorption first appears as a slight raggedness or blunting of the root apex and can proceed to severe loss of tooth substance **(Figure 2-52).** The condition is not reversible, but progression of the process can be avoided if the cause can be identified and removed. Resorption of impacted teeth can also occur. Generalized root resorption may also occur after orthodontic tooth movement.

Internal tooth resorption can occur in any tooth; usually only a single tooth is involved. In some cases no cause can be identified. However, it is usually associated with an inflammatory response in the pulp. If the process occurs in the coronal part of the

Figure 2-52 Tooth resorption. **A,** Root resorption of a mandibular anterior tooth associated with chronic inflammation. **B,** Resorption of tooth structure and bone because of chronic inflammation. **C,** Idiopathic resorption of an impacted tooth. **D,** Generalized root resorption associated with orthodontic tooth movement. (**A** courtesy Dr. Gerald P. Curatola.)

tooth, it may be seen clinically as a pinkish area in the crown. The dental hard tissue has resorbed and is thinner than normal, and the pink color results from the vascular, inflamed connective tissue that can be seen through the remaining enamel and dentin. When the process involves the root, it can be seen only radiographically. A round-to-ovoid, radiolucent area associated with the pulp is seen in the central portion of the tooth.

Root canal treatment can be successfully performed if internal resorption is discovered early. If not treated, the process can extend through the dental hard tissue and cause a perforation. After this perforation occurs, the tooth must be extracted.

FOCAL SCLEROSING OSTEOMYELITIS

Focal sclerosing osteomyelitis, also called **condensing osteitis,** is a change in bone near the apices of teeth that is thought to be a reaction to low-grade infection. Radiographically a radiopaque area is seen extending below the roots of the involved tooth **(Figure 2-53)**. The tooth most commonly associated with focal sclerosing osteomyelitis is the mandibular first molar. Occasionally the mandibular second molar and the mandibular premolars may also be involved.

Radiographically, focal sclerosing osteomyelitis appears as a radiopaque area extending below the roots of the tooth. The borders may be diffuse or well defined. Occasionally the periphery of the area is radiolucent; in other cases a central radiolucency surrounded by radiopacity is seen. Microscopically it is dense bone with little marrow or connective tissue. Generally very little inflammation is present. Focal sclerosing osteomyelitis is often associated with a carious or restored tooth. It is generally asymptomatic. However, pain may be associated if pulpal inflammatory disease is present. Focal sclerosing osteomyelitis may be present at any age, but it is typically first seen in young adults.

Diagnosis of focal sclerosing osteomyelitis can usually be made based on the characteristic radiographic appearance. Occasionally, biopsy may be necessary to rule out other radiopaque lesions such as osteoma, complex odontoma, or ossifying fibroma. Treatment is not necessary. The sclerotic bone remains even after treatment of the involved tooth.

Figure 2-53 Focal sclerosing osteomyelitis.

ALVEOLAR OSTEITIS ("DRY SOCKET")

Alveolar osteitis or **"dry socket"** is a postoperative complication of tooth extraction. The most frequently affected area is the socket of an extracted mandibular third molar. After the extraction of the tooth, the blood clot breaks down and is lost before healing has taken place. Pain develops several days after the extraction. On examination the tooth socket appears empty and the bone surfaces exposed. The patient complains of pain, bad odor, and bad taste. Because no infection exists, fever, swelling, and erythema are not present. Treatment of alveolar osteitis is directed at relief of pain and includes gentle irrigation and insertion of a medicated dressing.

Selected References

Books

Bath-Balogh M, Fehrenbach MJ: *Illustrated dental embryology, histology, anatomy,* Philadelphia, 1997, WB Saunders.

Fehrenbach MJ, Herring SW: *Illustrated anatomy of the head and neck,* ed 2, Philadelphia, 2002, WB Saunders.

Kumar V, Cotran RS, Robbins SL: *Basic pathology,* ed 6, Philadelphia, 1997, WB Saunders.

Neville BW et al: *Oral & maxillofacial pathology,* ed 2, Philadelphia, 2002, WB Saunders.

Peterson LJ, editor: *Principles of oral and maxillofacial surgery,* Philadelphia, 1992, JB Lippincott.

Peterson LJ et al, editors: *Contemporary oral and maxillofacial surgery,* St Louis, 1988, Mosby.

Regezi JA, Sciubba JJ: *Oral pathology: clinical-pathologic correlations,* ed 4, Philadelphia, 2003, WB Saunders.

Sittig M: *Handbook of toxic and hazardous chemicals,* Park Ridge, NJ, 1981, Noyes.

Sonis ST, Fazio RC, Fang L: *Principles and practice of oral medicine,* ed 2, Philadelphia, 1995, WB Saunders.

Towbridge HO, Emling RC: *Inflammation: a review of the process,* ed 5, Carol Stream, IL, 1997, Quintessence.

Journal Articles

Inflammation and Repair

Anderson I: The properties of hyaluronan and its role in wound healing, *Prof Nurse* 17(4):232, 2001.

Avidson JM: Wound repair, *J Hand Ther* 11:80, 1998.

Dalgleish AG, O'Byrne KJ: Chronic immune activation and inflammation in the pathogenesis of AIDS and cancer, *Adv Cancer Res* 84:231, 2002.

Kingsley A: Wound healing and potential therapeutic options, *Prof Nurse* 17(9):539, 2002.

Levy JH: The human inflammatory response, *J Cardiovasc Pharmacol* 27:S31, 1996.

Ley K: Molecular mechanisms of leukocyte recruitment in the inflammatory process, *Cardiovasc Res* 32:733, 1996.

Shaffer M, Barbul A: Lymphocyte function in wound healing and following injury, *Br J Surg* 85:444, 1998.

Slade JF, Chou KH: Bony tissue repair, *J Hand Ther* 11:118, 1998.

Smith KL, Dean SJ: Tissue repair of the epidermis and dermis, *J Hand Ther* 11:95, 1998.

Zoellner H, Chapple CC, Hunter N: Microvasculature in gingivitis and chronic periodontitis: disruption of vascular networks with protracted inflammation, *Microsc Res Tech* 56(1):15, 2002.

Lesions from Physical and Chemical Injuries to the Oral Tissues

Axell T, Hedin C: Epidemiologic study of excessive oral melanin pigmentation with special reference to the influence of tobacco habits, *Scand J Dent Res* 90:432, 1982.

Bouquot JE, Seime RJ: Bulimia nervosa: dental perspectives, *Pract Periodontics Aesthet Dent* 9:655, 1997.

Brady WF: The anorexia nervosa syndrome, *Oral Surg Oral Med Oral Pathol* 50:509, 1980.

Buchner A, Hansen LS: Amalgam pigmentation (amalgam tattoo) of the oral mucosa, *Oral Surg Oral Med Oral Pathol* 49:39, 1980.

Cash RC: Bruxism in children: review of the literature, *J Pedod* 12:107, 1988.

Ferguson MM et al: Enamel erosion related to wine making, *Occup Med* 46:159, 1996.

Gandara BK, Truelove EL: Diagnosis and management of dental erosion, *J Contemp Dent Pract* 1:16, 1999.

Geurtsen W: Rapid general dental erosion by gas-chlorinated swimming pool water. Review of the literature and case report, *Am J Dent* 13:291, 2000.

Gormley MB et al: Thermal trauma: a review of 22 electrical burns of the lip, *J Oral Surg* 30:531, 1972.

Greer RO, Paulsion TC: Oral tissue alterations associated with the use of smokeless tobacco by teenagers, *Oral Surg Oral Med Oral Pathol* 56:275, 1983.

Hanemura H et al: Periodontal status and bruxism. A comparative study of patients with periodontal disease and occlusal parafunctions, *J Periodontol* 58:173, 1987.

Imbery TA, Edwards P: Necrotizing sialometaplasia: literature review and case reports, *J Am Dent Assoc* 127:1087, 1996.

Järvinen V et al: Dental erosion and upper gastrointestinal disorders, *Oral Surg Oral Med Oral Pathol* 64:298, 1988.

Kapila YL, Kashani H: Cocaine-associated rapid gingival recession and dental erosion. A case report, *J Periodontol* 68:485, 1997.

Little, JW: Eating disorders: dental implications, *Oral Surg Oral Med Oral Pathol Oral Radiol Endod* 93:138, 2002.

Maron FS: Enamel erosion resulting from hydrochloric acid tablets, *J Am Dent Assoc* 127:781, 1996.

Mitchell-Lewis DA et al: Identifying oral lesions associated with crack cocaine use, *J Am Dent Assoc* 125:1104, 1994.

Needleman HL, Berkowitz RJ: Electric trauma to the oral tissues of children, *J Dent Child* 41:19, 1974.

Nemcovsky CE, Artizi Z: Erosion-abrasion lesions revisited, *Compend Contin Educ Dent* 17:416, 1996.

Owens BM, Gallien GS: Noncarious dental "abfraction" lesions in an aging population, *Compend Contin Educ Dent* 16:552, 1995.

Owens BM, Johnson WW, Schuman NJ: Oral amalgam pigmentation (tattoos): a retrospective study, *Quintessence Int* 23:805, 1992.

Owens BM, Schuman NJ, Johnson WW: Oral amalgam tattoos: a diagnostic study, *Compendium* 14:210, 1993.

Piotrowski BT, Gillette WB, Handcock EB: Examining the prevalence and characteristics of abfractionlike cervical lesions in a population of U.S. veterans, *J Am Dent Assoc* 132:1694, 2001.

Pollman L, Berger F, Pollman S: Age and dental abrasion, *Gerodontics* 3:94, 1987.

Pullinger AG, Seligman DA: The degree to which attrition characterizes differentiated patient groups of temporomandibular disorders, *J Orofac Pain* 7:196, 1990.

Rawlinson A: Case report. Labial cervical abrasion caused by misuse of dental floss, *Dent Health (London)* 26:3, 1987.

Richmond NL: Update on dental erosion. Office and home treatment for hypersensitive teeth, *J Indiana Dent Assoc* 66:29, 1987.

Roberts MW, Li SH: Oral findings in anorexia nervosa and bulimia nervosa: a study of 47 cases, *J Am Dent Assoc* 115:497, 1987.

Robertson PB, Walsh MM, Greene JC: Oral effects of smokeless tobacco use by professional baseball players, *Adv Dent Res* 11:307, 1997.

Rossie KM, Guggenheimer J: Thermally induced 'nicotine' stomatitis. A case report, *Oral Surg Oral Med Oral Pathol* 70:597, 1990.

Rugh JD, Harlan J: Nocturnal bruxism and temporomandibular disorders, *Adv Neurol* 49:329, 1988.

Rytomaa I et al: Bulimia and tooth erosion, *Acta Odontol Scand* 56:36, 1998.

Simmons MS, Thompson DC: Dental erosion secondary to ethanol-induced emesis, *Oral Surg Oral Med Oral Pathol* 64:731, 1987.

Sist T, Green G: Traumatic neuroma of the oral cavity, *Oral Surg Oral Med Oral Pathol* 51:394, 1981.

Tipton J: The selection of sun blocking topical agents to protect the skin, *Plast Reconstr Surg* 62:223, 1978.

Tylenda CA et al: Bulimia nervosa: its effect on salivary chemistry, *J Am Dent Assoc* 122:37, 1991.

Welsh RA, Donely C: The association between occlusion and attrition, *Aust Orthod J* 12:138, 1992.

Westergaard J et al: Exaggerated abrasion and erosion of human dental enamel surfaces. A case report, *Scand J Dent Res* 101:265, 1993.

Wray A, McGuirt F: Smokeless tobacco usage associated with oral carcinoma, *Arch Otolaryngol Head Neck Surg* 119:929, 1993.

Zimmers PL, Gobetti JP: Head and neck lesions commonly found in musicians, *J Am Dent Assoc* 125:1487, 1994.

Reactive Connective Tissue Hyperplasia

Bodner L et al: Growth potential of peripheral giant cell granuloma, *Oral Surg Oral Med Oral Pathol Oral Radiol Endod* 83:548, 1997.

Bonetti F et al: Peripheral giant cell granuloma: evidence for osteoclastic differentiation, *Oral Surg Oral Med Oral Pathol* 70:471, 1990.

Brown RS et al: Nitrendipine-induced gingival hyperplasia: first case report, *Oral Surg Oral Med Oral Pathol* 70:593, 1990.

Brunet L et al: Prevalence and risk of gingival enlargement in patients treated with anticonvulsant drugs, *Eur J Clin Invest* 31:781, 2001.

Daley TD, Nartey NO, Wysocki GP: Pregnancy tumor: an analysis, *Oral Surg Oral Med Oral Pathol* 72:196, 1991.

Daley T, Wysocki G, Day C: Clinical and pharmacologic correlations in cyclosporine-induced gingival hyperplasia, *Oral Surg Oral Med Oral Pathol* 62:417, 1986.

Gould A, Escobar V: Symmetrical gingival fibromatosis, *Oral Surg Oral Med Oral Pathol* 51:62, 1981.

Keith D: Side-effects of diphenylhydantosis: a review, *J Oral Surg* 36:206, 1978.

Lederman D et al: Gingival hyperplasia associated with nifedipine therapy. Report of a case, *Oral Surg Oral Med Oral Pathol* 57:620, 1984.

Miranda J et al: Prevalence and risk of gingival enlargement in patients treated with nifedipine, *J Periodontol* 72:605, 2001.

Parbatani R, Tinsley GF, Danford MH: Primary hyperparathyroidism presenting as a giant-cell epulis, *Oral Surg Oral Med Oral Pathol Oral Radiol Endod* 85:282, 1998.

Roberson JB, Crocker DJ, Schiller T: The diagnosis and treatment of central giant cell granuloma, *J Am Dent Assoc* 128:81, 1997.

Silverstein LH et al: The late development of oral pyogenic granuloma as a complication of pregnancy: a case report, *Compendium* 17:192, 1996.

Zain RB, Fei YJ: Fibrous lesions of the gingiva: a histopathologic analysis of 204 cases, *Oral Surg Oral Med Oral Pathol* 70:466, 1990.

Inflammatory Periapical Lesions

Gunraj MN: Dental root resorption, *Oral Surg Oral Med Oral Pathol Oral Radiol Endod* 88:647, 1999.

Harris EF, Butler MI: Patterns of incisor root resorption before and after orthodontic correction in cases with anterior open bites, *Am J Orthod Dentofacial Orthop* 101:112, 1992.

Harris EF, Robinson QC, Woods MA: An analysis of causes of apical root resorption in patients not treated orthodontically, *Quintessence Int* 24:417, 1993.

Review Questions

1. The initial response of the body to injury is:
   A. The immune response
   B. The inflammatory response
   C. Repair
   D. Hyperplasia
   E. Regeneration

2. What type of inflammation occurs if the injury is minimal and brief and the source is removed from the tissue?
   A. Fatal
   B. Acute
   C. Chronic
   D. Life threatening
   E. Granulomatous

3. In the inflammatory response, the first microscopic event is:
   A. Dilation of the microcirculation
   B. Increased permeability of the microcirculation
   C. Formation of exudate
   D. Constriction of the microcirculation
   E. Escape of white blood cells from the microcirculation

4. Which one of the following conditions is a chronic inflammatory lesion?
   A. Necrotizing sialometaplasia
   B. Periapical granuloma
   C. Acute necrotizing ulcerative gingivitis (ANUG)
   D. Aspirin burn
   E. Aphthous ulcer

5. The directed movement of white blood cells to the area of injury is called:
   A. Pavementing
   B. Margination
   C. Phagocytosis
   D. Hyperemia
   E. Chemotaxis

6. Which cells are most common in chronic inflammation?
   A. Neutrophils
   B. Macrophages and lymphocytes
   C. Neutrophils and macrophages
   D. Neutrophils and lymphocytes
   E. Lymphocytes and plasma cells

7. The macrophage has many functions. Which is not a function of the macrophage?
   A. Phagocytosis
   B. Removal of large foreign matter
   C. Removal of inhaled particles
   D. Formation of antibodies
   E. Helper in immune response

8. What term is used to describe blood plasma and proteins that leave the blood vessels and enter the surrounding tissues during inflammation?
   A. Hyperemia
   B. Hyperdrophy
   C. Margination
   D. Erythema
   E. Exudate

9. The process of phagocytosis directly involves the:
   A. Ingestion of foreign substances by white blood cells
   B. The escape of plasma fluids and proteins from the microcirculation into the surrounding tissues
   C. Displacement of white blood cells to the blood vessel walls
   D. Attachment of white blood cells to the blood vessel walls
   E. Margination and pavementing of white blood cells

10. Which of the following statements is correct concerning the neutrophil or PMN? It is a cell that:
    A. Makes up 60% to 70% of white blood cells
    B. Contains lysosomal enzymes
    C. Takes part in phagocytosis
    D. Has a multilobed nucleus
    E. Is also called a macrophage

11. During inflammation the second type of white blood cell to emigrate from the blood vessel into the injured tissue is the:
    A. Neutrophil
    B. Red blood cell
    C. Lymphocyte
    D. Monocyte
    E. Plasma cell

12. Components of the complement system mediate the inflammatory process by:
    A. Decreasing vascular permeability
    B. Releasing the neutrophil's histamine granules
    C. Causing cytolysis
    D. Decreasing phagocytosis
    E. Decreasing lysosomal enzymes

13. Two days after injury, granulation tissue can be described as:
    A. Immature vascular connective tissue
    B. Exudate
    C. Keloids

D. Ulceration

E. Scar tissue

14. The enlargement of superficial lymph nodes that occurs as a systemic sign of inflammation is:
    A. Called leukocytosis
    B. Regulated by the hypothalamus
    C. Caused by changes in their lymphocytes
    D. A process that involves only the lymph nodes in the submental area
    E. Caused by increased numbers of neutrophils

15. Which statement concerning repair in the body is true?
    A. Repair can be completed with the injurious agents present.
    B. Functioning cells and tissue components are always replaced by functioning scar tissue.
    C. Repair always results in regeneration.
    D. Replacement by live cells and new tissue components is a perfect process.
    E. The process of repair is initiated by the inflammatory response.

16. The clot that forms during repair:
    A. Consists of fibrous connective tissue
    B. Serves as a guide for migrating epithelial cells
    C. Forms after skin injury, but not after mucosal injury
    D. Only occurs with healing by secondary intention
    E. Only occurs with healing by primary intention

17. Healing by secondary intention refers to healing of an injury when:
    A. The incision has clean edges joined by sutures
    B. Only a small clot forms
    C. An infection forms in the injured area
    D. The patient has decreased formation of scar tissue
    E. The patient has increased formation of granulation tissue

18. An increase in the size of an organ or tissue resulting from an increase in the number of its cells is termed:
    A. Hyperemia
    B. Hyperplasia
    C. Inflammation
    D. Hypertrophy
    E. Hyperthermia

19. Normal bone tissue repair can be delayed by:
    A. Maintenance of osteoblast-producing tissues
    B. Inadequate movement of bone tissue
    C. Removal of an area of edema

D. Reduction in amount of tissue infection

E. Enhanced function of the immune response

20. Which one of the following would appear as a pigmented lesion?
    A. Amalgam tattoo
    B. Traumatic ulcer
    C. Frictional keratosis
    D. Aspirin burn
    E. Linea alba

21. Which statement is false?
    A. Attrition is the wearing away of tooth structure during mastication.
    B. Bruxism is the same as mastication.
    C. Erosion is the loss of tooth structure resulting from chemical action.
    D. Abrasion is due to mechanical, repetitive habits.
    E. Erosion can be associated with eating disorders.

22. Loss of tooth structure associated with bulimia is due to:
    A. Attrition
    B. Erosion
    C. Bruxism
    D. Abrasion
    E. Malnutrition

23. An aspirin burn:
    A. Occurs as a result of an overdose of aspirin
    B. Is usually painless
    C. Results from a misuse of aspirin
    D. Usually takes several weeks to heal
    E. Involves surgical tissue grafting

24. A patient has a generalized white appearance of the palate. Tiny erythematous dots can be seen, surrounded by a thickened white-to-gray area. Overall the palate appears wrinkled. This condition is most likely:
    A. Papillary hyperplasia of the palate
    B. Pseudopapillomatosis
    C. An aspirin burn
    D. Necrotizing sialometaplasia
    E. Nicotine stomatitis

25. The primary and most common cause of a mucocele is:
    A. Inflammation
    B. Tumor formation
    C. Severing of or trauma to a minor salivary gland duct
    D. Obstruction of a salivary gland duct
    E. A sialolith

26. A ranula is located on the:
    A. Lower lip
    B. Buccal mucosa
    C. Retromolar area
    D. Floor of the mouth
    E. Soft palate

27. Which one of the following would not occur on the gingiva?
    A. Irritation fibroma
    B. Pyogenic granuloma
    C. Giant cell granuloma
    D. Epulis fissuratum
    E. "Pregnancy tumor"

28. Generalized loss of tooth structure primarily on the lingual surfaces of maxillary teeth is associated with:
    A. Erosion
    B. Attrition
    C. Abrasion
    D. Bruxism
    E. Abfraction

29. External tooth resorption occurs as a result of:
    A. Caries
    B. Salivary gland dysfunction
    C. Chronic inflammation
    D. Medication
    E. Genetic factors

30. Which one of the following is considered to be the most likely cause of necrotizing sialometaplasia?
    A. Blocked salivary gland ducts
    B. Radiation therapy
    C. Smoking
    D. A sialolith
    E. Loss of blood supply

31. The most common site for a mucocele to occur is the:
    A. Floor of the mouth
    B. Tongue
    C. Buccal mucosa
    D. Retromolar area
    E. Lower lip

32. The peripheral giant cell granuloma only occurs on the:
    A. Gingiva
    B. Hard palate
    C. Buccal mucosa
    D. Floor of the mouth
    E. Tongue

33. A sialolith is:
    A. Chronic inflammation of a salivary gland
    B. Acute inflammation of a salivary gland
    C. A pooling of saliva in the connective tissue
    D. A salivary gland stone
    E. The most common cause of a mucocele

34. Which statement is false?
    A. A periapical cyst develops from a periapical granuloma.
    B. A periapical abscess always causes radiographic periapical changes.
    C. A periapical granuloma is a circumscribed area of chronically inflamed tissue.
    D. A periapical cyst is also called a radicular cyst.
    E. A radicular cyst most commonly occurs as a result of dental caries.

35. Epulis fissuratum results from irritation caused by:
    A. A denture flange
    B. Denture adhesive
    C. Poor suction from the denture in the palatal vault
    D. An allergic reaction to the acrylic in the denture
    E. Denture stomatitis

36. Which statement is true?
    A. A traumatic neuroma is never painful.
    B. Necrotizing sialometaplasia is considered a denture-related lesion.
    C. Chronic hyperplastic pulpitis is the same as gingival hyperplasia.
    D. Gingival enlargement may be caused by medication.
    E. Dilantin is a calcium channel blocker.

37. Loss of tooth structure caused by chemical action describes:
    A. Abrasion
    B. Drug allergy
    C. Erosion
    D. Attrition
    E. Bruxism

38. Which of the following cysts is characteristically associated with a tooth that is nonvital upon pulp testing?
    A. Residual cyst
    B. Radicular cyst
    C. Dentigerous cyst
    D. Dermoid cyst
    E. Traumatic bone cyst

39. Which cyst results when a tooth is extracted without removing the periapical cystic sac?
    A. Radicular
    B. Primordial
    C. Residual
    D. Periodontal
    E. Follicular

40. The most common cause of the radicular cyst is:
    A. Deep restorations without a base
    B. Caries
    C. Occlusal trauma
    D. Toothbrush abrasion at the cementoenamel junction
    E. A fistula

41. The wearing away of tooth structure through an abnormal mechanical action defines:
    A. Attrition
    B. Abrasion
    C. Erosion
    D. Germination
    E. Mastication

42. Which one of the following is not associated with attrition?
    A. Toothpaste
    B. Bruxism
    C. Mastication
    D. Diet
    E. Age

43. Heavy plaque and calculus, mouth breathing, orthodontic appliances, and overhanging restorations best describe some of the causative factors for:
    A. Phenytoin (Dilantin) hyperplasia
    B. A reaction from nifedipine (Procardia)
    C. Irritation fibromatosis
    D. Chemical fibromatosis
    E. Epulis fissuratum

44. The central giant cell granuloma:
    A. May occur on the tongue
    B. May present as a multilocular radiolucency
    C. Is histologically the same as a pyogenic granuloma
    D. Occurs primarily in men older than 60 years of age
    E. Originates from the periodontal ligament

45. During examination of the dentition, the dental hygienist notes the presence of active wear facets. This indicates that the patient is:
    A. Chewing too vigorously
    B. Bulimic
    C. A vegetarian
    D. Lip biting
    E. A bruxer

46. A patient has a loss of tooth structure on the labial surfaces of the anterior teeth and reports a high intake of citrus fruit juices. The hygienist would most likely suspect:
    A. Abrasion
    B. Bulimia
    C. Bruxism
    D. Attrition
    E. Erosion

47. The amalgam tattoo represents amalgam particles in the tissue and is most commonly observed in the oral cavity on the:
    A. Lateral borders of the tongue
    B. Anterior palate near the rugae
    C. Floor of the mouth
    D. Posterior gingiva and edentulous ridge
    E. Maxillary tuberosity

48. A pink protruding mass in the occlusal surface of a mandibular first or second molar is most likely:
    A. Pulpal granuloma
    B. Caused by caries
    C. A pulp polyp
    D. A mass of chronic inflammatory tissue
    E. All of the above

49. Which of the following drugs does not cause gingival enlargement?
    A. Dilantin
    B. Cyclosporine
    C. Procardia
    D. Cardizem CD
    E. Tetracycline

50. Traumatic ulcers are usually diagnosed based on a:
    A. Patient's medical history
    B. The clinical appearance and history of the ulcers
    C. Biopsy
    D. Therapeutic diagnosis
    E. Mucosal smear

Chapter 2 Synopsis

Condition/ Disease	Cause	Age/Race/Sex	Location
Injuries to Teeth			
Attrition	Mastication	>Age M>F	Occlusal/incisal surfaces Proximal
Abrasion	Repetitive mechanical habit	*	Dependent upon cause
Abfraction	Biomechanical forces on teeth	Adults	Cervical regions of teeth
Erosion	Chemical action	*	Dependent upon cause
Injuries to Soft Tissues			
Chemical Burn (e.g., aspirin, phenol)	Caustic chemical in contact with mucosa	*	Site of contact
Electric Burn	Live electric cord in contact with mucosa	Infants & young children	Site of contact
Thermal Burn	Hot food or liquid	*	Site of contact
Cocaine Use	Crack cocaine Cocaine hydrochloride	*	Midpalate Site of contact
Hematoma	Trauma	*	Site of trauma > Buccal/labial mucosa
Traumatic Ulcer	Trauma to mucosa	*	Site of trauma
Frictional Keratosis	Chronic friction against mucosal surface	*	Site of friction
Linea Alba	Teeth clenching/habit	*	Buccal mucosa at occlusal plane
Nicotine Stomatitis	Smoking	*	Hard palate
Tobacco Pouch Keratosis	Chewing tobacco	*	Site where tobacco is habitually placed

* No significant information.

Clinical Features	Radiographic Features	Microscopic Features	Treatment	Diagnostic Process
Flattening of tooth surfaces	N/A	N/A	Prevention Restoration	Clinical
Loss of tooth structure at site of wear	N/A	N/A	Prevention Restoration	Clinical
Wedge-shaped notching at cervical areas of involved teeth	N/A	N/A	Restoration May not require treatment	Clinical
Loss of tooth structure Smooth polished surface	N/A	N/A	Prevention Restoration	Clinical
Painful ulcer with necrotic surface	N/A	N/A	Palliative	Clinical
Tissue destruction	N/A	N/A	Tissue repair	Clinical
Painful erythema and superficial ulceration	N/A	N/A	None/palliative	Clinical
Painful ulceration and erythema Necrotic ulcers	N/A	N/A	Elimination of cause	Clinical
Red to purple to bluish-black mass lesion Size depends upon extent of trauma	N/A	N/A	None	Clinical
Painful, mucosal ulceration	N/A	Ulcer with eosinophils present in inflammatory infiltrate	Elimination of cause	Clinical
White mucosal surface	N/A	Hyperkeratosis	Elimination of cause	Clinical
Anterior to posterior white line	N/A	Epithelial hyperplasia and hyperkeratosis	None	Clinical
White, opacification of the palatal mucosa with raised red dots	N/A	Hyperkeratosis with inflamed minor salivary glands	Elimination of cause	Clinical
Granular to white, wrinkled appearance	N/A	Hyperkeratosis and epithelial hyperplasia Sometimes epithelial atypia	Elimination of cause	Clinical Microscopic

Continued

Chapter 2   Synopsis—cont'd

Condition/ Disease	Cause	Age/Race/Sex	Location
Injuries to Soft Tissues—cont'd			
Traumatic Neuroma	Injury to a peripheral nerve	*	Site of injured nerve
Amalgam Tattoo	Particles of amalgam in connective tissue	*	Most common on gingiva and edentulous alveolar ridge
Smoker's Melanosis	Smoking	*	Anterior labial gingiva
Solar (Actinic) Cheilitis	Sun exposure	>Adults	Vermilion of lips
Mucocele	Severed salivary gland duct	Any age	Most common—lower lip
Ranula	Obstruction/severing of salivary gland duct	*	Floor of mouth
Necrotizing Sialometaplasia	Compromised blood supply to area	*	Most common—junction of the hard and soft palate
Sialolith	Precipitation of calcified material around a central core	*	Major and minor salivary glands
Sialadenitis	Infection Obstruction of salivary gland duct	*	Symptomatic when involving major salivary glands
Reactive Connective Tissue Hyperplasia			
Pyogenic Granuloma	Response to injury Puberty Pregnancy	*	Most common—gingiva Also other areas

* No significant information.

Clinical Features	Radiographic Features	Microscopic Features	Treatment	Diagnostic Process
Painful, submucosal nodule	N/A	Mass of nerve	Surgical excision	Microscopic
Bluish-gray macule	Tiny radiopacity	Black granular material in connective tissue	No treatment after identification	Clinical Microscopic Radiographic
Diffuse grayish-brown color of gingiva	N/A	Melanin pigment in basal layer of epithelium and in underlying connective tissue	None Fades with decreased smoking	Clinical
Indistinct, fissured skin–mucosal interface	N/A	Degenerative changes in connective tissue	Protect lips and skin from sun exposure	Clinical
Localized tissue swelling that increases/decreases in size	N/A	Extravasated mucus in tissue surrounded by granulation tissue	Excision May spontaneously resolve	Clinical Microscopic
Fluid-filled swelling that increases/decreases in size	N/A	Resembles mucocele or mucous cyst	Surgery	Clinical
Moderately painful swelling and ulceration Acute onset	N/A	Necrosis of the salivary glands Replacement of salivary duct epithelium with squamous epithelium	Spontaneous resolution	Microscopic
Obstruction of the gland Hard nodule in soft tissue	Floor of the mouth—radiopaque structure	Calcified structure arranged in concentric rings	Surgical removal of stone	Clinical Radiographic Microscopic
Painful swelling of gland	N/A	Acute or chronic inflammatory infiltrate in salivary gland	Antibiotics if infection	Clinical Laboratory Microscopic
Deep red-purple exophytic lesion, usually ulcerated	N/A	Ulcerated granulation tissue	Surgical excision	Microscopic

Continued

Chapter 2 Synopsis—cont'd

Condition/ Disease	Cause	Age/Race/Sex	Location
Reactive Connective Tissue Hyper-plasia—cont'd			
Giant Cell Granuloma Peripheral	Unknown	>40-60 yrs F>M	Gingiva
Central	Unknown	Children & young adults F>M	Within bone of maxilla or mandible Usually anterior segments
Irritation Fibroma	Trauma	*	Common on the gingiva Many other oral locations
Denture-Induced Fibrous Hyperplasia (Epulis Fissuratum)	Ill-fitting denture Continuous wearing of denture	*	Vestibule along a denture border
Papillary Hyperplasia of the Palate	Removable prosthesis	*	Hard palate
Gingival Enlargement	Response to chronic inflammation Idiopathic Drug reaction Hormonal changes Genetic	*	Gingiva—generalized or localized
Chronic Hyperplastic Pulpitis	Dental caries	Children & young adults	Primary or permanent molars
Inflammatory Periapical Lesions Periapical Abscess	Inflammation of the dental pulp Preexisting periapical chronic inflammation	*	Roots of primary or permanent teeth

No significant information.

Clinical Features	Radiographic Features	Microscopic Features	Treatment	Diagnostic Process
Deep-red exophytic lesion	N/A	Many multinucleated giant cells in well-vascularized connective tissue	Surgical excision	Microscopic
Usually asymptomatic	Radiolucency may be multilocular	Many multinucleated giant cells in well-vascularized connective tissue	Surgical excision	Microscopic
Broad-based, pink, exophytic lesion	N/A	Dense fibrous connective tissue usually surfaced by normal epithelium	Surgical excision	Microscopic
Elongated folds of exophytic tissue surrounding denture phlange	N/A	Dense fibrous connective tissue surfaced by epithelium that may be hyperplastic and ulcerated	Surgical excision Fabrication of new denture	Clinical Microscopic
Mucosa surfaced by multiple, erythematous papillary projections	N/A	Papillary projections composed of fibrous connective tissue (usually inflamed) surfaced by squamous epithelium	Surgical removal of papillary tissue Fabrication of new denture	Clinical
Increase in the bulk of the free and attached gingiva No stippling Erythematous to normal color	N/A	Connective tissue (usually inflamed) surfaced by squamous epithelium	Gingivectomy Meticulous oral hygiene	Clinical Microscopic
Red or pink nodule protruding from the pulp chamber of a tooth with a large, open carious lesion	N/A	Granulation tissue surfaced by squamous epithelium	Extraction of tooth or endodontic treatment	Clinical
Pain, swelling, fistula, slight extrusion of tooth	None Thickening of periodontal ligament space Periapical radiolucency	Acute inflammatory infiltrate	Establish drainage	Clinical

Continued

Chapter 2 Synopsis—cont'd

Condition/ Disease	Cause	Age/Race/Sex	Location
Inflammatory Periapical Lesions—cont'd			
Periapical Granuloma	Pulpal inflammation and necrosis	*	Roots of primary or permanent teeth
Radicular Cyst (Periapical Cyst)	Nonvital tooth	*	Roots of primary or permanent teeth
Resorption of Teeth External Resorption	Chronic inflammation		Roots of primary or permanent teeth
Internal Resorption	Chronic pulpal inflammation		Dental hard tissue within root or crown
Focal Sclerosing Osteomyelitis	Low-grade chronic infection	*	Bone adjacent to any tooth Mandibular first molar most common
Aveolar Osteitis ("Dry Socket")	Postoperative complication of tooth extraction	*	Extraction site

* No significant information.

Clinical Features	Radiographic Features	Microscopic Features	Treatment	Diagnostic Process
Asymptomatic Tooth sensitive to percussion Slight extrusion of tooth	Slight thickening of periodontal ligament space Periodontal radiolucency	Chronic inflammatory infiltrate	Root canal therapy Extraction	Radiographic Microscopic
Most are asymptomatic	Radiolucency associated with the root of a nonvital tooth	Space lined by epithelium surrounded by an infiltrate of chronic inflammatory cells	Root canal therapy Apicoectomy Extraction and curettage of the extraction site	Radiographic Microscopic
Asymptomatic	Blunting of root apex to severe loss of root substance	N/A	Identify and remove cause	Radiographic
Asymptomatic May see pinkish color if crown involved	Round to avoid radiolucency in the central part of the tooth	N/A	Root canal therapy Extraction	Radiographic
Asymptomatic	Radiopaque area below roots of the tooth	Dense bone	None	Radiographic
Pain develops several days after extraction	N/A	N/A	Gentle irrigation Insertion of medicated dressing	Clinical

Immunity

Margaret J. Fehrenbach
Joan A. Phelan

Objectives

After studying this chapter, the student will be able to:

1. Define each of the words in the vocabulary list for this chapter.
2. Describe the primary difference between the immune response and the inflammatory response.
3. List and describe the two main types of lymphocytes, their origins, and their activities.
4. List the activities of macrophages.
5. Describe, using the cells involved, the difference between the humoral immune response and the cell-mediated immune response.
6. Describe the difference between passive and active immunity.
7. Give one example of passive immunity and one example of active immunity.
8. List and describe four types of hypersensitivity reactions, and give an example of each.
9. Define autoimmunity, and describe how it results in disease.
10. Define immunodeficiency, and describe how it results in disease.
11. Describe and contrast the clinical features of each of the three types of aphthous ulcers.
12. List three systemic diseases associated with aphthous ulcers.
13. Describe and compare the clinical features of urticaria, angioedema, contact mucositis, fixed drug eruption, and erythema multiforme.
14. Describe the clinical and histologic features of lichen planus.
15. List the triad of systemic signs that compose Reiter syndrome, and describe the oral lesions that occur in this syndrome.
16. Name the two cells that histologically characterize Langerhans cell disease. Describe the acute disseminated form, chronic disseminated form, and chronic localized form and state the names that have traditionally been used for each of these conditions.
17. Describe the oral manifestations of each of the following autoimmune diseases: Sjögren syndrome, lupus erythematosus (LE), pemphigus vulgaris, cicatricial pemphigoid, and Behçet syndrome.
18. Describe the clinical features of desquamative gingivitis, and list three diseases in which it may occur.
19. Describe the components of Behçet syndrome.

Vocabulary

Acantholysis (āk″an-thol′ĭ-sis) Dissolution of the intercellular bridges of the prickle cell layer of the epithelium.

Allergy (al′er-je) A hypersensitive state acquired through exposure to a particular allergen; reexposure to the same allergen elicits an exaggerated reaction.

Anaphylaxis (an″ah-fĭ-lak′sis) A severe type of hypersensitivity or allergic reaction in which the exaggerated immunologic reaction results from the release of vasoactive substances such as histamine; the reaction occurs on reexposure to a foreign protein or other substance after sensitization.

Antibody (an′tĭ-bod″e) A protein molecule, also called an immunoglobulin, which is produced by plasma cells and reacts with a specific antigen.

Antigen (an′tĭ-jen) Any substance able to induce a specific immune response.

Autoantibody (aw″to-an′tĭ-bod″e) An antibody that reacts against an antigenic constituent of the person's own tissues.

Autoimmune disease (aw″to-ĭ-mun′dĭ-zēz′) A disease characterized by tissue injury caused by a humoral or cell-mediated immune response against constituents of the body's own tissues.

B lymphocyte (B lim′fo-sīt) A lymphocyte, also called a B cell, that matures without passing through the thymus and later can develop into a plasma cell that produces antibodies.

Cell-mediated immunity (sel me′de-a″ted ĭ-mu′nĭ-te) Immunity in which the predominant role is played by T lymphocytes.

Humoral immunity (hu′mor-l ĭ-mu′nĭ-te) Immunity in which B lymphocytes and antibodies play the predominant role.

Hypersensitivity (hi″per-sen″sĭ-tiv′ĭ-te) A state of altered reactivity in which the body reacts to a foreign agent with an exaggerated immune response.

Immune complex (ĭ-m ū′n kom′pleks) A combination of antibody and antigen.

Immunodeficiency (ĭ-m″u-no-dĕ-fish′en-se) A deficiency of the immune response resulting from hypoactivity or decreased numbers of lymphoid cells.

Immunoglobulin (ĭ-m″u-no-glob′u-lin) A protein, also called an antibody, synthesized by plasma cells in response to a specific antigen.

LE cell A cell that is a characteristic of lupus erythematosus (LE) and other autoimmune diseases; it is a mature neutrophil that has phagocytized a spherical inclusion derived from another neutrophil.

Lymphoid tissue (lim′foid tish′u) Tissue composed of lymphocytes supported by a meshwork of connective tissue.

Macrophage (mak′ro-fāj) A large tissue-bound mononuclear phagocyte derived from monocytes circulating in blood; macrophages become mobile when stimulated by inflammation and interact with lymphocytes in an immune response.

Mucositis (mu″ko-si′tis) Mucosal inflammation.

Natural killer cell (NK cell) A lymphocyte that is part of the body's initial innate immunity, which by unknown mechanisms is able to directly destroy cells recognized as foreign.

Nikolsky sign (nĭ-kol′skē sīn) In some bullous diseases, such as pemphigus vulgaris and bullous pemphigus, the superficial epithelium separates easily from the basal layer on exertion of firm, sliding manual pressure.

Rheumatoid factor (roo′mah-toid fak′tor) A protein, immunoglobulin M (IgM), found in serum and detectable on laboratory tests; it is associated with rheumatoid arthritis and other autoimmune diseases.

T lymphocyte (T lim′fo-sīt) A lymphocyte that matures in the thymus before migrating to tissues; the T lymphocyte, also called a T cell, is responsible for cell-mediated immunity and may modulate the humoral immune response.

Thymus (thī′mus) A lymphoid organ located high in the chest, which is large in an infant and gradually shrinks in size.

Xerophthalmia (ze″rof-thal′me-ah) Abnormal dryness of the eyes.

Xerostomia (ze″ro-sto′me-ah) Dryness of the mouth caused by decreased salivary flow.

The acute inflammatory response, which is described in Chapter 2, is a rapid first line of defense against tissue injury and disease-producing microorganisms. The immune response, described in this chapter, occurs after the inflammatory response and is generally necessary for complete recovery. This chapter begins with a description of the immune response and includes those oral diseases that result from harmful effects of the immune response. Surveillance against neoplastic cells also requires the immune response. The neoplastic process is described in Chapter 7.

The Immune Response

The immune response, like the inflammatory response, defends the body against injury, particularly from foreign substances like microorganisms. The immune response differs from the inflammatory response in that it has the capacity to remember and respond more quickly to a foreign substance that enters the body a second time. It works amid the background of an already activated inflammatory response and a working repair process and involves a complex network of white blood cells, primarily lymphocytes, and their products. As with inflammation, the immune response may also result in an increased level of injury and disease.

Antigens

Antigens are the foreign substances against which the immune system defends the body. These substances are mainly proteins and are often microorganisms and their toxins. Transformed human cells, such as tumor cells or cells infected by viruses, can be antigens. Human tissue, as in the case of an organ transplant, tissue graft, or incompatible blood transfusion, can be an antigen. In diseases called **autoimmune diseases**, parts of an individual's own body become antigens.

Cells Involved in the Immune Response

The cells involved in the immune response are the following:

- B lymphocytes (associated plasma cells)
- T lymphocytes
- NK cells
- Macrophages

LYMPHOCYTES

The primary white blood cells involved in the immune response are **lymphocytes**. These cells are able to recognize and respond to an antigen.

Lymphocytes, like other white blood cells, are derived from a precursor cell called the stem cell, which is located in the bone marrow. Lymphocytes constitute 20% to 25% of the white blood cell population. They are antigen-sensitive cells that are long-lived and mobile. Different types of lymphocytes have different functions. The two main types of lymphocytes are called **B lymphocytes** (B cells) and **T lymphocytes** (T cells) **(Figure 3-1)**. A third type of lymphocyte is called the **natural killer cell (NK cell).** This type of lymphocyte is part of the body's innate immunity. NK cells have the ability to destroy cells (early in the immune response) that they recognize as foreign without first having to recognize specific antigens. In several immunodeficiency diseases, including acquired immunodeficiency syndrome (AIDS), NK cell function is abnormal.

B Lymphocytes

After developing from the stem cell in the bone marrow, the B lymphocyte matures and resides in lymphoid tissue, which is found in lymph nodes and many other body locations including tonsillar tissues. When antigen stimulates lymphocytes, they travel to the site of injury. Two main types of B lymphocytes exist: (1) The first type becomes the **plasma cell** when stimulated by antigen (the plasma cells produce the specific antibody needed to fight the antigen); (2) the second type is the B memory cell. This type of B lymphocyte retains the memory of previously encountered antigens. In the presence of an antigen, this cell duplicates or clones itself. All the

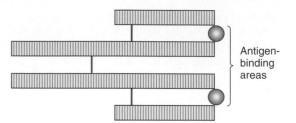

Figure 3-2 The basic structure of an antibody includes four protein chains consisting of two identical heavy polypeptide chains and two identical light chains, shaped to form a Y. The sections that make up the tips of the Y's arms vary greatly, creating a pocket uniquely shaped to enfold a specific antigen. This is called the variable (V) region. The stem of the Y serves to link the antibody to other participants in the immune response. This area is identical in all antibodies of the same class and is called the constant (C) region.

Figure 3-3 The five types of antibodies include the same basic structure arranged differently. This variation in structure allows them to function differently.

Figure 3-1 The differentiation of B and T lymphocytes. The primary cell of the immune response is the lymphocyte. The two main types of lymphocytes are (1) the B lymphocyte and (2) the T lymphocyte. Lymphocytes, like other white blood cells, are derived from a stem cell in the bone marrow. *PMN,* Polymorphonuclear leukocytes or neutrophils.

newly formed cells retain the capacity to remember the previously encountered antigen.

Plasma cells produce proteins called **antibodies.** Antibodies, also called **immunoglobulins (Igs),** are carried in blood serum. Specific antibodies are produced in response to specific antigens. Five different types of antibodies exits: (1) produced IgG, (2) IgM, (3) IgE, (4) IgA, and (5) IgD. They all have the same basic structure **(Figure 3-2):** two identical, heavy polypeptide chains and two identical light chains, shaped to form a *Y*. However, in each type of antibody the sections that make up the tips of the *Y*'s arms vary greatly, creating a pocket called the variable (*V*) region. This region is uniquely shaped to enfold a specific antigen, allowing the antibody to function differently **(Figure 3-3).** The stem of the *Y* serves to link the antibody to other participants in the immune response. This area is identical in all antibodies of the same class and is called the constant (*C*) region. Antibodies combine with antigen, forming an **immune complex,** also called an antigen-antibody complex. The formation of an immune complex usually renders the antigen inactive. The level of a specific antibody in the blood is called the **antibody titer** and can be measured by laboratory tests. This is helpful in the diagnosis of some infectious diseases.

T Lymphocytes

After they develop from the bone marrow stem cell, the T lymphocytes travel to the **thymus** and then are processed to maturity. The thymus is a primary lymphoid organ located high in the chest. It is quite large in infants and shrinks as an individual matures. Different types of T lymphocytes have different functions. Some are memory cells; others are **T-helper cells** that increase the functioning of the B lymphocytes (enhancing the antibody response) and are easily identifiable by the T4 cell marker **(Figure 3-4). T-suppressor cells** suppress or "turn off" the functioning of the B lymphocytes. **T-cytotoxic cells,** which usually carry the T8 marker, are active in surveillance against virally infected cells or tumor cells by directly attacking these cells.

Cell products or cytokines of either B or T lymphocytes are called lymphokines. Different cytokines have different functions **(Table 3-1).** They can activate macrophages and enhance the ability of macrophages to destroy foreign cells. Cytokines may also be involved in various other functions concerning leukocytes, fibroblasts, and endothelial cells. One of the first cytokines to be discovered was interferon. Produced by T lymphocytes and macrophages (as

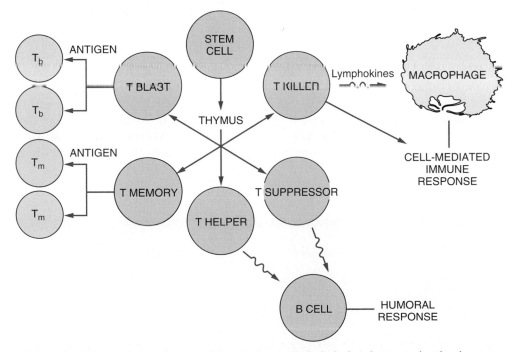

Figure 3-4 The various types of T lymphocytes and their involvement in the immune response.

Table 3-1 Cytokines and Their Functions During the Immune Response

Cytokine	Function
Interleukins (ILs)	Stimulates leukocyte proliferation and other functions
Macrophage chemotactic factor (MCF)	Stimulates macrophage emigration
Migration inhibitory factor (MIF)	Inhibits macrophage activity
Macrophage-activating factor (MAF)	Activates macrophages to produce and secrete lysosomal enzymes
Lymphotoxin (LT)	Destroys fibroblasts
Interferons (IFNs)	Various functions involving leukocytes, fibroblasts, and endothelial cells
Tumor necrosis factor (TNF)	Various functions involving leukocytes and fibroblasts

well as by cells outside the immune system), interferons are a family of proteins with antiviral properties.

MACROPHAGES

Macrophages are involved in the immune response to an antigen. They are present in the connective tissue during inflammation (see Chapter 2). Macrophages are active in phagocytosis of foreign substances and also help both the B lymphocytes and T lymphocytes; they produce cytokines called monokines. After phagocytosis of an antigen at the injury site, the macrophages process and present the antigen to the lymphocytes. This stimulates the lymphocytes to travel from the lymphoid tissue to the injury site. Macrophages serve as a link between the inflammatory and immune responses. In addition to phagocytosis, macrophages can also act as antigen-presenting cells. When activated, macrophages can function in many different ways, always amplifying the immune response. Unlike lymphocytes, macrophages do not remember the encountered antigen and need to be reactivated during each encounter.

Major Divisions of the Immune Response

The immune response to an antigen can take one of two forms **(Figure 3-5):** (1) the **humoral response** and (2) the **cell-mediated response.** The humoral response involves the production of antibodies. The B lymphocytes are the primary cells of the humoral response. The immune system's other main mechanism, the cell-mediated immune response (cell-mediated immunity [CMI]), involves lymphocytes working alone (usually T lymphocytes) or assisted by macrophages. The cell-mediated portion of the immune system regulates both major responses. Thus the humoral and cell-mediated responses are interrelated.

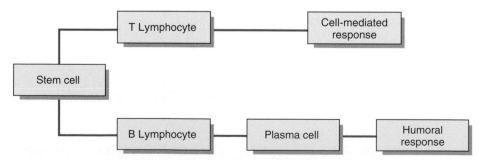

Figure 3-5 The major divisions of the immune response.

Memory and Immunity

Memory is an important function of the immune system. This is different from the inflammatory response, which is not capable of memory. Certain lymphocytes retain the memory of an antigen after an initial encounter. For this reason, the immune response to that antigen is much faster and stronger the next time it enters the body. The increased responsiveness that results from the retained memory of an already encountered antigen is called immunity.

Types of Immunity

PASSIVE IMMUNITY

Two types of immunity occur: (1) passive and (2) active. Using antibodies produced by another person to protect an individual against infectious disease is called **passive immunity.** This type of immunity can occur naturally or it can be acquired. Natural passive immunity occurs when antibodies from a mother pass through the placenta to the developing fetus. These antibodies protect a newborn infant from disease until the immune system matures. Passive immunity can be acquired through an injection of antibodies against a microorganism to which the person has not previously developed antibodies.

Acquired passive immunity is used to confer immediate protection against the disease caused by that microorganism. These antibodies are collected from individuals who have already had the disease and have naturally produced antibodies to the disease-causing microorganism. This type of passive immunity is short lived but can act immediately. It is used because the unprepared immune system of an individual takes longer to produce antibodies, and in the meantime the disease may develop. Acquired passive immunity, using hepatitis B immunoglobulin (HBIg), may be provided to dental personnel after needlestick or other occupational exposure incidents that do not have immunity to hepatitis B.

ACTIVE IMMUNITY

Active immunity can occur naturally or can be acquired. It occurs naturally when a a microorganism causes the disease. Protection against further attack by that microorganism is conferred to the individual if the body recovers from the disease. A less risky way of achieving active immunity is by an acquired or artificial means. A person is injected with or ingests either altered pathogenic microorganisms or products of those microorganisms. This is called a vaccine, and the process is called vaccination. When the pathogenic microorganism is encountered after vaccination, the immune system produces a stronger, faster response and prevents development of the disease. This production of acquired immunity is called immunization. Immunization lowers the risk of an antigen causing disease because it safely prepares the immune system to fight future attacks by the disease-causing microorganism. In some cases more than one exposure to the antigen is needed to ensure adequate immunity. A repeated exposure by way of a vaccination is called a booster. Immunization by vaccination is used to protect children and adults against many diseases. Dental personnel should be vaccinated against the hepatitis B virus because of their high risk of occupational exposure to that virus.

Immunopathology

Immunopathology is the study of immune reactions involved in disease. The immune response helps defend the body against disease-producing antigens, but it can also malfunction and cause tissue damage. Immunopathology includes those diseases caused by malfunctioning of the immune system. Hypersensitivity reactions and autoimmune diseases are examples of conditions in which damage is caused by the immune response.

HYPERSENSITIVITY

Hypersensitivity reactions are also called allergic reactions and comprise the same types of reactions that occur when the immune response is fighting microorganisms and protecting the body against disease. However, hypersensitivity reactions are exaggerated responses, and tissue destruction occurs as a result of the immune response. Four main types of hypersensitivity reactions occur, and they are classified by the nature of the immune response that causes the disease **(Table 3-2).**

Type I Hypersensitivity

Type I hypersensitivity is a reaction that occurs immediately (within minutes) after exposure to a previously encountered antigen (from pollen to latex to penicillin). Plasma cells produce IgE as a response to

Table 3-2   Hypersensitivity Reactions

Type of Reaction	Examples
Type I (anaphylactic type)	Hay fever
	Asthma
	Anaphylaxis
Type II (cytotoxic type)	Autoimmune hemolytic anemia
Type III (immune complex type)	Autoimmune disease
Type IV (cell-mediated type)	Granulomatous disease (for example, tuberculosis)

the antigen. IgE causes mast cells to release their granules containing histamine, which results in increased dilation and permeability of blood vessels and constricting smooth muscle in the bronchioles of the lungs. This type of hypersensitivity ranges from everyday hay fever to the more serious asthma and then finally to **anaphylaxis,** which can be life threatening because the individual may not be able to breathe as a result of the tissue swelling and constriction of the bronchioles.

Type II Hypersensitivity

In **type II hypersensitivity,** antibody combines with an antigen bound to the surface of tissue cells, usually a circulating red blood cell. Activated complement components, IgG and IgM antibodies in blood, participate in this type of hypersensitivity reaction. The result is the destruction of the tissue that has the antigen on the surface of its cells. This type of reaction occurs in incompatible blood transfusions and in Rhesus (Rh) incompatibility. In this condition, the mother's antibodies cross the placenta and destroy the newborn's red blood cells (hemolytic anemia).

Type III Hypersensitivity

In **type III hypersensitivity,** immune complexes are formed between microorganisms and antibody in the circulating blood. The complexes leave the blood and are deposited in various body tissues or in a localized area. In either case the deposition results in the initiation of an acute inflammatory response. Neutrophils are attracted to the tissues in which the complexes have been deposited. As a result of phagocytosis and death of the neutrophils, lysosomal enzymes are released, causing tissue destruction. This type of hyper-

sensitivity occurs in autoimmune diseases such as systemic lupus erythematosus (SLE) (discussed later).

Type IV Hypersensitivity

Type IV hypersensitivity, also called **delayed hypersensitivity,** involves a cell-mediated immune response rather than a humoral (antibody) response. T lymphocytes that have previously been introduced to an antigen cause damage to the tissue cells themselves or they recruit other cells. This type of hypersensitivity reaction is put to use in the tuberculin test, called a purified protein derivative (PPD [discussed in Chapter 4]), used to diagnose tuberculosis. A skin reaction occurs if the individual tested has previously been exposed to the organism that causes tuberculosis. This type of hypersensitivity is responsible for the rejection of tissue grafts and transplanted organs.

Hypersensitivity to Drugs

Drugs can act as antigens and cause an immunologically induced inflammatory response. Many factors influence the risk of an allergic (hypersensitivity) reaction to a drug. The route of administration influences how the reaction will be manifested and the severity of the reaction. Topical administration may cause a greater number of reactions than oral and parenteral (administered by injection) routes of administration. However, when a reaction occurs after parenteral administration, it may be more widespread and severe because the allergen (the antigen eliciting the response) can be carried quickly to many parts of the body in the blood stream. The presence of infection may increase the risk of an allergic reaction. Patients with multiple allergies are more likely to have allergic reactions to drugs, and patients with autoimmune diseases such as SLE commonly have adverse reactions to medication. Children are less likely than adults to have an allergic reaction to a drug.

Drugs can cause any of the previously described hypersensitivity reactions. Type I allergy to a drug can include anaphylaxis, urticaria, and angioedema. A systemic anaphylactic reaction is more likely to occur with an injected drug but can also occur with a drug administered orally and can be fatal. For example, penicillin can cause a systemic anaphylactic reaction in approximately 1 in 10,000 patients. It causes about 300 deaths per year in the United States, although the overall toxicity of penicillin in all patients is low.

A classic example of a Type III allergy is **serum sickness.** This name was given to a reaction that occurred frequently when patients were given large amounts of horse antitoxin serum to provide passive immunity in the treatment of diphtheria and tetanus. This reaction can occur in response to other foreign agents as well. Penicillin is the single most common cause of serum sickness. However, other drugs, such as barbiturates, can cause this reaction as well. The symptoms of serum sickness include fever, painful swelling of the joints (arthritis), renal disturbance or failure, edema around the eyes, carditis, and skin lesions.

Drugs can also cause a type IV hypersensitivity reaction. This cell-mediated allergic reaction can occur in response to topically applied substances and can produce contact dermatitis and mucositis.

AUTOIMMUNE DISEASES

The immune system learns early to differentiate between the body's own cells and tissues and foreign substances. This recognition and the nonresponsiveness of the immune system to the body's own cells and tissues is called immunologic tolerance. In autoimmune diseases, also called connective tissue diseases, the recognition mechanism breaks down and certain body cells are no longer tolerated, with the immune system treating them as antigens. An autoimmune disease may involve a single cell type or a single organ or may be even more extensive, involving multiple organs. Tissues and even entire organs may be damaged. Genetic factors may play a role in the predisposition of an individual to autoimmune disease, and viral infection may be involved. An example is the T cells that attack pancreatic cells contributing to diabetes mellitus. Several autoimmune diseases have oral manifestations, which are described later in this chapter.

IMMUNODEFICIENCY

Immunodeficiency is a type of immunopathologic condition that involves a deficiency in number, function, or interrelationships of the involved white blood cells and their products. This condition may be congenital (present at birth) or acquired (develops after birth). Immunodeficiency may be genetically inherited or can be caused by numerous other factors. When a person's immune system is not functioning adequately, infections and tumors may develop. AIDS, which is discussed in Chapter 4, is an example of an immunodeficiency that has numerous oral manifestations.

Oral Diseases with Immunologic Pathogenesis

APHTHOUS ULCERS

Aphthous ulcers, also known as **canker sores** or **aphthous stomatitis,** are painful oral ulcers for which the cause remains unclear. They frequently recur in episodes. Three forms of recurrent aphthous ulceration exist: (1) minor, (2) major, and (3) herpetiform. The three forms differ in the size and duration of the ulcers. Aphthous ulcers are common ulcers in the oral cavity, occurring in about 20% of the general population. However, a dramatic variation in occurrence takes place, from as high as 57% of a professional school population to 5% of patients studied in a large innercity hospital. The first episode of these ulcers usually occurs in adolescence, and they are somewhat more common in females than in males. The clinical appearance and location are important in establishing the diagnosis.

Trauma is the most commonly reported precipitating factor in the development of aphthous ulcers. They are often reported to occur after trauma to the oral mucosa during dental procedures, for example, in the area of film placement or at the site of injection of local anesthetics. Some patients may experience aphthous ulcers as a result of manipulation of oral tissues during dental hygiene treatment. Emotional stress has also been suggested as a contributing factor. Some patients associate the initiation of aphthous ulcers with eating certain foods such as citrus fruits. However, it is possible that patients perceive these foods as causative because of the sensitivity of the ulcers to foods with a high acid content. The recurrence of aphthous ulcers has been associated with menstruation, whereas pregnancy has been found to produce a decrease in the episodes. These ulcers occur in association with certain systemic diseases, such as:

- Behçet syndrome
- Crohn disease
- Ulcerative colitis
- Cyclic neutropenia
- Sprue (gluten intolerance)
- Intestinal lymphoma

Substantial evidence indicates that aphthous ulcers have an immunologic pathogenesis. Patients in whom aphthous ulcers develop have slightly elevated levels of antibodies to oral mucous membranes. Histologically an infiltrate of lymphocytes is present in the lesion, suggesting that CMI may be important in development of the ulcers. The infiltrate contains primarily T-helper cells in the prodromal stage, T-cytotoxic cells in the ulcerative phase, and T-helper cells again in the healing stage. The T-cytotoxic cells are probably responsible for the ulceration. However, the specific antigen they are responding to has not yet been identified.

Minor Aphthous Ulcers

Minor aphthous ulcers are the most commonly occurring type. They appear as discrete, round to oval ulcers that are up to 1 cm in diameter and exhibit a yellowish-white fibrin surface surrounded by a halo of erythema **(Figure 3-6).** The ulcers occur on the movable mucosa of the oral cavity (the mucosa not covering bone) and occasionally extend onto the gingiva. They occur on the labial and buccal mucosa, the maxillary and mandibular vestibular mucosa, the ventral and lateral borders of the tongue, and the soft palate and oropharynx. Minor aphthous ulcers are more common in the anterior part than the posterior part of the mouth. The ulcers often have a prodromal period of 1 to 2 days, which is characterized by a burning sensation or soreness in the area in which the ulcer will form. Aphthous ulcers are exquisitely painful, and single or multiple lesions may be present. The ulcers heal spontaneously in 7 to 10 days.

Major Aphthous Ulcers

Major aphthous ulcers (Sutton disease, periadenitis mucosa necrotica recurrens) are larger than 1 cm in diameter and are deeper and last longer than minor aphthous ulcers **(Figure 3-7).** They are also painful and often occur in the posterior part of the mouth. Major aphthous ulcers may require biopsy for diagnosis to rule out other causes of ulceration. They can take several weeks to heal and frequently result in scarring. Ulcers that resemble major aphthous ulcers have been reported to occur in patients with human immunodeficiency virus (HIV) infection (see Chapter 4).

A   B

Figure 3-6 **A,** Example of a minor aphthous ulcer. **B,** Minor aphthous ulcer on the buccal mucosa on the papilla of Stenson duct.

Figure 3-7 Examples of major aphthous ulcers. **A,** Labial mucosa. **B,** Soft palate. **C,** Buccal mucosa.

Herpetiform Aphthous Ulcers

Herpetiform aphthous ulcers are very tiny (1 to 2 mm) **(Figure 3-8).** They are called herpetiform because they resemble ulcers caused by the herpes simplex virus (see Chapter 4). They are painful, may develop anywhere in the oral cavity, and generally occur in groups.

Diagnosis

The diagnosis of minor aphthous ulcers is made based on their distinctive clinical appearance, the location of the lesions, and a complete patient history. **Table 3-3** summarizes the clinical features of each of the three types of aphthous ulcers. Laboratory results are not specific for any form of aphthous ulcer.

The location of the ulcers is important in differentiating between recurrent aphthous ulcers and recurrent intraoral ulceration caused by the herpes simplex virus (see Table 4-2). When they occur intraorally, ulcers resulting from the herpes simplex virus appear on mucosa fixed to bone (that is, the palate and gingiva).

A biopsy is frequently necessary for diagnosing major aphthous ulcers because they may clinically resemble squamous cell carcinoma or deep fungal infections.

Herpetiform aphthous ulcers may be difficult to distinguish clinically from primary herpetic gingivostomatitis. However, no systemic signs or symptoms

Figure 3-8 Herpetiform aphthous ulcers.

Table 3-3   Clinical Features of the Three Types of Recurrent Aphthous Ulcers

Feature	Minor	Major	Herpetiform
Size	Small, 3-5 mm	Large, 5-10 mm	Very small, 1-2 mm
Location	Unattached mucosa	Unattached mucosa	Unattached mucosa
Most common area	Anterior	Posterior	Anywhere
Number	1-5	1-10	1-100
Scarring	No	Yes	No
Pain	Yes	Yes	Yes
Appearance	Shallow	Deep	Ulcers coalesce

exist as in primary herpes simplex infection. Herpetiform aphthous ulcers have been reported to respond to topical application of liquid tetracycline. This response may be helpful in confirming the diagnosis of herpetiform aphthous ulcers because true herpes simplex ulceration does not respond to this treatment.

Treatment

The local application of topical steroids is helpful in the treatment of aphthous ulcers. Topical steroids are most effective when applied during the prodromal period. Occasionally, systemic steroids may be necessary for managing patients with major aphthous ulcers. Topical application of liquid tetracycline is also helpful, particularly in herpetiform ulceration for when the diagnosis is not clear. The use of topical steroids is contraindicated for viral ulcers; therefore accurate diagnosis is important. Topical anesthetics can be helpful in decreasing the pain of aphthous ulcers.

URTICARIA AND ANGIOEDEMA

Urticaria and angioedema are similar lesions. **Urticaria,** also called **hives (Figure 3-9),** appears as multiple areas of well-demarcated swelling of the skin, usually accompanied by itching (pruritus). The lesions are caused by localized areas of vascular permeability in the superficial connective tissue beneath the epithelium. **Angioedema (Figure 3-10)** is a similar lesion that appears as a diffuse swelling of tissue caused by permeability of deeper blood vessels. The

Figure 3-9 Urticaria.

Figure 3-10 Angioedema. (Courtesy Dr. Edward V. Zegarelli.)

skin covering the swelling appears normal, and angioedema is usually not accompanied by itching. Urticaria and angioedema may both occur in acute self-limited episodes. Chronic or recurrent forms may occasionally occur.

In many cases of urticaria and angioedema, the cause cannot be identified. Infection, trauma, emotional stress, and certain systemic diseases have been reported to cause these lesions. Ingested allergens are frequent causes of urticaria.

Several mechanisms are capable of causing the increased vascular permeability that results in urticaria and angioedema, including the release of the chemical mediator histamine from mast cells stimulated by IgE antibodies (type I hypersensitivity) and the activation of IgG or IgM antibodies along with trauma, causing vascular permeability. Acetylsalicylic acid (aspirin) and nonsteroidal antiinflammatory drugs such as ibuprofen can produce a nonspecific effect that can cause vascular permeability. A rare hereditary form of angioedema exists in which uncontrolled activation of the complement cascade occurs, resulting in prolonged vascular permeability.

The diagnoses of urticaria and angioedema are based on the clinical appearance of the lesions and the patient's history. Avoidance of the causative agent, if identified, is important in managing patients with recurring urticaria and angioedema. Immediate treatment is essential. Antihistaminic drugs are the principal method of treatment. Angioedema involving the larynx and pharynx can cause asphyxiation and therefore may be fatal.

CONTACT MUCOSITIS AND DERMATITIS

Contact mucositis and **dermatitis** are lesions that result from the direct contact of an allergen with the skin or mucosa. The development of these conditions involves CMI and is an example of type IV hypersensitivity. The exact underlying immunologic basis is not always clear.

In contact mucositis the mucosa becomes erythematous and edematous, often accompanied by burning and pruritus (**Figure 3-11,** *A*). The mucositis occurs at the point at which the offending agent has contacted the mucosa, giving it a smooth, shiny appearance that is firm to palpation. Small vesicles and ulcers may appear in the affected areas. In contact dermatitis, the initial lesion may be erythematous,

Figure 3-11 A, Contact mucositis from acrylic. **B,** Contact dermatitis from latex gloves (seen here on the skin between the thumb and index finger). (**A** courtesy Dr. Edward V. Zegarelli.)

with swelling and vesicles. Later the area becomes encrusted with a scaly, white epidermis.

Topical antibiotics, antihistamines, preservatives in local anesthetics, and components of topical medication are common causes of allergic reactions. Acrylics, metal-based alloys, epoxy resins, and the flavoring agents in chewing gum and dentifrices have all been reported to cause contact mucositis.

Contact dermatitis, particularly that affecting the hands, may occur in response to the materials used in dentistry. The routine use of gloves in dental care has decreased the incidence of this type of dermatitis, but gloves and glove powder have also been responsible for contact dermatitis in some individuals (**Figure 3-11**, *B*).

Skin testing for sensitivity to a particular substance can help confirm the agent that caused the lesion. However, first the substance has to be identified. Topical and systemic corticosteroids may be used in the management of these lesions in some patients.

FIXED DRUG ERUPTIONS

Fixed drug eruptions are lesions that appear in the same site each time a drug is introduced. The lesions generally appear suddenly after a latent period of several days and subside when the drug is discontinued. They appear again when the drug is reintroduced, usually with greater intensity. Clinically there may be single or multiple slightly raised, reddish patches or clusters of macules on the skin or, rarely, the mucous membranes. Pain and pruritus may be associated with these lesions.

The fixed drug eruption is a type of allergic reaction (type III hypersensitivity) in which immune complexes are deposited along the endothelial wall of blood vessels. The ensuing inflammatory reaction causes vasculitis and subsequent damage to the vessel wall, giving rise to erythema and edema of the superficial layers of the skin or mucosa. If possible, the drug causing the reaction should be identified and its use discontinued.

ERYTHEMA MULTIFORME

Erythema multiforme is an acute, self-limited disease that affects the skin and mucous membranes. The cause is not clear, but some evidence exists that it is a hypersensitivity reaction.

Erythema multiforme most commonly occurs in young adults and affects men more commonly than women. The characteristic skin lesion is called a target, iris, or bull's eye lesion and consists of concentric rings of erythema alternating with normal skin color. The color is darkest at the center of the lesion **(Figure 3-12)**. The term erythema multiforme refers to the variety of skin lesions that can occur, which range from macules to plaques to bullae. Erythema multiforme can affect the oral mucosa either alone or in association with skin lesions. Skin lesions can occur without oral lesions. The oral lesions are usually ulcers (**Figure 3-13**, *A* to *C*). However, erythematous areas may also occur. The ulcers frequently form on the lateral borders of the tongue. Crusted and bleeding lips are frequently seen in erythema multiforme, and gingival involvement is rare. The

Figure 3-12 Skin lesions of erythema multiforme. **A,** Target lesion *(arrow)*. **B,** Bullae. (**A** courtesy Dr. Edward V. Zegarelli.)

disease usually has an explosive onset, and systemic symptoms are mild or lacking. The disease may be chronic on occasion, or there may be recurrent acute episodes. The most severe form of erythema multiforme is called **Stevens-Johnson syndrome** (see Figure 3-13, *C*). Mucosal lesions are more extensive and painful; genital mucosa and the mucosa of the eyes may be involved; and lips are generally encrusted and bloody.

Although the cause of erythema multiforme is not clear, triggering factors can be identified in some cases. Infections such as herpes simplex, tuberculosis, and histoplasmosis have been associated with episodes of erythema multiforme, as have malignant tumors and drugs such as barbiturates and sulfonamides.

Diagnosis

The diagnosis of erythema multiforme is made based on the clinical features and the exclusion of other diseases. The microscopic appearance is nonspecific. Biopsy and histologic examinations are sometimes helpful in excluding other diseases with similar clinical features but more distinctive histologic features.

A

B

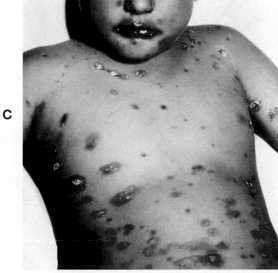

C

Figure 3-13 Oral lesions of erythema multiforme. **A,** Crusted lip lesions with edema, ulceration, and erythema. **B,** Erythematous and ulcerated lesions of the lips and buccal mucosa. **C,** Stevens-Johnson syndrome. (**C** courtesy Dr. Sidney Eisig.)

Treatment and Prognosis

Topical corticosteroids may be helpful in mild cases of erythema multiforme, but systemic corticosteroid treatment is usually needed. Eye lesions in Stevens-Johnson syndrome may lead to scarring and blindness. Systemic antiviral medication is sometimes used to attempt to decrease recurrent episodes thought to be stimulated by herpes simplex virus infection.

LICHEN PLANUS

Lichen planus is a benign, chronic disease affecting the skin and oral mucosa. In some patients this disease may affect both the skin and the oral mucosa. In others either oral mucosa or skin alone may be affected. The lesions have a characteristic pattern of interconnecting lines called striae, resembling the pattern of the plant lichen as it grows on rocks and trees.

The classic appearance of lichen planus affecting the oral mucosa is an arrangement of interconnecting white lines and circles **(Figure 3-14).** The slender white lines are called Wickham striae. The fundamental lesion is a small, papular, pinhead-sized, domed or hemispheric, glistening, white nodule on the mucosa. The clinical appearance depends on the arrangement of these minute papules and striae. The most common location is the buccal mucosa. However, lichen planus also occurs on the tongue, lips, floor of the mouth, and gingiva. Lesions of lichen planus are frequently distributed symmetrically in the oral cavity.

The prevalence of lichen planus in the general population of the United States has been reported to be about 1%. In one study of 100 cases, the age of individuals affected ranged from 13 to 78 years. However, the disease is most common in middle age. A slight female predominance has been suggested. In another reported study of 200 cases, most were found to be asymptomatic and were discovered on routine oral examination.

Many factors have been implicated in lichen planus; however, the cause remains unknown. Erosive lesions do tend to worsen with emotional stress. Many drugs and chemicals have been shown to produce lichenoid lesions. However, these have a different histologic appearance from true lichen planus.

Types of Lichen Planus

Several forms of lichen planus have been described. The most common is **reticular lichen planus.** In this form the lesions are composed of Wickham striae along with white, slightly raised white plaquelike areas. Those in which the epithelium separates from the connective tissue and erosions, bullae, or ulcers form are called **erosive** and **bullous lichen planus (Figure 3-15).**

Gingival lesions clinically described as **desquamative gingivitis** can also be caused by lichen planus **(Figure 3-16).** In addition to the gingival lesions, striated lesions generally occur elsewhere.

The skin lesions of lichen planus are 2 to 4 mm papules **(Figure 3-17).** Wickham striae may also be present, as may pruritus. Lesions can occur anywhere

A   B

Figure 3-14 A and **B,** Two examples of the oral lesions of lichen planus. (**A** courtesy Dr. Edward V. Zegarelli.)

on the skin, but the most common sites are the lumbar region, the flexor surfaces of the wrist, and the anterior surface of the ankles. Some patients have only skin lesions, some have only oral lesions, and others have both skin and oral lesions.

Diagnosis

The diagnosis of lichen planus is made based on the distinctive clinical appearance and the histologic appearance of biopsy tissue **(Figure 3-18)**. The epithelium is generally parakeratotic and may be either hyperplastic or atrophic. The characteristic microscopic features include degeneration of the basal cell layer of the epithelium in small to extensive areas, saw tooth-shaped rete ridges, and a broad band of lymphocytes in the connective tissue immediately subjacent to the epithelium. In erosive areas the separation of the epithelium from the connective tissue occurs at the interface of the epithelium and connective tissue. Epithelial atypia and dysplasia may also occur in lesions that appear clinically as lichen planus, and it has been suggested that these lesions may be premalignant.

Figure 3-15 Lichen planus. Erosion of the mucosa appears as erythema adjacent to white striae.

Figure 3-17 Skin lesions of lichen planus.

Figure 3-16 Lichen planus. The gingival lesions of lichen planus are described clinically as desquamative gingivitis. (Courtesy Dr. Edward V. Zegarelli.)

Figure 3-18 Lichen planus seen by low-power microscopy. The reader should note the degeneration of the basal cell layer of the epithelium *(B)* and the bandlike infiltrate of lymphocytes *(L)*.

Treatment and Prognosis

Lichen planus is a chronic disease. Treatment is indicated only when lesions are symptomatic. Erosive lesions usually respond quickly when topical corticosteroid medication is applied. Improvement of gingival lesions with meticulous oral hygiene has been reported. If a drug can be identified as the causative agent of lichenoid-appearing lesions, discontinuation of the drug should cause the lesions to disappear. At times, however, it is not possible to discontinue the drug.

Studies have been reported that suggest that patients with lichen planus may be at increased risk for the development of squamous cell carcinoma. Therefore regular oral soft tissue examination and biopsy of any lesions not consistent with lichen planus are recommended.

REITER SYNDROME

Classically, Reiter syndrome comprises the triad of arthritis, urethritis, and conjunctivitis. However, all the components of the syndrome may not be present. The cause of this syndrome is not clear. (A **syndrome** is a group of signs and symptoms that occur together. Other syndromes are described elsewhere in this text.)

An antigenic marker called HLA-B27 is present in most patients with Reiter syndrome, suggesting a genetic influence. An abnormal immune response to a microbial antigen is considered the most likely mechanism of occurrence. Reiter syndrome is far more prevalent in men (10:1) than in women (15:1). Reiter syndrome characteristically develops 1 to 4 weeks after venereal or gastrointestinal infection. The syndrome is usually benign and self-limited.

The arthritis of Reiter syndrome usually involves the joints of the lower extremities (knees and ankles). It may be asymmetric and migratory, chronic and recurrent.

Radiographically a periosteal proliferation can be detected on the heels, ankles, metatarsals, phalanges, knees, and elbows. Fever, malaise, and weight loss may be associated with the arthritis. The urethritis usually precedes the other lesions. No infectious organisms can be identified. The conjunctivitis is usually mild, but some individuals experience iritis (inflammation of the iris).

Skin and mucous membrane lesions are seen in many patients with Reiter syndrome. Oral lesions occur almost anywhere in the oral cavity **(Figure 3-19)**. Aphthouslike ulcers, erythematous lesions, and geographic tonguelike lesions have been described in patients with Reiter syndrome.

Figure 3-19 A and **B,** Lesions are present on the palate and tongue in this patient with Reiter syndrome.

Diagnosis

The diagnosis of Reiter syndrome is made based on the clinical signs and symptoms along with identification of the HLA-B27 antigenic marker.

Treatment and Prognosis

The disease lasts from weeks to months. The patient may experience spontaneous remission, but recurrent attacks are common. Aspirin or other nonsteroidal antiinflammatory drugs are generally used for treatment.

LANGERHANS CELL DISEASE

Langerhans cell disease was formerly called histiocytosis X. Three entities were traditionally grouped under the category of histiocytosis X: (1) Letterer-Siwe disease, (2) Hand-Schüller-Christian disease, and (3) solitary eosinophilic granuloma. Histologically all are characterized by a combination of Langerhans cells (the histiocytic cells responsible for the name histiocytosis X) and eosinophils **(Figure 3-20)**. However, in all three diseases the proliferating cell is the Langerhans cell. The presence of eosinophils is thought to result from the production of an eosinophilic chemotactic factor produced by the macrophage.

The Langerhans cell (a type of macrophage) is an immunologically competent cell of the mononuclear phagocyte series and participates in CMI. The cause and pathogenesis of Langerhans cell disease remains unclear. A reactive process, a primary immunodeficiency disease, and a neoplastic process have all been suggested.

Letterer-Siwe disease (acute disseminated form) is an acute fulminating disorder that usually affects children younger than 3 years of age. The course of the disease is usually so rapid that significant oral involvement does not often occur. The disease resembles a lymphoma in that it generally has a rapidly fatal course that sometimes responds to chemotherapy.

The chronic disseminated or multifocal form of Langerhans cell disease has been called **Hand-Schüller-Christian disease.** This form occurs in children, usually less than 5 years of age. A classic triad is seen in about 25% of patients. All changes are caused by localized collections of Langerhans cells. The triad includes single to multiple well-defined or "punched-out" radiolucent areas in the skull (may also occur in the jawbones), unilateral or bilateral exophthalmos, and diabetes insipidus that is due to collections of macrophages in the sella turcica area, affecting the pituitary gland.

Oral manifestations of the chronic disseminated form of the disease include sore mouth with or without ulcerative lesions, halitosis, gingivitis, unpleasant taste, loose and sore teeth, early exfoliation of teeth, and nonhealing extraction sites. A characteristic loss of supporting alveolar bone occurs, mimicking advanced periodontal disease **(Figure 3-21).**

A solitary or chronic localized form has been called **eosinophilic granuloma of bone.** This form primarily affects older children and young adults. Males are affected twice as commonly as females. The skull and mandible are commonly involved with eosinophilic granuloma. The radiographic appearance varies, and the lesion may resemble periodontal disease or periapical inflammatory disease; or it may appear as a well-circumscribed radiolucency with or without a sclerotic border **(Figure 3-22).** Cases of multifocal eosinophilic granuloma have also been reported.

Treatment

Eosinophilic granuloma is treated by conservative surgical excision; recurrence is rare. Low-dose radiation therapy may also be used for treatment.

Figure 3-20 Langerhans cell disease seen by high-power microscopy.

Figure 3-22 Radiograph of eosinophilic granuloma. (Courtesy Drs. Paul Freedman and Stanley Kerpel.)

Figure 3-21 Langerhans cell disease. Chronic disseminated form also known as *Hand-Schüller-Christian disease*. **A,** Skull radiograph. **B,** Ulcerated lesion of the mandible. (Courtesy Dr. Sidney Eisig.)

Autoimmune Diseases That Affect the Oral Cavity

Several autoimmune diseases affect the oral cavity **(Table 3-4)**. In this type of disease, tissue damage occurs because the immune system treats the person's own cells and tissues as antigens. An individual with one autoimmune disease has an increased risk of developing another autoimmune disease. Although these are systemic diseases, they are included in this chapter because of their relationship to immunity.

SJÖGREN SYNDROME

Sjögren syndrome is an autoimmune disease that affects the salivary and lacrimal glands, resulting in a decrease in saliva and tears. This combination of dry mouth and dry eyes is sometimes called **sicca** (dry)

syndrome. Decreased salivary flow results in dry mouth **(xerostomia);** decreased lacrimal flow results in dry eyes **(xerophthalmia).** The eye damage that occurs in Sjögren syndrome is called **keratoconjunctivitis sicca.** Other secretory glands, such as sweat glands and glands that lubricate the vagina, can also be affected. The specific cause of Sjögren syndrome is not known. Both cellular immunity and humoral immunity are involved.

In some patients only the mouth and eyes are involved. In others the autoimmune process can be more extensive. Many patients (about 50%) with Sjögren syndrome have another autoimmune disease, such as rheumatoid arthritis or SLE. Lacrimal and salivary gland involvement without the presence of another autoimmune disease is called **primary Sjögren syndrome.** When another autoimmune disease accompanies salivary and lacrimal gland involvement, the combination is called **secondary Sjögren syndrome.**

The oral manifestation of Sjögren syndrome is xerostomia (dry mouth), which occurs as a result of decreased salivary flow and causes the mucosa to become erythematous. Patients complain of oral discomfort. Lack of saliva causes the mouth to feel sticky. Lips are cracked and dry, and a generalized

Table 3-4 Autoimmune Diseases That Affect the Oral Region

Disease	Oral Manifestation
Sjögren syndrome	Xerostomia
Lupus erythematosus (LE)	White, erosive lesions of the oral mucosa
Pemphigus vulgaris	Mucosal ulceration, bullae
Benign mucous membrane pemphigoid	Mucosal ulceration, desquamative gingivitis
Behçet syndrome	Aphthous ulcers
Pernicious anemia*	Mucosal atrophy, mucosal ulceration, loss of filiform and fungiform papillae

*Described in Chapter 9.

Figure 3-23 Sjögren syndrome. This patient had severe xerostomia. The filiform papillae are lacking.

Figure 3-24 Bilateral parotid gland swelling seen in Sjögren syndrome. (Courtesy Dr. Louis Mandel.)

loss of filiform and fungiform papillae occurs on the dorsum of the tongue **(Figure 3-23)**. Patients with xerostomia are at high risk for the development of caries, periodontal disease, and oral candidiasis.

Both major and minor salivary glands are affected. Parotid gland enlargement, usually bilateral and symmetric, occurs in about 50% of patients **(Figure 3-24)**. The characteristic histologic appearance of these enlarged glands consists of replacement of the glands by lymphocytes and the presence of islands of epithelium called epimyoepithelial islands. Biopsy of the minor salivary glands is often performed to confirm a diagnosis of Sjögren syndrome. The minor glands show aggregates of lymphocytes surrounding the salivary gland ducts **(Figure 3-25)**.

Figure 3-25 Microscopy of a minor salivary gland from a patient with Sjögren syndrome. (Courtesy Dr. Harry Lumerman.)

In addition to the oral findings, patients with decreased lacrimal flow that results in xerophthalmia complain of burning and itching of the eyes and photophobia (abnormal visual intolerance to light). Severe eye involvement may lead to ulceration and opacification of the cornea. Twenty percent of patients with Sjögren syndrome also have **Raynaud phenomenon,** which is a disorder affecting the fingers and toes. Cold and emotional stress trigger the reaction, which is characterized by an initial pallor of the skin that results from vasoconstriction and reduced blood flow. The initial pallor is followed by cyanosis, which occurs because of the decreased blood flow. When the skin is rewarmed, the blood vessels dilate and the hyperemia results in a reddening of the skin. Finally, in minutes to hours, the color returns to normal. Raynaud phenomenon can occur alone or in association with other autoimmune diseases, as well as in Sjögren syndrome. Patients with Sjögren syndrome might also complain of myalgia, arthralgia, and chronic fatigue.

Laboratory abnormalities are commonly found in patients with this syndrome. Ninety percent of patients with Sjögren syndrome have a positive reaction to rheumatoid factor, which is an antibody to IgG that is present in serum. It is an antibody to an antibody. Patients with other autoimmune diseases, such as rheumatoid arthritis, also react positively to rheumatoid factor. Other autoantibodies, called anti-Sjögren syndrome A (anti-SS-A) and anti-Sjögren syndrome B (anti-SS-B), are also found in patients with Sjögren syndrome. Other laboratory abnormalities include mild anemia, a decreased white blood cell count, an elevated erythrocyte sedimentation rate, and a diffuse elevation of serum Igs.

Diagnosis and Management

The diagnosis of Sjögren syndrome is made when at least two of its three components are present: (1) xerostomia, (2) keratoconjunctivitis sicca, and (3) rheumatoid arthritis or another autoimmune disease. Xerostomia can result from conditions other than autoimmune disease. Measurement of stimulated and unstimulated salivary flow and biopsy of minor salivary glands (see Figure 3-25) can be helpful in the diagnosis of Sjögren syndrome. A characteristic pattern is seen in a parotid sialogram **(Figure 3-26).** The pattern reflects the lack of functioning glandular elements.

Keratoconjunctivitis is confirmed by eye examination. Lacrimal flow is measured using filter paper. Special examination techniques are necessary to demonstrate the corneal erosions.

The course of the disease for the majority of patients is chronic and benign. However, patients with Sjögren syndrome are at risk for the development of other, more serious autoimmune diseases, lymphoma, and Waldenström macroglobulinemia (a disorder characterized by a high concentration of IgM in serum) and should therefore be monitored by a physician.

Treatment

Sjögren syndrome is usually treated symptomatically. Nonsteroidal antiinflammatory agents are used for the arthritis. In severe cases, corticosteroids and other immunosuppressive drugs may be necessary. Saliva substitutes are helpful, and for some patients the use of a humidifier at night makes the xerostomia more tolerable. Sugarless gum or lozenges may be used to stimulate saliva production. However, the

Figure 3-26 Sialogram of Sjögren syndrome. (Courtesy Dr. Louis Mandel.)

greater the destruction of salivary gland tissue, the less saliva will be stimulated. An "artificial tears" formula containing methylcellulose helps to protect the eye from the drying effects of the disease. Glasses provide shielding and are helpful to minimize the drying effects of wind. Pilocarpine may also be used in some patients to increase salivary flow.

Maintaining good oral hygiene and using fluoride toothpaste and daily fluoride rinses can minimize the effects of xerostomia. The interval between recall appointments should be sufficiently short to ensure early detection and treatment of root caries. The toothbrush and other oral hygiene aids may need modification if arthritis affects the movement of hands and arms.

SYSTEMIC LUPUS ERYTHEMATOSUS

SLE is an acute and chronic inflammatory autoimmune disease of unknown cause. The disorder affects women eight times more frequently than it does men, predominantly during the childbearing years. It occurs three times more frequently in black women than in white women. SLE is a syndrome rather than a specific disease entity and includes a wide spectrum of disease activity and signs and symptoms that range from lesions confined to the skin, such as discoid LE,

to a widespread, debilitating, life-threatening disease with multiple-organ involvement. SLE is usually chronic and progressive, with periods of remission and exacerbation.

Both cellular immunity and humoral immunity are impaired in SLE. It has been suggested that cellular immunity is primarily affected, resulting in deregulation of the humoral response. Antigen and antibody complexes are deposited in various organs and stimulate an inflammatory response, which may be responsible for the tissue damage that occurs in SLE. Autoantibodies to the patient's deoxyribonucleic acid (DNA) (antinuclear antibodies) are present in serum. These circulating antibodies are responsible for the positive antinuclear antibody (ANA) and LE laboratory test results. Production of these antibodies is enhanced by estrogen. Antibodies to lymphocytes are present in some patients. Evidence exists for a genetic component in the pathogenesis of SLE.

Clinical Features

Skin lesions are among the most common signs of the disease, occurring in 85% of individuals **(Figure 3-27).** The most common skin lesion is an erythematous rash involving areas of the body exposed to sunlight. The classic "butterfly" rash occurs over the

Figure 3-27 A and **B,** Two examples of skin lesions in lupus erythematosus (LE). (**B** courtesy Dr. Edward V. Zegarelli.)

bridge of the nose, and there may be erythematous lesions on the fingertips. The lesions can heal with scarring in the center as they continue to spread at the periphery. The skin lesions tend to worsen when exposed to sunlight. Atrophy and hypo- or hyperpigmentation can follow these lesions. Other skin lesions such as bullae, purpura, a discoid rash, vitiligo, or subcutaneous nodules can also occur.

Arthritis and arthralgia are common manifestations of SLE. Any joint can be involved, and symptoms resemble rheumatoid arthritis but without severe deformities. Raynaud phenomenon occurs in 15% of patients. Myalgia and myositis also occur. A retinal vasculitis causes degeneration of the nerve fiber layer of the retina and can cause loss of vision. Psychoses and depression are signs of central nervous system involvement, and seizures can be present. Involvement of the pleura may cause shortness of breath and chest pain. Pericarditis, cardiac arrhythmias, and endocarditis may be seen late in the disease. Kidney involvement is common. Thrombocytopenia may also occur in patients with LE.

Oral lesions accompany skin lesions in about 25% of patients with discoid LE, which is the mildest form of LE. Oral lesions appear as erythematous plaques or erosions. White striae radiating from the center of the lesion are usually present. The lesions may resemble lichen planus but are less symmetric in their distribution. The involvement of the oral mucosa in this disease is usually mild **(Figure 3-28).**

Petechiae and gingival bleeding may be present in patients with severe thrombocytopenia. Sjögren syndrome may be present in some patients with SLE.

Diagnosis

The diagnosis of SLE is usually based on the classic multiorgan involvement and the presence of antinuclear antibodies in serum. The diagnosis of SLE is difficult if the onset is slow and insidious. The histologic appearance of oral lesions resembles that of lichen planus. Microscopically, destruction of the basal cells is seen, as in lichen planus. However, the inflammatory infiltrate is distributed around blood vessels in the connective tissue rather than in a subepithelial band. Direct immunofluorescence and immunohistochemical testing of skin and mucosal lesions shows granular and linear deposits of immunoglobins along the basement membrane area.

Treatment and Prognosis

Once the diagnosis of SLE is made, the decision as to whether treatment is indicated depends on the degree of disease activity. This once-fatal disease is now managed with several drugs. Aspirin and nonsteroidal antiinflammatory agents are used for mild signs and symptoms. Hydroxychloroquine, an antimalarial agent, and corticosteroids combined with other immunosuppressive agents, such as azathio-

A   **B**

Figure 3-28 A and **B,** Oral lesions in lupus erythematosus (LE). (**B** courtesy Dr. Edward V. Zegarelli.)

prine and cyclophosphamide, are also used. If the course of the disease is mild and only a few organs are involved, the prognosis is excellent. The disease can also be fatal. Kidney involvement can be associated with severe hypertension and rapid onset of renal failure, which is a cause of death in patients with SLE. Other common causes of death include hemorrhage secondary to thrombocytopenia, nervous system involvement, and infection.

SLE is an extremely complex disease. A consultation with the patient's physician should take place before initiating dental treatment. Antibiotic prophylaxis to prevent bacterial endocarditis may be necessary. The extent of systemic involvement and the drugs being used for treatment should be clarified.

PEMPHIGUS VULGARIS

Pemphigus vulgaris is a severe, progressive autoimmune disease that affects the skin and mucous membranes. It is characterized by intraepithelial blister formation that results from breakdown of the cellular adhesion between epithelial cells. This type of epithelial cell separation is called **acantholysis.** The patient with pemphigus vulgaris has circulating autoantibodies that are reactive against components of the epithelial cell attachment mechanism. The higher the titer of circulating antibodies, the greater the epithelial destruction. These autoantibodies are also found in surrounding epithelial cells. Pemphigus vulgaris is the type of pemphigus seen most frequently. Three other forms of pemphigus are (1) pemphigus vegetans, (2) pemphigus foliaceus, and (3) pemphigus erythematosus. These are much rarer conditions, but all are characterized by epithelial acantholysis. No sex predilection exists. A broad age range has been reported, including both children and elderly individuals. Most cases occur in the fourth and fifth decades of life. Genetic and ethnic factors have been reported. Although it is a relatively rare condition, pemphigus vulgaris is often seen in Ashkenazic Jews.

In more than 50% of cases of pemphigus vulgaris, the first signs of disease occur in the oral cavity. Oral lesions can precede cutaneous lesions by many months. The appearance of oral lesions ranges from shallow ulcers to fragile vesicles or bullae.

Because the bullae are so fragile, they rupture soon after they form; the detached epithelium remains as a gray membrane **(Figure 3-29)**. Ulcers are painful and range in size from small to very large. Gentle finger pressure with movement on clinically normal mucosa can produce a cleavage in the ep-

Figure 3-29 A to **C,** Examples of oral lesions in pemphigus vulgaris. (**B** courtesy Dr. Fariba Younai; **C,** courtesy Dr. Sidney Eisig.)

ithelium and result in the formation of a bulla. This is called **Nikolsky sign.**

Skin lesions in pemphigus vulgaris include erythema, vesicles, bullae, erosions, and ulcers. Microscopic examination of tissue shows an intact basal layer of epithelium attached to the underlying connective tissue **(Figure 3-30).** The loss of attachment between the epithelial cells results in detached cells that appear rounded. These rounded cells are called **acantholytic cells** or **Tzanck cells** and are present in the area of separation. Tzanck cells may also be seen on cytologic smear, but the diagnosis must be confirmed by biopsy.

Diagnosis

The diagnosis of pemphigus vulgaris is made by biopsy and microscopic examinations, and direct or indirect immunofluorescence. Direct immunofluorescence is performed on biopsy tissue and identifies autoantibodies present in the tissue. The tissue is viewed through a special microscope (in pemphigus vulgaris, fluorescence is seen surrounding the cells in the prickle cell layer). In indirect immunofluorescence, the patient's serum is used to detect the presence of circulating autoantibodies. Eighty percent of patients with pemphigus vulgaris have the identifiable circulating autoantibodies.

Treatment and Prognosis

Treatment generally involves high doses of corticosteroids. Other immunosuppressive drugs, such as azathioprine and methotrexate, are often used in addition to systemic corticosteroids. The amount of autoantibodies present in the patient's serum correlates with the severity of lesions; therefore this concentration of autoantibodies is used to monitor the success of drug treatment. Pemphigus vulgaris was at one time a life-threatening disease. Today the mortality rate is about 8% to 10% in 5 years and is related to the complications of corticosteroid treatment rather than to the disease itself.

Other autoimmune diseases may occur in association with pemphigus vulgaris. Among them are LE, rheumatoid arthritis, and Sjögren syndrome.

CICATRICIAL PEMPHIGOID

Cicatricial pemphigoid is also called **mucous membrane pemphigoid** and **benign mucous membrane pemphigoid.** It is a chronic autoimmune disease that affects the oral mucosa, conjunctiva, genital mucosa, and skin. It is not as severe as pemphigus vulgaris. Lesions may heal with scarring. *Cicatricial pemphigoid* refers to this healing with scarring. Autoantibodies and complement components have been identified at the basement membrane of the epithelium. Lesions occur as a result of cleavage of the epithelium from the underlying connective tissue in this area.

The most common site for cicatricial pemphigoid lesions is the gingiva. The appearance ranges from erythema to ulceration and involves both the free and the attached gingiva.

The gingival lesions have been called **desquamative gingivitis (Figure 3-31).** However, desquamative gingivitis is a clinical and descriptive term, and similar lesions can be seen in lichen planus and pemphigus

Figure 3-30 Pemphigus vulgaris seen by microscopy. The reader should note the acantholysis of the epithelium and the intact basal layer attached to the connective tissue.

Figure 3-31 Cicatricial pemphigoid (desquamative gingivitis). (Courtesy Dr. Victor M. Sternberg.)

vulgaris. Nikolsky sign can be produced on normal-appearing tissue. Bullae, erosions, and ulcers can also occur in other locations in the oral cavity. Bullae are thick walled and much less fragile than those of pemphigus vulgaris, and they may persist for 24 to 48 hours.

Diagnosis

The diagnosis of cicatricial pemphigoid is made by biopsy and histologic examination. On microscopic examination, the epithelium appears to detach from the connective tissue at the basement membrane **(Figure 3-32)**. No degeneration of the epithelium occurs. An inflammatory infiltrate, usually with prominent plasma cells and eosinophils, is seen in the connective tissue. Direct immunofluorescence shows a linear pattern of fluorescence at the basement membrane. Indirect immunofluorescence (identifying autoantibodies in serum) is usually not helpful in the diagnosis of cicatricial pemphigoid.

Treatment and Prognosis

Cicatricial pemphigoid is a chronic disease that follows a benign course. Gingival involvement can occur alone, or more extensive lesions can be present. Topical corticosteroid application is helpful in the management of mild cases. In more severe cases, high doses of systemic corticosteroids may be necessary. The disease may be difficult to control and slow to respond to therapy.

Patients may experience episodes of exacerbation followed by periods of remission. An ophthalmologic consultation to rule out the presence of eye lesions should be considered. If eye lesions are present, severe damage to the cornea, conjunctiva, and eyelid can occur.

BULLOUS PEMPHIGOID

Some investigators have suggested that bullous and cicatricial pemphigoid are variants of a single disease. However, differences exist between the two diseases that make this questionable. Eighty percent of patients with bullous pemphigoid are older than 60 years of age, and no sex predilection exists. Unlike cicatricial pemphigoid, circulating autoantibodies are usually detectable but do not correlate with disease activity. Oral lesions are less common in bullous pemphigoid than in cicatricial pemphigoid, occurring in only about one third of patients. When they occur, the gingival lesions are very similar to those of cicatricial pemphigoid, and other mucosal lesions are more extensive and painful. As in cicatricial pemphigoid, the microscopic appearance of bullous pemphigoid shows a cleavage of the epithelium from the connective tissue at the basement membrane.

High doses of systemic corticosteroids and nonsteroidal antiinflammatory drugs are used in the management of bullous pemphigoid. The disease is chronic with periods of remission and is usually not life threatening.

BEHÇET SYNDROME

Behçet syndrome is a chronic, recurrent autoimmune disease consisting primarily of oral ulcers, genital ulcers, and ocular inflammation. No sex predilection exists, and the mean age of onset is 30 years. Evidence for an autoimmune pathogenesis includes the identification of antibodies to human mucosa in patients with Behçet syndrome.

The oral ulcers that occur in Behçet syndrome are very similar in appearance to aphthous ulcers **(Figure 3-33)**. They are painful and recurrent. The lesions range in size from a few millimeters to several centimeters. The genital ulcers are usually small and are located on the scrotum or base of the penis and on the labia majora. The ocular lesions usually begin with photophobia and can develop into conjunctivitis and uveitis. The skin lesions show a papular pattern of pustules and are most common on the trunk and limbs.

Figure 3-32 Cicatricial pemphigoid seen by microscopy. Note the separation of the epithelium from the connective tissue at the basement membrane area.

Figure 3-33 Oral lesion seen in Behçet syndrome. Aphthouslike oral mucosal ulcer.

Diagnosis

The diagnosis of Behçet syndrome requires that two of the three principal manifestations (oral, genital, and ocular) be present. A pustular lesion that develops after a needle puncture is highly suggestive of Behçet syndrome.

Treatment and Prognosis

Systemic and topical corticosteroids are used in the management of Behçet syndrome. Chlorambucil is used for the ocular lesions. Occasionally, other immunosuppressive drugs are needed.

Selected References

Books

Bath-Balogh M, Fehrenbach MJ: *Illustrated dental embryology, histology, anatomy*, Philadelphia, 1997, WB Saunders.

Cruse J, Lewis RE: *Illustrated dictionary of immunology*, New York, 1995, CRC Press.

Fehrenbach MJ, Herring SW: *Illustrated anatomy of the head and neck*, ed 2, Philadelphia, 2002, WB Saunders.

Kumar V: *Basic pathology*, ed 6, Philadelphia, 1997, WB Saunders.

Neville BW et al: *Oral and maxillofacial pathology*, ed 2, Philadelphia, 2002, WB Saunders.

Parham P: *The immune system*, New York, 2000, Garland Publishing.

Regezi JA, Sciubba JJ: *Oral pathology. Clinical-pathologic correlations*, ed 4, Philadelphia, 2003, WB Saunders.

Sonis ST, Fazio RC, Fang L: *Principles and practice of oral medicine*, ed 2, Philadelphia, 1995, WB Saunders.

Peakman M, Vergani D, Britton R: *Basic and clinical immunology*, London, 1997, Churchill Livingstone.

Trowbridge HO, Emling RC: *Inflammation: a review of the process*, ed 5, Chicago, 1997, Quintessence.

Journal Articles

Ahmed R, Gray D: Immunological memory and protective immunity: understanding their relation, *Science* 272:54, 1996.

Anderson KE et al: Contact dermatitis: a review, *Contact Dermatitis* 16:55, 1987.

Antoon JW, Miller RL: Aphthous ulcers: a review of the literature of etiology, pathogenesis, diagnosis and treatment, *J Am Dent Assoc* 101:803, 1980.

Ardekian L et al: Clinical and radiographic features of eosinophilic granuloma in the jaws: review of 41 lesions treated by surgery and low-dose radiotherapy, *Oral Surg Oral Med Oral Pathol Oral Radiol Endod* 87:238, 1999.

Atkinson JC, Fox PC: Sjögren's syndrome: oral and dental considerations, *J Am Dent Assoc* 124:74, 1993.

Barnard NA et al: Oral cancer development in patients with oral lichen planus, *J Oral Pathol Med* 22:241, 1993.

Barrett AW, Scully CM, Eveson JW: Erythema multiforme involving gingiva, *J Periodontol* 64:910, 1993.

Baudet-Pommel M et al: Early dental loss in Sjögren's syndrome, *Oral Surg Oral Med Oral Pathol* 78:181, 1994.

Cooper MD: B lymphocytes: normal development and function, *N Engl J Med* 317:1452, 1987.

Dinarello C, Mier J: Lymphokines, *N Engl J Med* 317:940, 1987.

Eisenberg E: Lichen planus and oral cancer: is there a connection between the two? *J Am Dent Assoc* 123:104, 1992.

Eversole LR: Immunopathology of oral mucosal ulcerative, desquamative, and bullous diseases, *Oral Surg Oral Med Oral Pathol* 77:555, 1994.

Gabriel SA et al: Lichen planus: possible mechanisms of pathogenesis, *J Oral Med* 40:56, 1985.

Gawkrodger DJ, Stephenson TJ, Thomas SE: Squamous cell carcinoma complicating lichen planus: a clinico-pathological study of three cases, *Dermatology* 188:36, 1994.

Gosling P: The cellular, immune and metabolic response to trauma, *Crit Rev Clin Lab Sci* 35:59, 1998.

Holmstrup P, Schiotz AW, Westergaard J: Effect of dental plaque control on gingival lichen planus, *Oral Surg Oral Med Oral Pathol* 69:585, 1990.

Jorizzo JL et al: Oral lesions in systemic lupus erythematosus. Do ulcerative lesions represent a necrotizing vasculitis? *J Am Acad Dermatol* 27:389, 1992.

Katz RW, Brahim JS, Travis WD: Oral squamous cell carcinoma arising in a patient with long-standing lichen planus: a case report, *Oral Surg Oral Med Oral Pathol* 70:282, 1990.

Krippaehne JA, Montgomery MT: Erythema multiforme: a literature review and case report, *Spec Care Dentist* 12:125, 1992.

Loh HS, Quah TC: Histiocytosis X (Langerhans-cell histiocytosis) of the palate. Case report, *Aust Dent J* 35:117, 1990.

Lozada-Nur F, Gorsky M, Silverman S Jr: Oral erythema multiforme: clinical observations and treatment of 95 patients, *Oral Surg Oral Med Oral Pathol* 67:36, 1989.

MacPhail LA et al: Recurrent aphthous ulcers in association with HIV infection. Description of ulcer types and analysis of T-lymphocyte subsets, *Oral Surg Oral Med Oral Pathol* 71:678, 1991.

Manton SL, Scully C: Mucous membrane pemphigoid: an elusive diagnosis? *Oral Surg Oral Med Oral Pathol* 66:37, 1988.

Miller MF, Ship II, Ram C: A retrospective study of the prevalence and incidence of recurrent aphthous ulcers in a professional population, 1958-1971, *Oral Surg Oral Med Oral Pathol* 43:532, 1977.

Miller RL, Gould AR, Bernstein ML: Cinnamon-induced stomatitis venenata, *Oral Surg Oral Med Oral Pathol* 73:708, 1992.

Nossal GJV: The basic components of the immune system, *N Engl J Med* 316:1320, 1987.

Porter SR, Scully C, Standen GR: Autoimmune neutropenia manifesting as recurrent oral ulceration, *Oral Surg Oral Med Oral Pathol* 78:178, 1994.

Raghoebar GM, Brouwer TJ, Schoots CJ: Pemphigus vulgaris of the oral mucosa: report of two cases, *Quintessence Int* 22:199, 1991.

Rodu B, Mattingly G: Oral mucosal ulcers: diagnosis and management, *J Am Dent Assoc* 123:83, 1992.

Schofield JK, Tatnall FM, Leigh IM: Recurrent erythema multiforme: clinical features and treatment in a large series of patients, *Br J Dermatol* 34:63, 1993.

Sciubba JJ: Sjögren's syndrome: pathology, oral presentation and dental management, *Compend Contin Educ Dent* 15:1084, 1994.

Scully C, El-Kom M: Lichen planus: review and update on pathogenesis, *J Oral Pathol* 14:431, 1985.

Shaw L, Glenwright HD: Histiocytosis X: an oral diagnostic problem, *J Clin Periodontol* 15:312, 1988.

Spina AM, Levine HJ: Latex allergy: a review for the dental professional, *Oral Surg Oral Med Oral Pathol Oral Radiol Endod* 87:5, 1999.

Turjanmaa K: Incidence of immediate allergy to latex gloves in hospital personnel, *Contact Dermatitis* 17:270, 1987.

Unanue E: Cooperation between mononuclear phagocytes and lymphocytes in immunity, *N Engl J Med* 303:997, 1980.

Vincent SD, Lilly GE, Baker KA: Clinical, historical and therapeutic features of cicatricial pemphigoid. A literature review and open therapeutic trial with corticosteroids, *Oral Surg Oral Med Oral Pathol* 76:453, 1993.

Vincent SD et al: Oral lichen planus: the clinical, historical and therapeutic features of 100 cases, *Oral Surg Oral Med Oral Pathol* 70:165, 1990.

Woo S-B, Sonis ST: Recurrent aphthous ulcers: a review of diagnosis and treatment, *J Am Dent Assoc* 127:1202, 1996.

Yazici H, Barnes CG: Practical treatment recommendations for pharmacotherapy of Behçet's syndrome, *Drugs* 42:796, 1991.

Zegarelli DJ: The treatment of oral lichen planus, *Ann Dent* 52:3, 1993.

Review Questions

1. The immune system usually defends the body against foreign substances that are called:
   A. Plasma cells
   B. Antibodies
   C. Antigens
   D. Lymphocytes
   E. Immunoglobulins

2. Memory is an important function of the immune system because:
   A. It retains the memory of the antibody.
   B. It allows faster future immune responses.
   C. It allows faster inflammatory responses.
   D. It weakens future immune responses.
   E. It functions the same as the inflammatory response.

3. Immunization with a vaccine works by:
   A. Increasing the risk of an antigen-causing disease
   B. Using antibodies produced by another person
   C. Passing antibodies from the mother to the fetus
   D. Producing active acquired immunity
   E. Producing passive immunity

4. A B-lymphocyte cell is a cell in the immune system that:
   A. Is derived from a precursor stem cell
   B. Matures and resides in the thymus
   C. Is produced from plasma cells
   D. Is active in foreign-substance surveillance
   E. Never duplicates itself

5. A macrophage is a cell in the immune system that:
   A. Retains the memory of the encountered antigen
   B. Produces antibodies
   C. Undergoes B-cell phagocytosis initially during inflammation
   D. Is derived from T lymphocytes
   E. Can be activated by lymphokines

6. Which statement is *true* of NK cells?
   A. NK cells do not circulate.
   B. NK cells secrete antibodies.
   C. NK cells are part of the body's innate immunity.
   D. NK cells are T-lymphocytes.
   E. NK cells are the macrophages.

7. The cells of the body are no longer tolerated, and the immune system treats them as antigens in which type of immunopathologic disease?
   A. Hypersensitivity
   B. Immunodeficiency
   C. Hyperplasia
   D. Autoimmune disease
   E. Anaphylaxis

8. During the anaphylactic type of hypersensitivity reaction, the plasma cells:
   A. Produce antibody called IgE
   B. React with lymphocytes
   C. Combine with antigen
   D. Form immune complexes with antigen
   E. Directly produce histamine

9. Which type of hypersensitivity reaction involves activated complement?
   A. Type I
   B. Type II
   C. Type III
   D. Anaphylaxis
   E. Delayed hypersensitivity

10. What type of lymphocyte matures in the thymus, produces lymphokines, and can increase or suppress the humoral immune response?
    A. B lymphocyte
    B. Plasma cell
    C. NK cell
    D. Macrophage
    E. T lymphocyte

11. In the immune system, antibodies are proteins that are:
    A. Also termed immunoglobins
    B. Directly produced by lymphocytes
    C. Directly produced by neutrophils
    D. Directly produced from mast cells
    E. Also called antigens

12. Which immunopathology involves a decreased number or activity of lymphoid cells?
    A. Autoimmunity
    B. Hypersensitivity
    C. Immunodeficiency
    D. Immunization
    E. Anaphylaxis

13. The humoral immune response involves the production of:
    A. Antigens
    B. Antibodies
    C. Autoimmune cells
    D. Toxins
    E. T lymphocytes

14. Measurement of a specific antibody level in the blood is called:
    A. Phagocytosis
    B. Margination
    C. Titer
    D. Pavementing
    E. Immunization

15. Which type of immunity may be immediately provided to dental personnel after needle-stick accidents?
    A. Natural passive immunity
    B. Acquired passive immunity
    C. Natural active immunity
    D. Acquired active immunity
    E. Artificial active immunity

16. All of the following are examples of hypersensitivity reactions *except*:
    A. Systemic lupus erythematosus
    B. Urticaria
    C. Angioedema
    D. Contact mucositis
    E. Anaphylaxis

17. Reiter syndrome is:
    A. An infectious disorder
    B. An immunodeficiency disease
    C. An immunologic disorder
    D. More common in women than in men
    E. Diagnosed using a routine complete blood count

18. The "target lesion" on the skin is associated with which disease?
    A. Behçet syndrome
    B. Systemic lupus erythematosus
    C. Lichen planus
    D. Erythema multiforme
    E. Pemphigus vulgaris

19. Tzanck cells are seen in which condition?
    A. Pemphigus vulgaris
    B. Erythema multiforme
    C. Systemic lupus erythematosus
    D. Behçet syndrome
    E. Cicatricial pemphigoid

20. The oral lesions in Reiter syndrome may resemble:
    A. Nicotine stomatitis
    B. Lichen planus
    C. Angioedema
    D. Geographic tongue
    E. Desquamative gingivitis

21. Which of the following systemic diseases is *not* associated with aphthous ulcers?
    A. Behçet syndrome
    B. Langerhans cell disease
    C. Ulcerative colitis
    D. Crohn disease
    E. Cyclic neutropenia

22. The two cells that histologically characterize Langerhans cell disease are:
    A. Lymphocytes and plasma cells
    B. Fibroblasts and lymphocytes
    C. Eosinophils and mononuclear cells
    D. Neutrophils and lymphocytes
    E. B and T lymphocytes

23. Which one of the following is the form of Langerhans cell disease that is characterized by a triad of symptoms?
    A. Letterer-Siwe disease
    B. Acute disseminated reticulosis
    C. Eosinophilic granuloma
    D. Behçet syndrome
    E. Hand-Schüller-Christian disease

24. The most benign type of Langerhans cell disease is:
    A. Hand-Schüller-Christian disease
    B. Eosinophilic granuloma
    C. Letterer-Siwe disease
    D. Chronic disseminated reticulosis
    E. Acute disseminated reticulosis

25. The most characteristic oral manifestation of Sjögren syndrome is:
    A. Leukoplakia
    B. Geographic tongue
    C. Erythema multiforme
    D. Arthritis of the temporomandibular joint
    E. Xerostomia

26. Which of the following statements is *false*?
    A. The bullae of pemphigus vulgaris are more fragile than those of bullous pemphigoid.
    B. Acantholysis of the epithelium is seen in pemphigus vulgaris.
    C. In pemphigoid, the separation of the epithelium from the connective tissue occurs in the area of the basement membrane.
    D. Skin lesions are common in cicatricial pemphigoid.
    E. Pemphigus vulgaris is a severe progressive autoimmune disease.

27. Which is the most distinct and definitive characteristic that distinguishes pemphigus from pemphigoid?
    A. Size of the ulcerations
    B. Age and sex of the patient
    C. The histologic findings
    D. The amount of hyperkeratosis
    E. Observation of Nikolsky sign

28. Desquamative gingivitis may be seen in:
    A. Cicatricial pemphigoid
    B. Pemphigus vulgaris
    C. Lichen planus
    D. Bullous pemphigoid
    E. All of the above

29. In angioedema, involvement of which of the following tissues could create a life-threatening situation for the patient?
    A. Lips
    B. Mucosa
    C. Eyelids
    D. Skin
    E. Epiglottis

30. Which of the following is a pathologic condition that produces a characteristic butterfly-shaped lesion on the face and oral ulcers, occurs more frequently in females than males, and for which the result of a blood test is important to diagnosis?
    A. Pemphigus
    B. Erosive lichen planus
    C. Desquamative gingivitis
    D. Lupus erythematosus
    E. Reiter syndrome

Chapter 3 Synopsis

Condition/ Disease	Cause	Age/Race/Sex	Location
Oral Diseases with Immunologic Pathogenesis			
Minor Aphthous	Unclear immunologic pathogenesis involving cell-mediated immunity Trauma is most common precipitating factor	More common in younger than older individuals More common in women than men	Oral mucosa not covering bone Anterior > posterior
Major Aphthous Ulcers	Unclear immunologic pathogenesis involving cell-mediated immunity	*	Oral mucosa not covering bone Often occur in the posterior oral cavity
Herpetiform Aphthous Ulcers	Unclear immunologic pathogenesis involving cell-mediated immunity	*	Anywhere in oral cavity
Urticaria (Hives)	Type I hypersensitivity Release of IgG, IgM—often to ingested allergen Infection, trauma, emotional stress also associated with urticaria Localized vascular permeability in superficial connective tissue	*	Skin
Angioedema	Type I hypersensitivity Trauma, release of IgG or IgM Permeability of deeper blood vessels	*	Skin or mucosa
Contact Mucositis	Direct contact of allergen with mucosa	*	Mucosa in contact with allergen
Contact Dermatitis	Direct contact of allergen with skin	*	Skin in contact with allergen

*No significant information.
†Not covered in this text.

Clinical Features	Radiographic Features	Microscopic Features	Treatment	Diagnostic Process
Painful, discrete, round to oval, yellowish white ulcers Halo of erythema Up to 1 cm in diameter Spontaneous healing in 7-10 days	N/A	Ulcer with lymphocytic infiltrate	Topical corticosteroids	Clinical
Painful Greater than 1 cm in diameter Often deeper than minor aphthous ulcers May last several weeks Often heal with scarring	N/A	May require biopsy for diagnosis to rule out other causes of ulceration	Topical or systemic corticosteroids Biopsy to rule out ulceration from other cause	Clinical Microscopic
Painful, very tiny 1 to 2 mm ulcers Often occur in groups Resolve spontaneously	N/A	Unclear	Topical corticosteroids Topical tetracycline	Clinical
Multiple areas of well-demarcated swelling accompanied by itching (pruritus) Self-limiting episodes	N/A	†	Identification and avoidance of causative agent Antihistaminic drugs	Clinical
Diffuse swelling of tissue Usually no itching Self-limiting episodes	N/A	†	Identification of causative agent Antihistaminic drugs	Clinical
Smooth, shiny, firm mucosa with erythema and edema May form vesicles Often itching or burning sensation	N/A	†	Identification of causative agent Topical and systemic corticosteroids	Clinical
Erythema, swelling, vesicles to encrusted, scaly, white appearance	N/A	†	Identification of causative agent Topical and systemic corticosteroids	Clinical

Continued

Chapter 3 Synopsis—cont'd

Condition/ Disease	Cause	Age/Race/Sex	Location
Fixed Drug Eruptions	Type III hypersensitivity	*	Same site each episode Usually skin Occasionally oral mucosa
Erythema Multiforme	Unclear Evidence for hypersensitivity reaction that in some cases may be associated with infectious agents	Most frequent in young adults Men more frequent than women	Skin and mucous membranes
Lichen Planus	Unknown	Broad age range Increased prevalence in middle age Women more than men	Skin and oral mucosal lesions Oral mucosa—buccal mucosa, tongue, labial mucosa, floor of mouth, gingiva
Reiter Syndrome	Abnormal immunologic response to infectious agent Genetic influence presence of HLA-B27	Much greater frequency in men than women (10 to 15:1)	Conjunctiva Urethra Oral mucosa Skin Knee and ankle joints
Langerhans Cell Disease	Unclear—suggested reactive process, immunologic disease, neoplastic process		
Acute disseminated form (Letterer-Siwi disease)		Affects children under 3 years of age	Disseminated disease
Chronic disseminated multifocal form (Hand-Shüller-Christian disease)		Affects children under 5 years of age	Multiple locations

*No significant information.
†Not covered in this text.

Clinical Features	Radiographic Features	Microscopic Features	Treatment	Diagnostic Process
Lesions appear when drug is introduced and subside when drug is discontinued with increasing intensity Single to multiple raised reddish patches or clusters of macules Pain/pruritis may be present	N/A	†	Identification and discontinuation of causative drug	Clinical
Skin—characteristic target lesion, also macules, plaques, bullae Mucosa—erythema, ulcers, crusted, bleeding lips Severe form—Stevens-Johnson syndrome Explosive onset	N/A	Nonspecific	Identification of causative agent if possible Topical/systemic corticosteroids	Clinical

Oral lesions
   Wickham striae
   Erosive and plaquelike lesions may occur
Gingival lesions—desquamative gingivitis
	N/A	Degeneration of the basal layer of the epithelium
		Broad band of lymphocytes in the connective tissue subjacent to the epithelium
			None if asymptomatic
			Topical corticosteroids if symptomatic
			Follow-up evaluations
				Clinical
				Microscopic

Syndrome triad
   Arthritis
   Urethritis
   Conjunctivitis
Skin lesions
Oral lesions
   Aphthouslike ulcers
   Lesions resembling geographic tongue
 	
Erythematous lesions
	N/A	†	ASA and NSAIDs	Clinical

†	N/A	†	Chemotherapy Poor prognosis	Clinical Microscopic

Classic triad
   Skull radiolucencies
   Exophthalmos
   Diabetes insipidus
	Radiolucencies ("punched out") of skull
	Max/Mand radiolucencies including alveolar bone
		Infiltrate of Langerhans cells (macrophages) and eosinophils	†	Clinical
				Microscopic

Continued

Chapter 3 Synopsis—cont'd

Condition/ Disease	Cause	Age/Race/Sex	Location
Langerhans Cell Disease—cont'd			
Solitary disseminated (multifocal form)			
Solitary (chronic) localized form (Eosinophilic granuloma)	Unclear—suggested reactive process, immunologic disease, neoplastic process	Affects older children and young adults Affects males more than females (2:1)	Bone—skull and mandible are commonly involved
Sjögren Syndrome	Autoimmune disease Decreased lacrimal flow Decreased salivary flow	*	Eyes Oral cavity
Systemic Lupus Erythematosus (SLE)	Autoimmune disease	Affects women more frequently than men (8:1) Black more frequent than white (3:1)	Multiple sites Skin Mucous membranes Joints Eyes CNS Kidneys Heart + others
Pemphigus Vulgaris	Autoimmune disease	Affects children and adults Most common in fourth to fifth decade More common in Ashkenazic Jews	Mucous membranes Skin

*No significant information.
†Not covered in this text.

Clinical Features	Radiographic Features	Microscopic Features	Treatment	Diagnostic Process
Oral—sore mouth with or without ulceration halitosis, gingivitis, unpleasant taste, loose, sore teeth, early exfoliation of teeth				
N/A	Radiolucency May resemble periodontal disease or may be well-circumscribed radiolucency May be multifocal	Infiltrate of Langerhans cell (macrophages) and eosinophils	Conservative surgical excision Low-dose radiation treatment	Microscopic
Primary S. syndrome Dry eyes (xerophthalmia) Dry mouth (xerostomia) Secondary S. syndrome Dry eyes (xerophthalmia) Dry mouth (xerostomia) Another autoimmune disease	Sialogram shows characteristic features (see text)	Salivary gland changes—lymphocytic infiltration and epimyoepithelial islands	Xerostomia Saliva substitutes Saliva stimulation Pilocarpine	Clinical Radiographic Microscopic Laboratory
Oral lesions Erythematous plaques or erosions White striations radiating from center of lesion	N/A	Destruction of the basal layer of the epithelium with inflammatory infiltrate around blood vessels Immunohistochemical testing Granular and linear deposits of immunoglobulins along basement membrane zone	Antiinflammatory and immunosuppressive agents	Laboratory Microscopic Clinical
Progressive involvement of mucous membranes and skin Oral lesions Painful, erythema, vesicles, bullae, erosions Positive Nikolsky sign	N/A	Intact basal layer attached to the underlying connective tissue Acantholysis of the prickle cell layer Tzanck cells	Corticosteroids and other immuno-suppressive agents	Laboratory Microscopic

Continued

Chapter 3 Synopsis—cont'd

Condition/ Disease	Cause	Age/Race/Sex	Location
Cicatrical Pemphigoid (mucosal pemphigoid, benign mucous membrane pemphigoid)	Autoimmune disease	Adults	Mucous membranes most common—gingiva May affect eyes
Bullous Pemphigoid	Autoimmune disease	80% affected are over 60 years old	Mucous membranes Skin
Behçet Syndrome	Autoimmune disease	Mean age of onset 30 years	Mucous membranes Oral Genital Ocular

*No significant information.
†Not covered in this text.

Clinical Features	Radiographic Features	Microscopic Features	Treatment	Diagnostic Process

Oral lesions
  Desquamative
    gingivitis
  Bullae, erosions,
    ulcers
  Lesions heal with
    scarring
	N/A	Epithelium detaches
		  from the connective
		  tissue at the basement
		  membrane
			Topical/systemic
			  corticosteroids
				Microscopic

Oral lesions as in
  cicatricial pemphigoid
  but less common
	N/A	Epithelium detaches
		  from the connective
		  tissue at the basement
		  membrane
			Systemic
			  corticosteroids
			  and other
			  antiinflammatory
			  agents
				Microscopic

Oral lesions
  Aphthouslike ulcers
	N/A	†	Corticosteroids and
			  other immuno-
			  suppressive
			  agents
				Clinical

Infectious Diseases

Joan A. Phelan

Objectives

After studying this chapter, the student will be able to:

1. State the difference between the inflammatory and immune response to infection.
2. Describe the factors that allow opportunistic infection to develop.
3. List two examples of opportunistic infections that can occur in the oral cavity.
4. For each of the following infectious diseases, name the organism causing it, list the route or routes of transmission of the organism and the oral manifestations of the disease, and describe how the diagnosis is made: impetigo, tuberculosis, actinomycosis, syphilis (primary, secondary, tertiary), verruca vulgaris, condyloma acuminatum, and primary herpetic gingivostomatitis.
5. Describe the relationship between streptococcal tonsillitis and pharyngitis and the need for antibiotic prophylaxis for dental hygiene treatment.
6. List and describe four forms of oral candidiasis.
7. Describe the clinical features of herpes labialis.
8. Describe the clinical features of recurrent intraoral herpes simplex infection, and compare them with the clinical features of minor aphthous ulcers.
9. Describe the clinical characteristics of herpes zoster when it affects the skin of the face and oral mucosa.
10. List two oral infectious diseases for which a cytologic smear may assist in confirming the diagnosis.
11. List four diseases associated with the Epstein-Barr virus.
12. List two diseases caused by coxsackieviruses that have oral manifestations.
13. Describe the spectrum of human immunodeficiency virus (HIV) disease, including initial infection and the development of acquired immunodeficiency syndrome (AIDS).
14. List and describe the clinical appearance of five oral manifestations of HIV infection.

Vocabulary

Granuloma (gran″u-lo′mah) A tumorlike mass of inflammatory tissue consisting of a central collection of macrophages, often with multinucleated giant cells, surrounded by lymphocytes.

Granulomatous disease (gran″u-lom′ah-tus dĭ-zēz′) A disease characterized by the formation of granulomas.

Incubation period (in″ku-ba′shĕn pir-ē-ĕd) The period between the infection of an individual by a pathogen and the manifestation of the disease it causes.

Malaise (mah-lāz′) A vague, indefinite feeling of discomfort, debilitation, or lack of health.

Opportunistic infection (op″or-tu-nis′tik in-fek′shun) A disease caused by a microorganism that does not or-

dinarily cause disease but becomes pathogenic under certain circumstances.

Parenteral (pah-ren′ter-al) Administered by injection.

Paresthesia (par″ĕs-the′zhĕ) An abnormal sensation such as prickling or tingling.

Pathogenic microorganism (path-o-jen′ik mi″kro-or′gan-izm) A microorganism that causes disease.

Pruritus (proo-ri′tĕs) Itching.

Subclinical infection (sĕb-klinĭ-kel) An infectious disease not detectable by the usual clinical signs.

Whitlow (hwit′lo) An infection involving the distal phalanx of a finger.

Human beings are surrounded and inhabited by an enormous number of microorganisms. The ability of these organisms to cause disease depends on both the microorganism and the state of the body's defenses. The organism must be capable of causing disease and the individual must be susceptible to the disease. Microorganisms are traditionally divided into those that produce disease (pathogenic) and those that do not (nonpathogenic). To cause disease the organism must gain access to the body, accommodate to growth in the human environment, and avoid multiple host defenses. These defense mechanisms include intact skin and mucosal surfaces, antimicrobial secretory and excretory products on the skin and mucosa, the normal competition of microbial flora, the inflammatory response, and the immune response.

Numerous infectious diseases can affect the tissues of the oral cavity. Bacterial, fungal, and viral infections are the most common, but even protozoan and helminthic infections, though extremely rare, have been reported.

The oral cavity can be the primary site of involvement of an infectious disease, or a systemic infection can have oral manifestations. These infections are usually transmitted from one individual to another by several different routes. Organisms can be transferred through the air on dust particles or water droplets. Some organisms require intimate and direct contact to be transferred. Some can be transferred on hands and objects, and others, such as hepatitis B, must be transferred from one person to another in blood or other body fluids. Microorganisms initially invading the oral tissues can cause a local infection, systemic infection, or both. Microorganisms circulating in the blood stream can cause lesions in the oral cavity, and microorganisms causing infection in the lungs can be transferred to oral tissues when they are present in sputum. The oral cavity contains numerous microorganisms that make up the normal oral flora. Changes such as a decrease in salivary flow, antibiotic administration, and immune system alterations affect the oral flora so that organisms that are usually nonpathogenic are able to cause disease. This type of infection is called an **opportunistic infection.**

Microorganisms penetrating epithelial surfaces act as foreign bodies and stimulate the inflammatory response (see Chapter 2). The inflammatory response is a nonspecific response and results in edema and the accumulation of a large number of white blood cells at the site. The responses of the immune system are highly specific (see Chapter 3). Specific antibodies are formed in response to specific antigens; microorganisms are antigens.

Humoral immunity (antibodies) is an effective defense against some microorganisms, and cell-mediated immunity is the primary defense against others, such as intracellular bacteria (tuberculosis), viruses, and fungi. Microbial infections are responsible for many more diseases than those included in this chapter. The diseases discussed here are common, cause specific oral lesions, and help to illustrate principles of infectious disease. Dental caries and periodontal disease are clearly important to dental hygienists. However, they are not included in this text because they are usually studied in courses other than oral pathology. The dental hygienist frequently encounters oral infectious diseases and must be able to recognize their clinical features and significance for control of infection.

Bacterial Infections

IMPETIGO

Impetigo is a bacterial skin infection caused by *Streptococcus pyogenes* and *Staphylococcus aureus.* Impetigo most commonly involves the skin of the face or extremities and is usually seen in young children. The organisms are present on skin, and nonintact skin is necessary for infection. Therefore areas of trauma, such as cuts and abrasions, and areas of dermatitis are likely sites of this infection. The lesions of impetigo are either vesicles that rupture, resulting in thick, amber-colored crusts, or longer-lasting bullae. The lesions may itch (pruritus) and regional lymphadenopathy may be present. Systemic manifestations such as fever and malaise generally do not occur with this infection. The lesions may resemble recurrent herpes simplex infection (see Figure 4-18, p. 141). However, recurrent herpes simplex infection is much less common than impetigo in small children. The diagnosis is made based on the clinical presentation or by identification of the bacteria from cultures of the lesions. Topical or systemic antibiotics are used for treatment.

TONSILLITIS AND PHARYNGITIS

Tonsillitis and **pharyngitis** are inflammatory conditions of the tonsils and pharyngeal mucosa. Many different organisms cause them, including streptococci, adenoviruses, influenza viruses, and Epstein-Barr virus. The clinical features include sore throat, fever, tonsillar hyperplasia, and erythema of the oropharyngeal mucosa and tonsils.

Streptococcal tonsillitis and pharyngitis is a common bacterial infection that is spread by contact with infectious nasal or oral secretions. The appearance of streptococcal tonsillitis and pharyngitis, "strep throat," closely resembles tonsillitis and pharyngitis caused by other infections such as viral infections. Specific laboratory tests are available for diagnostic confirmation of streptococcal cause. Antibiotics are used to treat streptococcal infection.

Tonsillitis and pharyngitis caused by group A, β (beta) hemolytic streptococci are significant because of their relationship to scarlet fever and rheumatic fever. **Scarlet fever** usually occurs in children. In addition to fever, patients with scarlet fever develop a generalized red skin rash that is caused by a toxin released by the bacteria. In addition to streptococcal tonsillitis and pharyngitis, oral manifestations of scarlet fever include petechiae on the soft palate and an appearance of the tongue that has been called **strawberry tongue.** The fungiform papillae are red and prominent, with the dorsal surface of tongue either exhibiting a white coating or erythema. Throat culture is helpful in confirming the diagnosis of scarlet fever.

Rheumatic fever is a childhood disease that follows a group A, β hemolytic streptococcal infection, usually tonsillitis and pharyngitis. Rheumatic fever is characterized by an inflammatory reaction involving the heart, joints, and central nervous system. A history of rheumatic fever is particularly important in the dental treatment setting because of the relationship between the heart valve damage that may occur as a result of rheumatic fever and the development of bacterial endocarditis subsequent to dental treatment procedures. Patients with rheumatic heart disease require antibiotic prophylaxis for dental hygiene treatment.

TUBERCULOSIS

Tuberculosis is an infectious chronic granulomatous disease usually caused by the organism *Mycobacterium tuberculosis.* The chief form of the disease is a primary infection of the lung (inhaled droplets containing bacteria lodge in the alveoli of the lungs). After undergoing phagocytosis by macrophages, the organisms are resistant to destruction and multiply in the macrophages. They then disseminate in the blood stream. After a few weeks, dissemination ceases. The signs and symptoms of this lung infection include fever, chills, fatigue and malaise, weight loss, and persistent cough. The bacteria can be carried to widespread areas of the body and cause involvement of organs such as the kidneys and liver. This is called **miliary tuberculosis.** Involvement of the submandibular and cervical lymph nodes causes enlargement of those nodes and is called **scrofula** or **tuberculous lymphadenitis.** The lung infection can occur at any age. Most commonly, foci of infection in the lungs become completely walled off and heal by fibrosis and calcification. A reactivation of the primary lesion can occur years after the initial infection.

Oral lesions associated with tuberculosis occur but are rare. They most likely appear when organisms are carried from the lungs in sputum and are transmitted to the oral mucosa **(Figure 4-1).** The tongue and palate are the most common sites for oral lesions of tuberculosis, but they may occur anywhere in the oral cavity, even in bone as in osteomyelitis. Oral lesions appear as painful, nonhealing, slowly enlarging ulcers that can be either superficial or deep.

Diagnosis

Oral lesions of tuberculosis are identified by biopsy and microscopic examination of the tissue. They are chronic granulomatous inflammatory lesions composed of areas of necrosis surrounded by macrophages, multinucleated giant cells, and lymphocytes. Similar lesions occur in sarcoidosis, deep fungal infections, and foreign-body reactions. Staining the tissue to be examined microscopically with a special stain may reveal the organisms. Tissue culture to diagnose tuberculosis requires a specialized laboratory.

A skin test is used to determine if an individual has been exposed and infected with *Mycobacterium tuberculosis.* An antigen called **purified protein derivative (PPD)** is injected into the skin. If the individual's cell-mediated immune system has previously encountered the antigen, a positive inflammatory skin reaction occurs (a type IV hypersensitivity reaction). This skin reaction indicates previous infection

Figure 4-1 Ulcer on tongue seen in tuberculosis.

with the bacteria but not necessarily active disease. To determine if active disease is present after a positive skin test result, chest radiographs are generally taken.

Effective drug treatment for tuberculosis became available in the 1940s. In the United States, most tuberculosis treatment centers had closed by the mid-1970s. State health departments reported a dramatic increase in new cases in the mid-1980s, particularly in densely populated urban areas. This increase was suggested to be related to HIV infection and to the noncompliance of patients with therapy. Recent public health efforts have focused on ensuring compliance with antituberculosis drug treatment; as a result the number of new cases reported is decreasing.

Tuberculosis is an infectious disease that can be occupationally transmitted to dental health care personnel. Routine use of universal precautions, including eye protection, mask, or facial shield, is important in preventing the transmission of airborne droplet infections such as tuberculosis. However, for patients with active tuberculosis, routine dental treatment is deferred. When emergency dental treatment is needed, the use of a special mask is recommended to ensure prevention of transmission of the tuberculosis organism.

Treatment and Prognosis

Oral lesions resolve with treatment of the patient's primary (usually pulmonary) disease. Several different combination medications, including isoniazid (INH) and rifampin, are used to treat tuberculosis. Treatment continues for many months and may continue for as long as 2 years. Patients usually become noninfectious shortly after treatment begins. Consultation with the patient's physician should confirm that treatment is ongoing and the patient is no longer infectious.

ACTINOMYCOSIS

Actinomycosis is an infection caused by a filamentous bacterium called *Actinomyces israelii*. These organisms were at one time thought to be fungi and therefore the name ends in the suffix "mycosis," which usually indicates a fungal infection.

The most characteristic form of the disease is the formation of abscesses that tend to drain by the formation of sinus tracts (see **Figure 4-2**). The colonies or organisms appear in the pus as tiny, bright yellow-

grains and are called sulfur granules because of their yellow color. They can also be identified by microscopic examination. These organisms are common inhabitants of the oral cavity. It is not clear why these organisms only occasionally cause disease. Predisposing factors have not been identified. The infection is often preceded by tooth extraction or an abrasion of the mucosa.

Generally the clinician makes a diagnosis of actinomycosis by identifying the colonies in the tissue from the lesion. Actinomycosis is treated with long-term high doses of antibiotics.

SYPHILIS

Syphilis is a disease caused by the spirochete *Treponema pallidum*. The organism is transmitted from one person to another by direct contact. The spirochete, a corkscrew-like organism, can penetrate mucous membranes but requires a break in the continuity of the skin surface to invade through the skin. The organisms die quickly when exposed to air and changes in temperature. Syphilis is usually transmitted through sexual contact with a partner who has active lesions. It can also be transmitted by transfusion of infected blood or by transplacental inoculation of a fetus from an infected mother.

Figure 4-2 Actinomycosis. Skin lesion over mandible. Incision and drainage site seen below lesion. "Sulfur granules" were noted in the laboratory report, and the condition was treated with long-term antibiotic therapy.

The disease occurs in three stages: (1) primary, (2) secondary, and (3) tertiary **(Table 4-1)**. The lesion of the primary stage, called the **chancre,** is highly infectious and forms at the site at which the spirochete enters the body **(Figure 4-3)**. Regional lymphadenopathy accompanies the chancre. The lesion heals spontaneously after several weeks without treatment, and the disease enters a latent period.

The secondary stage occurs about 6 weeks after the primary lesion appears. In the secondary stage, diffuse eruptions of the skin and mucous membranes occur. The skin lesions have many forms. The oral lesions are called **mucous patches** and appear as multiple, painless, grayish-white plaques covering ulcerated mucosa. The lesions of secondary syphilis are the most infectious. They undergo spontaneous remission but can recur for months or years. After remission the disease may remain latent for many years.

The tertiary lesions occur years after the initial infection if treatment for the infection has not been given. They chiefly involve the cardiovascular system and the central nervous system. The localized tertiary lesion is called a *gumma* and is noninfectious. A gumma can occur in the oral cavity; the most common sites are the tongue and palate. The lesion appears as a firm mass that eventually becomes an ulcer. The gumma is a destructive lesion and can lead to perforation of the palatal bone.

Congenital Syphilis

Syphilis can be transmitted from an infected mother to the fetus because the organism can cross the placenta and enter the fetal circulation. Congenital syphilis often causes serious and irreversible damage to the child, such as facial and dental abnormalities. The developmental disorders that result from fetal and neonatal syphilis are described in Chapter 5.

Diagnosis and Treatment

The diagnosis of syphilitic lesions occurring on skin can be made using a special microscopic technique called a **dark-field examination** to identify the spirochetes. However, other spirochetes are present in the oral cavity; therefore this examination is not reliable for oral lesions. Two serologic (blood) tests are commonly used to confirm the diagnosis of syphilis: (1) the Venereal Disease Research Laboratory (VDRL)

Table 4-1 Stages of Syphilis

Stage	Oral Lesion
Primary	Chancre
Secondary	Mucous patch
Latent	None
Tertiary	Gumma

Figure 4-3 **A,** Chancre on tongue seen in primary syphilis. **B,** Chancre on lip. (**A** courtesy Dr. Norman Trieger; **B** courtesy Dr. Edward V. Zegarelli.)

test and (2) the fluorescent treponemal antibody absorption (FTA-ABS) test. These tests may produce negative results in primary syphilis because sufficient antibodies may not have formed for the test result to be positive.

Syphilis is generally treated with penicillin. The VDRL test is used again to evaluate the success of treatment. The antibody titer decreases if treatment has been successful.

NECROTIZING ULCERATIVE GINGIVITIS

Necrotizing ulcerative gingivitis (NUG) is also called **acute necrotizing ulcerative gingivitis (ANUG).** It is a painful erythematous gingivitis with necrosis of the interdental papillae **(Figure 4-4).** NUG is most likely caused by both a fusiform bacillus and a spirochete *(Borrelia vincentii)* and is associated with decreased resistance to infection.

The gingiva is painful and erythematous, with necrosis of the interdental papillae generally accompanied by a foul odor and metallic taste. The necrosis results in cratering of the interdental papillae area. Sloughing of the necrotic tissue presents as a pseudomembrane over the tissues. Systemic manifestations of infection, such as fever and cervical lymphadenopathy, may be present. Clinical features distinguish NUG from acute marginal gingivitis and the gingival component of acute primary herpes simplex infection (see Figure 4-17, *B,* p. 140).

Figure 4-4 Necrotizing ulcerative gingivitis (NUG).

PERICORONITIS

Pericoronitis is an inflammation of the mucosa around the crown of a partially erupted, impacted tooth. The soft tissue around the mandibular third molar is the most common location for pericoronitis. The inflammation is usually the result of infection by bacteria that are part of the normal oral flora, which proliferate in the pocket between the soft tissue and the crown of the tooth. Compromised host defenses, ranging from minor illnesses to immunodeficiency, are associated with an increased risk of pericoronitis. Trauma from an opposing molar and impaction of food under the soft tissue flap (operculum) covering the distal portion of the third molar may also precipitate pericoronitis.

Diagnosis

The diagnosis of pericoronitis is made based on the clinical presentation. The tissue around the crown of a partially erupted tooth is swollen, erythematous, and painful.

Treatment and Prognosis

Treatment of pericoronitis includes mechanical débridement and irrigation of the pocket and systemic antibiotics. Extraction of the impacted molar is usually necessary to prevent recurrence.

ACUTE OSTEOMYELITIS

Acute osteomyelitis involves acute inflammation of the bone and bone marrow **(Figure 4-5,** *A).* Acute osteomyelitis of the jaws is most commonly a result of the extension of a periapical abscess. It may follow fracture of the bone or surgery and may also result from bacteremia.

Diagnosis

The diagnosis of the specific organism causing acute osteomyelitis is based on culture results, and treatment is based on antibiotic sensitivity testing. Microscopic examination shows nonviable bone, necrotic debris, acute inflammation, and bacterial colonies in the marrow spaces. No change is seen on the radiograph unless the disease has been present for more than 1 week.

Treatment and Prognosis

The treatment of acute osteomyelitis involves drainage of the area and the use of appropriate antibiotics.

CHRONIC OSTEOMYELITIS

Chronic osteomyelitis is a long-standing inflammation of bone. It may follow inadequately treated acute osteomyelitis, long-term inflammation with no recognized acute phase, Paget disease, sickle cell disease, or bone irradiation that results in decreased vascularity. The involved bone is painful and swollen, and radiographic examination reveals a diffuse and irregular radiolucency that can eventually become radiopaque (**Figure 4-5,** *B*). When radiopacity develops, the condition is called **chronic sclerosing osteomyelitis.**

A

B

Figure 4-5 A, Low-power microscopy of acute osteomyelitis showing nonviable bone. Bacterial colonies and inflammatory cells are seen between trabeculae of bone. **B,** Chronic osteomyelitis as seen radiographically.

Diagnosis

The diagnosis of chronic osteomyelitis is based on biopsy results and the histologic examination, which shows chronic inflammation of bone and marrow. Bacterial culture may be helpful, but bacteria may be difficult to identify.

Treatment

Treatment of chronic osteomyelitis involves débridement and administration of systemic antibiotics. In some patients, the use of hyperbaric oxygen may be needed to successfully treat this condition.

Fungal Infections

CANDIDIASIS

Candidiasis, also called **moniliasis** and **thrush,** occurs as a result of an overgrowth of the yeastlike fungus *Candida albicans.* It is the most common oral fungal infection. This fungus is part of the normal oral flora in many individuals, particularly those who wear dentures. Overgrowth of *Candida albicans* can result from many different conditions. Some of these include the following:

- Antibiotic therapy
- Cancer chemotherapy
- Corticosteroid therapy
- Dentures
- Diabetes mellitus
- HIV infection
- Hypoparathyroidism
- Infancy (newborn)
- Multiple myeloma
- Primary T-lymphocyte deficiency
- Xerostomia

Newborn infants are particularly susceptible to an overgrowth of this fungus because they do not have either an established oral flora or a fully developed immune system. Pregnant women often have *Candida vaginitis,* and the organism is transmitted to the infant while passing through the birth canal. Antibiotics can alter the bacteria of the oral flora, which can allow the overgrowth of *Candida albicans.* Systemic and topical corticosteroids, diabetes, and cell-mediated immune system deficiency are other factors that allow the overgrowth of this fungus. Candidiasis is one of the most common oral lesions that occur in association with immunodeficiency. Candidiasis generally affects the superficial layers of the epithelium; therefore when it is present, the proliferating organisms are easily identified in a scraping (smear) of the lesion.

Types of Oral Candidiasis

Several forms of oral candidiasis exist; recognition of their clinical features is important so that candidiasis is included in the differential diagnosis of a variety of clinical presentations. The types of oral candidiasis are:

- Pseudomembranous
- Erythematous
- Chronic atrophic (denture stomatitis)
- Chronic hyperplastic (candidal leukoplakia)
- Angular cheilitis

Pseudomembranous Candidiasis. A white curdlike material is present on the mucosal surface in **pseudomembranous candidiasis (Figure 4-6).** The underlying mucosa is erythematous. Occasionally a burning sensation is felt, and the patient may complain of a metallic taste

Erythematous Candidiasis. An erythematous, often painful, mucosa is the presenting complaint in **erythematous candidiasis (Figure 4-7).** This type of candidiasis may be localized to one area of the oral mucosa or may be more generalized.

Chronic Atrophic Candidiasis. The most common type of candidiasis affecting the oral mucosa is called **chronic atrophic candidiasis,** also known as **denture stomatitis (Figure 4-8).** This type of candidiasis also presents as erythematous mucosa, but the erythematous change is limited to the mucosa covered by a full or partial denture. The lesions may vary from petechiae-like to more generalized and granular. It is most common on the palate and maxillary alveolar ridge and is usually asymptomatic, being dis-

Figure 4-7 Erythematous candidiasis. **A,** Recent onset and erythematous lesions elsewhere in the oral cavity differentiate this from median rhomboid glossitis. **B,** Response to antifungal treatment confirmed the diagnosis of oral candidiasis in this patient.

Figure 4-6 Pseudomembranous candidiasis.

A

B

Figure 4-8 Chronic atrophic candidiasis (denture stomatitis). **A,** Full denture. **B,** Partial denture.

Figure 4-9 Chronic hyperplastic candidiasis. The white appearance of the tongue did not wipe off, and it disappeared with antifungal treatment.

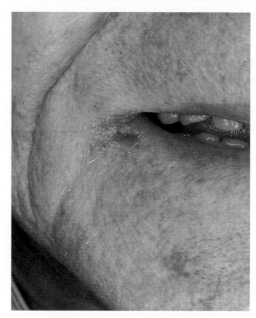

Figure 4-10 Angular cheilitis.

covered on examination by the dental hygienist or dentist.

Chronic Hyperplastic Candidiasis. **Candidal leukoplakia** and **hypertrophic candidiasis** are other names for this type of oral candidiasis **(Figure 4-9)**. It appears as a white lesion that does not wipe off the mucosa. An important diagnostic feature of this type of candidiasis is its response to antifungal medication: when leukoplakia is caused by candidiasis, it disappears when treated with antifungal medication. If the lesion does not respond to antifungal therapy, biopsy should be considered.

Angular Cheilitis. *Candida* organisms often cause **angular cheilitis (Figure 4-10)**. It appears as erythema or fissuring at the labial commissures. Angular cheilitis may be caused by other factors, such as nutritional deficiency; however, it most commonly results from *Candida* infection. Angular cheilitis frequently accompanies intraoral candidiasis.

Chronic Mucocutaneous Candidiasis. A severe form of candidiasis that usually occurs in patients who are severely immunocompromised is called **chronic mucocutaneous candidiasis.** The patient has chronic oral and genital mucosal candidiasis and has skin lesions as well. Oral involvement may appear as pseudomembranous, erythematous, or hyperplastic candidiasis and angular cheilitis is common. The skin lesions usually involve the nails and skin folds.

Median Rhomboid Glossitis. Several studies have reported an association between **median rhomboid glossitis (Figure 4-11)** and candidiasis. It appears as an erythematous, often rhombus-shaped, flat-to-raised area on the midline of the posterior dorsal tongue. *Candida* organisms have been identified in some lesions, and some lesions disappear with antifungal treatment. However, the response to antifungal treatment is not consistent; therefore although this lesion has been associated with candidiasis, the cause is not yet clear.

Diagnosis and Treatment

Because *Candida* is part of the oral flora in many individuals, the use of a culture for diagnosis is not particularly helpful. A positive culture result indicates that the organisms are present but not that they are causing infection. The use of the mucosal smear **(Figure 4-12)** is usually more helpful. The surface of the lesion is vigorously scraped with a tongue blade, wooden spatula, or specially designed brush, and the scrapings are spread on a glass slide and fixed with alcohol. The slide is then sent to an oral pathology laboratory for staining and examination. In addition to the smear, the response of the lesion to antifungal treatment is important in confirming the diagnosis of candidiasis. Lesions caused by *Candida* should resolve with antifungal treatment. Both topical and systemic medications are used for candidiasis. However, in some patients, particularly those who are immunocompromised, candidiasis is persistent and recurrent.

Although the final diagnosis and management of a patient with oral candidiasis is the responsibility of the dentist, dental hygienists are often the first to recognize the oral changes characteristic of this condition. Recurrent oral candidiasis may be an early sign of a severe underlying medical problem.

DEEP FUNGAL INFECTIONS

Oral lesions occur in some deep fungal infections, for example, histoplasmosis, coccidioidomycosis, blastomycosis, and cryptococcosis. They are all characterized by primary involvement of the lungs. Oral lesions are caused by implantation of the organism carried by sputum from the lungs to the oral mucosa.

Infections caused by some of these organisms are more common in certain areas of the United States than in others. Histoplasmosis is widespread in the midwestern United States, and coccid-

Figure 4-11 Median rhomboid glossitis.

Figure 4-12 Photomicrograph of a smear showing epithelial cells and *Candida* organisms.

ioidomycosis is more prevalent in parts of the western United States, particularly the San Joaquin Valley of California. Blastomycosis is common in the Ohio-Mississippi river basin area. Therefore oral lesions caused by these organisms are most likely seen in areas of the country in which the infection is most common.

Cryptococcosis is transmitted through inhalation of organisms contained in dust from bird droppings, particularly from pigeons. In addition to the regional distribution of these infections, reactivation, including the development of oral lesions, can also occur in patients who are immunocompromised.

Diagnosis

The initial signs and symptoms of these deep fungal infections are usually related to the primary lung infection. Oral lesions are preceded by pulmonary involvement. These oral lesions are chronic, nonhealing ulcers that can resemble squamous cell carcinoma. Diagnosis is made by biopsy and microscopic examination. Special staining of the tissue reveals the organisms, which can be identified by their microscopic appearance. Culture of the tissue can also be done and is useful in establishing the diagnosis.

Treatment

Systemic antifungal medications, such as amphotericin B or ketoconazole, are used to treat these infections. However, latent infections may remain even after treatment and may reappear if the individual's immune system becomes deficient.

MUCORMYCOSIS

Mucormycosis, also called **phycomycosis,** is a rare fungal infection. The organism is a common inhabitant of soil and is usually nonpathogenic. However, infection with this organism occurs in diabetic and debilitated patients. The disease often involves the nasal cavity, maxillary sinus, and hard palate and can present as a proliferating or destructive mass in the maxilla. The diagnosis is made by biopsy and identification of the organisms in the tissue.

Viral Infections

PAPILLOMAVIRUS INFECTION

Many types of human papillomaviruses (HPVs) have been identified. Several have been identified in oral lesions, and some have been identified in normal oral mucosa. HPVs have also been implicated in neoplasia.

Verruca Vulgaris

The **verruca vulgaris,** or **common wart,** is a papillary oral lesion caused by a papillomavirus. It is a common skin lesion. Oral lesions are less common than skin lesions, but they do occur. The virus is inoculated by direct contact and may be transmitted from skin to oral mucosa. The lips are one of the most common intraoral sites for this lesion. Autoinoculation occurs through finger sucking or fingernail biting in patients with verrucae on the hands or fingers **(Figure 4-13).** The verruca vulgaris is usually a white, papillary, exophytic lesion **(Figure 4-14)** that closely resembles the benign tumor of squamous epithelium called the **papilloma** (see Chapter 7).

Histologically the verruca vulgaris consists of fingerlike projections of markedly keratotic, stratified squamous epithelium that exhibits a prominent granular cell layer, and numerous cells with clear cytoplasm are present in the upper spinous layer of the

Figure 4-13 A and **B,** Verruca vulgaris on the tongue of a child with a similar lesion on the thumb. (Courtesy Dr. Edward V. Zegarelli.)

epithelium. These cells contain the viral particles that are visible by electron microscopic examination. Each of the projections contains a central core of fibrous connective tissue containing many blood vessels. The vacuolated cells in the epithelium contain the viral particles.

Diagnosis. Biopsy and histologic examination reveal the light microscopic features of this lesion. Immunologic staining is also useful in identifying these viruses.

Treatment and Prognosis. Conservative surgical excision is the treatment of choice for verruca vulgaris. These lesions may recur. In addition, patients with skin lesions should be instructed to refrain from finger sucking or fingernail biting to prevent reinoculation and development of new lesions.

Condyloma Acuminatum

The **condyloma acuminatum** is a benign papillary lesion that is caused by another papillomavirus. The virus is generally transmitted by sexual contact and is most common in the anogenital region. It is transmitted to the oral cavity through oral-genital contact or self-inoculation.

Oral condylomas appear as papillary, bulbous masses and can occur anywhere in the oral mucosa **(Figure 4-15)**. Multiple lesions may be present.

They have been reported to occur on the tongue, buccal mucosa, palate, gingiva, and alveolar ridge. The oral condyloma tends to be more diffuse than the papilloma or verruca vulgaris and is generally not as well keratinized as the verruca vulgaris. The condyloma is pink, whereas the verruca vulgaris is usually white.

Histologically the condyloma acuminatum is composed of fingerlike (papillary) projections of epithelium covering cores of connective tissue. The epithelium is thickened, and cells with clear cytoplasm are seen throughout the epithelium. These clear cells contain viral particles that can be identified through immunologic staining.

When the condyloma acuminatum occurs in the oral cavity, it is generally treated by conservative surgical excision. However, recurrence is common, and multiple lesions make management difficult. Patients should be instructed to avoid oral-genital contact with an infected partner to prevent reinoculation.

Focal Epithelial Hyperplasia

Focal epithelial hyperplasia, also called **Heck disease,** is characterized by the presence of multiple whitish to pale-pink nodules distributed throughout the oral mucosa **(Figure 4-16)**. The disease is most common in children and was first described in Native Americans, but it has since been described in many different areas of the world. This disease is caused by

Figure 4-14 Verruca vulgaris on the lateral aspect of the tongue in an adult.

Figure 4-15 Condyloma acuminatum. The presence of condyloma acuminatum in a child is strongly suggestive of sexual abuse. (Courtesy Dr. Sidney Eisig.)

Figure 4-16 Focal epithelial hyperplasia. (Courtesy Dr. Stanley Kerpel.)

another HPV. The lesions are generally asymptomatic and do not require treatment. They resolve spontaneously within a few weeks. Histologically the lesions show thickened epithelium with broad, connected rete ridges. Cells in the epithelium have clear cytoplasm, which is a common finding in lesions caused by HPV.

HERPES SIMPLEX INFECTION

Two major forms of the herpes simplex virus exist: (1) type 1 and (2) type 2. Oral infections are generally caused by type 1, and genital infections are most commonly caused by type 2. Oral infection with the herpes simplex virus occurs in an initial (primary) form and a recurrent (secondary) form. The herpes simplex virus is one of a group of viruses called human herpes viruses (HHVs). Other herpes viruses include varicella-zoster virus, Epstein-Barr virus, cytomegalovirus, and human herpes virus 8 (HHV-8). Herpes simplex viruses have the ability to persist in an individual in a clinically quiescent or latent state. The primary infection undergoes remission without the virus being completely eliminated.

Primary Herpetic Gingivostomatitis

The oral disease caused by initial infection with the herpes simplex virus is called **primary herpetic gingivostomatitis (Figure 4-17).** Painful, erythematous, and swollen gingiva and multiple tiny vesicles on the perioral skin, vermilion border of the lips, and oral

Figure 4-17 **A,** Example of primary herpetic gingivostomatitis in a child. **B** and **C,** Primary herpetic gingivostomatitis in an adolescent. (**A** courtesy Dr. Edward V. Zegarelli.)

mucosa characterize the disease. These vesicles progress to form ulcers. Systemic symptoms such as fever, malaise, and cervical lymphadenopathy generally occur first, followed by gingival involvement and the appearance of mucosal vesicles and ulcers. The disease most commonly occurs in children between the ages of 6 months and 6 years. However, it may

Figure 4-18 Herpes labialis. **A,** Twelve hours after onset. **B,** Forty-eight hours after onset.

Figure 4-19 **A** and **B,** Recurrent intraoral herpes simplex.

occur at any age if an individual who has not been previously exposed to the virus comes into contact with it or if a sufficient level of antibodies has not developed to confer protection against reinfection. Because many more individuals have antibodies to herpes simplex than have a history of the disease, the majority of infections are thought to be subclinical. The disease is usually self-limited. The lesions heal spontaneously in 1 to 2 weeks.

Recurrent Herpes Simplex Infection

The herpes simplex virus tends to persist in a latent state, usually in the nerve tissue of the trigeminal ganglion, and causes localized recurrent infections. It has been estimated that one third to one half of the pop-

ulation of the United States experiences recurrent herpes simplex infection. The most common type of recurrent oral herpes simplex infection occurs on the vermilion border of the lips and is called **herpes labialis (Figure 4-18),** which is also called a **cold sore** or **fever blister.** Recurrent infections are often produced by certain stimuli, such as sunlight, menstruation, fatigue, fever, and emotional stress. These stimuli are thought to trigger the viral replication and immunologic changes that result in clinical lesions.

Recurrent herpes simplex infection can also occur intraorally **(Figure 4-19).** The appearance and location of these lesions are important to distinguish them from aphthous ulcers **(Table 4-2).** Recurrent intraoral herpes simplex occurs on keratinized mucosa that is fixed to bone, most commonly the hard palate and gingiva. The lesions appear as painful crops of tiny vesicles or ulcers that can coalesce to form a single ulcer with an irregular border. Usually patients experience prodromal symptoms such as pain, burning, or tingling in the area in which the vesicles develop. The lesions heal without scarring in 1 to 2 weeks. Episodes of recurrence vary from once a month in some individuals to once a year in others.

Herpes simplex virus is transmitted by direct contact with an infected individual, and the lesions of the primary infection occur at the site of inoculation. The herpes simplex virus can be isolated from both primary and recurrent lesions. The amount of virus present is highest in the vesicle stage. In some individuals, the virus is present in the oral cavity, even when no lesions are present. Herpes simplex virus can cause a painful infection of the fingers, called **herpetic whitlow,** in dentists and dental hygienists **(Figure 4-20).** Herpetic whitlow can be either a primary or a recurrent infection. Herpes simplex can also cause eye infection **(Figure 4-21).** Routine barrier infection control procedures (mask, eye protection, and gloves) are important in preventing the transmission of the herpes simplex virus to dental health care providers.

Table 4-2 Comparison of the Clinical Features of Recurrent Minor Aphthous Ulcers and Recurrent Herpes Ulceration

Feature	Minor Aphthous Ulcers	Herpes Simplex Ulceration
Location	Nonkeratinized mucosa	Keratinized mucosa
Number	One to several	Multiple (crops)
Vesicle precedes ulcer	No	Yes
Pain	Yes	Yes
Size	<1 cm	1-2 mm
Borders	Round to oval	Crops of ulcers coalesce to form a large irregular ulcer
Recurrent	Yes	Yes

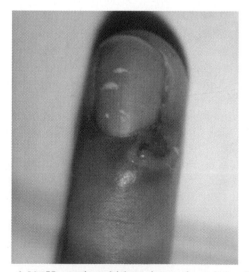

Figure 4-20 Herpetic whitlow in a dental hygienist. (Courtesy Susan Rod Graham.)

Figure 4-21 Herpetic eye infection. (Courtesy Dr. Sidney Eisig.)

Diagnosis. The diagnosis of herpes simplex infection, both primary and recurrent, is generally based on the clinical characteristics of the disease (see Table 4-2). In immunocompromised patients the characteristic clinical features may be lacking. A viral culture can be performed to confirm the diagnosis. This procedure requires a special culture medium and at least 2 days before results are available.

Herpes simplex virus causes changes in epithelial cells that can be seen microscopically. These virally altered cells can be seen in tissue obtained by biopsy or on a smear taken by scraping the basal cells of the lesion and spreading them on a glass slide, fixing them with alcohol, and submitting them to a pathology laboratory for staining and examination **(Figure 4-22)**. Smears of herpes simplex ulceration have been reported to be positive for virally altered cells only about 50% of the time.

Treatment. Antiviral drugs, such as acyclovir, are available for the treatment of herpes simplex infection and are used for treating genital herpes simplex infection. Antiviral drugs have not been consistently shown to be effective in treating the oral lesions of herpes simplex infection except in immunocompromised patients. Prevention of the development of herpes labialis may involve the use of sunscreens.

VARICELLA-ZOSTER VIRUS

The **varicella-zoster virus** causes both chickenpox (varicella) and shingles (herpes zoster). Respiratory aerosols and contact with secretions from skin lesions transmit the virus. Both chickenpox and herpes zoster are contagious.

Figure 4-22 Smear of virally altered cells resulting from herpes simplex. (Courtesy Dr. Harry Lumerman.)

Chickenpox

Chickenpox is a highly contagious disease that causes vesicular and pustular eruptions of the skin and mucous membranes, along with systemic symptoms such as headache, fever, and malaise **(Figure 4-23)**. The incubation period is about 2 weeks. Chickenpox usually occurs in children; although oral lesions occur, they generally do not cause severe discomfort. Usually an individual has only a single episode of chickenpox, but second, milder forms have also been described. Recovery generally occurs in 2 to 3 weeks.

Herpes Zoster

Although chickenpox has been described in adults, the virus usually causes a different form of disease in this population. The form that usually occurs in adults is called **herpes zoster** or **shingles**. It is characterized by a unilateral, painful eruption of vesicles along the distribution of a sensory nerve **(Figure 4-24)**. Whether or not the varicella-zoster virus is harbored in the sensory ganglia (during the interval between chickenpox and herpes zoster) in a manner similar to that of the herpes simplex virus is not clear. However, herpes zoster often occurs in association

A

B

Figure 4-23 Chickenpox. **A,** Skin lesions. **B,** Gingival lesion. (Courtesy Dr. Roger S. Kitzis.)

A

B

Ophthalmic branch
Maxillary branch
Mandibular branch

Figure 4-25 Diagram of the branches of the trigeminal nerve.

Figure 4-24 Herpes zoster. **A,** Unilateral distribution of vesicles along the distribution of a sensory nerve. **B,** Many vesicles coalesce to form large lesions.

with immunodeficiency or certain malignancies such as Hodgkin disease and leukemia.

The depression of cell-mediated immunity (CMI) appears to be important in the development of herpes zoster. Any of the three branches of the trigeminal nerve may be affected: (1) the ophthalmic branch, (2) the maxillary branch, or (3) the mandibular branch **(Figure 4-25)**. Oral lesions occur when the maxillary or mandibular branches are affected **(Figure 4-26)**. The oral lesions, like the skin lesions, are characterized by their unilateral distribution. Prodromal symptoms of pain, burning, or paresthesia often precede the development of vesicles. Oral lesions are painful and begin as vesicles that progress to ulcers. The disease usually lasts for several weeks, and in some patients neuralgia that takes months to resolve may follow the resolution of the lesions.

Diagnosis. The diagnosis of varicella and herpes zoster is generally made based on the clinical features. Biopsy or a smear of the lesion may show the same type of virally altered epithelial cells that are seen in herpes simplex infection. Viral cultures may take weeks to grow.

Treatment. Varicella generally requires only supportive treatment. Antiviral drugs are used for immunocompromised patients and for patients with herpes zoster. In some patients, corticosteroids have been used in an attempt to prevent the pain of postherpetic neuralgia.

EPSTEIN-BARR VIRUS INFECTION

The **Epstein-Barr virus** has been implicated in several diseases that occur in the oral region, including infectious mononucleosis, nasopharyngeal carcinoma, Burkitt lymphoma, and hairy leukoplakia. Nasopharyngeal carcinoma and Burkitt lymphoma are rare malignant neoplasms. Infectious mononucleosis and hairy leukoplakia are discussed here.

Figure 4-27 Hairy leukoplakia.

A

B

Figure 4-26 Herpes zoster. **A,** Unilateral facial lesions occurring along the distribution of the maxillary branch of the trigeminal nerve. **B,** Intraoral lesions in the same patient illustrate the unilateral distribution of herpes zoster.

Infectious Mononucleosis

Infectious mononucleosis is an infectious disease caused by the Epstein-Barr virus. It is characterized by sore throat, fever, generalized lymphadenopathy, enlarged spleen, malaise, and fatigue. Palatal petechiae occur in **infectious mononucleosis,** usually appearing early in the course of the disease. The mechanism for the development of these petechiae is unclear. The diagnosis is confirmed by the identification in the blood of mononucleosis cells, which are atypical activated T lymphocytes. Severe complications such as hepatitis occur in some patients. In developed countries, infectious mononucleosis occurs principally in late adolescents and young adults in

upper socioeconomic classes. The virus is transmitted by close contact. Contact with saliva during kissing is a frequent route of transmission of Epstein-Barr virus. In most patients, infectious mononucleosis is a benign, self-limited disease that resolves within 4 to 6 weeks. In some patients, fatigue lasts much longer.

Hairy Leukoplakia

This irregular, corrugated, white lesion most commonly occurs on the lateral border of the tongue **(Figure 4-27).** Epstein-Barr virus has been identified in the epithelial cells of hairy leukoplakia and is considered to be the cause of the lesion. Hairy leukoplakia was first identified in patients infected with HIV and occurs most commonly in those patients, it has also been reported in patients not infected with HIV.

COXSACKIEVIRUS INFECTIONS

The **coxsackieviruses,** named for the town in New York where the virus was first discovered, cause several different infectious diseases. Three of these have distinctive oral lesions and are discussed here. Fecal-oral contamination, saliva, and respiratory droplets can be the means of transmission.

Herpangina

Herpangina characteristically includes vesicles on the soft palate **(Figure 4-28),** along with fever, malaise, sore throat, and difficulty swallowing (dysphagia). An erythematous pharyngitis is also present. The disease is usually mild to moderate and resolves in less than 1 week without treatment.

Hand-Foot-and-Mouth Disease

Hand-foot-and-mouth disease usually occurs in epidemics in children less than 5 years of age. Oral lesions are generally painful vesicles and ulcers that can occur anywhere in the mouth. Multiple macules or papules occur on the skin, typically on the feet, toes, hands, and fingers. Lesions resolve spontaneously within 2 weeks.

Diagnosis. Although the oral lesions may resemble herpes simplex infection, the distribution of the skin lesions and the mild systemic symptoms usually help to differentiate the two conditions. Viral culture and measurement of circulating antibodies to the type of coxsackievirus that causes hand-foot-and-mouth disease may help to confirm the diagnosis but are generally not necessary.

Treatment. The disease is generally mild and of short duration. Treatment is generally not required.

Acute Lymphonodular Pharyngitis

Acute lymphonodular pharyngitis is another coxsackievirus infection that is characterized by fever, sore throat, and mild headache. Hyperplastic lymphoid tissue of the soft palate or tonsillar pillars appears as yellowish or dark pink nodules. The disease generally lasts several days to 2 weeks and does not usually require treatment.

Figure 4-28 Herpangina.

OTHER VIRAL INFECTIONS THAT MAY HAVE ORAL MANIFESTATIONS

Measles

Measles is a highly contagious disease causing systemic symptoms and a skin rash that results from a type of virus called a *paramyxovirus.* The disease most commonly occurs in childhood. Early in the disease, Koplik spots, which are small erythematous macules with white necrotic centers, may occur in the oral cavity.

Mumps

Mumps, or **epidemic parotitis,** is a viral infection of the salivary glands that is also caused by a paramyxovirus. The disease most commonly occurs in children and is characterized by painful swelling of the salivary glands, most commonly bilateral swelling of the parotid glands.

HUMAN IMMUNODEFICIENCY VIRUS (HIV) AND ACQUIRED IMMUNODEFICIENCY SYNDROME (AIDS)

The virus associated with AIDS was identified in 1983; in 1986 it was designated as **HIV.** The HIV virus is transmitted by sexual contact with infected persons, by contact with infected blood and blood products, and to infants of infected mothers. HIV infects cells of the immune system. The most important of the cells of the immune system that the virus infects is the CD4 T-helper lymphocyte. This lymphocyte is important both in cell-mediated immunity and in regulating the immune response. As the disease progresses, this lymphocyte becomes depleted. Other cells that may be infected with HIV include macrophages, Langerhans cells, and cells of the nervous system.

THE SPECTRUM OF HIV

Many individuals experience an acute disease that occurs shortly after infection with HIV, whereas other individuals remain asymptomatic. The acute disease resolves, and infected individuals may have no signs or symptoms of disease for some time. In most patients infected with HIV, a progressive immunodeficiency eventually develops. As the immune system begins to fail, the number of CD4 lymphocytes decreases. Patients have nonspecific problems such as fatigue, and opportunistic infections such as oral candidiasis may develop. As the immune system becomes profoundly deficient, life-threatening opportunistic infections and cancers occur. The most severe result of infection with HIV is AIDS.

DIAGNOSING AIDS

The diagnosis of AIDS is well defined. The definition of AIDS has been established by the Centers for Disease Control and Prevention (CDC) and is given in **Table 4-3**. Since it was identified in the early 1980s, the definition of AIDS has been changed several times as knowledge of the disease has grown. The most recent definition of AIDS in

Table 4-3 Definitions of Acquired Immunodeficiency Syndrome (AIDS)

AIDS is an illness characterized by one or more of the following diseases or conditions.

HIV Laboratory Tests Not Performed or Results Inconclusive and the Patient Has No Other Cause of Immunodeficiency

1. Candidiasis of the esophagus, trachea, bronchi, or lungs
2. Cryptococcosis, extrapulmonary
3. Cryptosporidiosis with diarrhea persisting longer than 1 month
4. Cytomegalovirus disease of an organ other than liver, spleen, or lymph nodes in a patient older than 1 month of age
5. Herpes simplex virus infection causing a mucocutaneous ulcer that persist longer than 1 month or bronchitis, pneumonitis, or esophagitis for any duration affecting a patient older than 1 month of age
6. Karposi sarcoma affecting a patient less than 60 years of age
7. Lymphoma of the brain affecting a patient less than 60 years of age
8. Lymphoid interstitial pneumonia, pulmonary hyperplasia, or both, affecting a child less than 13 years of age
9. *Mycobacterium avium* or *M. kansasii* disease, disseminated
10. *Pneumocystis carinii* pneumonia
11. Progressive multifocal leukoencephalopathy
12. Toxoplasmosis of the brain affecting a patient older than 1 month of age

With Laboratory Evidence of HIV Infection

Less than 200 CD4+ T lymphocytes/μl or a CD4+ T-lymphocyte percentage of total lymphocytes less than 14

Any of the preceding diseases listed or those that follow:

1. Multiple bacterial infections of certain types affecting a child less than 13 years of age
2. Coccidioidomycosis, disseminated
3. HIV encephalopathy (HIV dementia)
4. Histoplasmosis, disseminated
5. Isosporiasis with diarrhea persisting longer than 1 month
6. Lymphoma of the brain at any age
7. Kaposi sarcoma
8. Certain types of lymphoma
9. Mycobacterial disease other than tuberculosis, disseminated
10. Extrapulmonary tuberculosis
11. *Salmonella* septicemia, recurrent
12. HIV-related wasting syndrome
13. Pulmonary tuberculosis
14. Recurrent pneumonia
15. Invasive cervical cancer

Even if HIV laboratory test results are negative, if other causes of immunodeficiency are not ruled out, a diagnosis of AIDS can be made if certain of these diseases are diagnosed.

Adapted from Centers for Disease Control and Prevention: 1993 revised classification system for HIV infection and expanded surveillance case definition for AIDS among adolescents and adults, MMWR Recomm Rep 41(RR-17):1, 1992.

adults and adolescents includes HIV infection with severe CD4 lymphocyte depletion (less than 200 CD4 lymphocytes per microliter [μl] of blood). The normal CD4 lymphocyte count is between about 550 and 1000 lymphocytes/μl blood. The revised definition continues to include a number of opportunistic diseases, such as *Pneumocystis carinii* pneumonia, esophageal candidiasis, and Kaposi sarcoma. Also included is HIV-related wasting syndrome. In addition to including the CD4 lymphocyte count, the revised definition includes pulmonary tuberculosis, recurrent pneumonia, and invasive cervical cancer.

HIV TESTING

Two antibody tests are now generally used to determine if a person has been infected with HIV. The first test is an enzyme-linked immunosorbent assay (ELISA). When this test is positive twice, it is followed by a more specific test called the **Western blot test**. To be considered seropositive for HIV, a person must have two positive ELISA test results followed by a positive Western blot test result. Other tests, such as the polymerase chain reaction (PCR), identify virus rather than antibody. Informed consent by the patient and pretest counseling may be required before HIV testing can be done.

CLINICAL MANIFESTATIONS

As mentioned, the initial infection with HIV may be completely asymptomatic. In some individuals, lymphadenopathy may develop; in still others an acute illness, resembling infectious mononucleosis and lasting 8 to 14 days, can occur. When this acute illness develops, the patient may have sore throat, general malaise, myalgia and arthralgia, lymphadenopathy, and fever. Patients with acute infection can also have a skin rash, nausea, and diarrhea. After this acute illness, some individuals have persistent lymphadenopathy, but many become completely asymptomatic.

The virus infects cells of the immune system; as a result this system stops protecting the individual against certain infections and tumors. In time, as the immune system becomes deficient, a variety of signs and symptoms can develop, signaling changes in the immune system. Several of these signs and symptoms occurring together are sometimes called AIDS-related complex (ARC). These symptoms include oral candidiasis, fatigue, weight loss, and lymphadenopathy. HIV can also infect cells of the nervous system, resulting in dementia in some patients.

Antibodies to HIV generally begin to be detectable in blood about 6 weeks after the initial infection. However, in some individuals antibodies may not be detectable for 6 months and occasionally for up to 1 year or more.

The spectrum of HIV infection includes the full range of problems that result from infection with this virus from asymptomatic infection to AIDS **(Figure 4-29)**. AIDS represents terminal HIV infection in this spectrum. It is not yet known how many of the persons who become infected with HIV go on to experience immunodeficiency, opportunistic diseases, or dementia. Some patients who are HIV-seropositive appear to remain immunocompetent for many

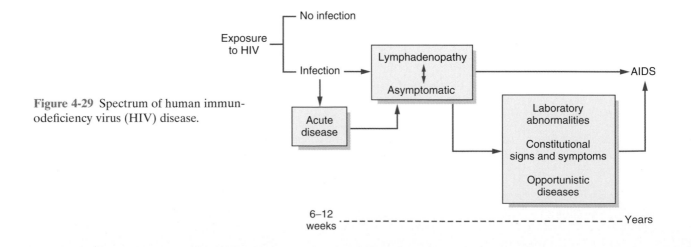

Figure 4-29 Spectrum of human immunodeficiency virus (HIV) disease.

years. Cofactors that can contribute to the development of the immunodeficiency are being studied. Each year the results of natural history studies show an increase in the percentage of HIV-infected individuals in whom AIDS develops.

MEDICAL MANAGEMENT

Tests such as PCR are used to measure the amount of HIV circulating in serum. This is called viral load. Measurement of viral load along with the CD4 lymphocyte count is used to assess HIV infection. Patients with HIV infection are managed with combinations of different types of antiretroviral (anti-HIV) drugs and with drugs that prevent and treat opportunistic diseases. Measurement of viral load is used to evaluate the effectiveness of antiretroviral therapy. Management of HIV infection is continually changing in response to the results of ongoing clinical drug trials.

ORAL MANIFESTATIONS

Oral lesions are prominent features of AIDS and HIV infection **(Table 4-4).** Some of these lesions are known to be indicators of developing immunodeficiency and predictors of the development of AIDS in individuals who are HIV seropositive. The oral lesions that occur develop because of the deficiency in CMI and because of the deregulation of immunologic responses that occurs when the T-helper cells become depleted. Oral lesions include opportunistic infections, tumors, and autoimmune-like diseases.

Oral Candidiasis

This oral lesion occurs frequently in individuals with cell- mediated immunodeficiency and is one of the most common oral lesions seen in persons with HIV infection **(Figure 4-30).** It is also called **thrush.** All of the different types of oral candidiasis described earlier in this chapter, including mucocutaneous candidiasis, can occur. It is important to remember that candidiasis can be associated with a variety of conditions other than HIV infection, such as uncontrolled diabetes, other immunodeficiency diseases, antibiotic treatment, and xerostomia. Both topical and systemic antifungal treatment can be used to control oral candidiasis in the patient with immunodeficiency caused by HIV infection. Recurrence is common.

In persons who are known to be infected with HIV, the development of oral candidiasis is worrisome because it generally signals the beginning of a progressively severe immunodeficiency. Persons with unexplained oral candidiasis should be referred to a physician for evaluation if the cause of the candidia-

Figure 4-30 Candidiasis in a patient with human immunodeficiency virus (HIV) infection. Removable white plaques are present on the mucosa of the soft palate.

Table 4-4 Oral Lesions Associated with Human Immunodeficiency Infection

Candidiasis
Herpes simplex infection
Herpes zoster
Hairy leukoplakia
Human papillomavirus (HPV) lesions
Atypical gingivitis and periodontitis
Other opportunistic infections reported
   Mycobacterium avium, M. intracellulare
   Cytomegalovirus
   Cryptococcus neoformans
   Klebsiella pneumoniae
   Enterobacter cloacae
   Histoplasma capsulatum
Kaposi sarcoma
Non-Hodgkin lymphoma
Aphthous ulcers
Mucosal pigmentation
Bacterial salivary gland enlargement and xerostomia
Spontaneous gingival bleeding resulting from thrombocytopenia

sis cannot be determined. Studies have shown oral candidiasis to be a very early sign of developing immunodeficiency and predictive of the development of AIDS in a person who is infected with HIV. Oral lesions caused by other fungal infections, such as histoplasmosis and coccidioidomycosis, have also been reported in persons with HIV infection, but they are rare.

Herpes Simplex Infection

Ulcers caused by the herpes simplex virus occur in persons with HIV infection **(Figure 4-31)**. Herpes labialis and lesions consistent with intraoral recurrent herpes simplex infection can develop in persons with HIV infection. The clinical characteristics of these lesions are the same as those occurring in immunocompetent individuals. However, when the immune system, particularly cell-mediated immunity, becomes deficient, HIV-infected individuals are at risk for the development of ulcers caused by the herpes simplex virus that do not have the same clinical characteristics as those seen in immunocompetent persons. These appear as persistent, superficial, painful ulcers that can be located anywhere in the oral cavity. Small, characteristic herpes simplexlike ulcers can be seen surrounding larger ulcers, but their presence cannot be depended on for diagnosis. The diagnosis of these ulcers is made by several methods, including viral culture, cytologic smear, biopsy, and response to the antiviral medication acyclovir.

Ulceration of the oral mucosa from herpes simplex infection that has been present for more than 1 month is an oral lesion that meets the criteria for the diagnosis of AIDS. This can occur only when a person has profound immunodeficiency. Oral ulcers caused by cytomegalovirus may also occur in HIV-infected individuals who are severely immunodeficient. These ulcers are much rarer than those caused by herpes simplex virus.

Herpes Zoster

Herpes zoster is caused by the varicella-zoster virus and is described earlier in this chapter. When herpes zoster occurs in a person with HIV infection, it generally follows the usual pattern (see Figures 4-24, 4-25, 4-26). Although the infection can disseminate, most cases are self-limited. In the facial and oral area, the lesions appear as distinctly unilateral ones following the distribution of one or more branches of the trigeminal nerve. The development of herpes zoster in a person infected with HIV is a sign of developing immunodeficiency.

Hairy Leukoplakia

Hairy leukoplakia is caused by Epstein-Barr virus and was discussed earlier in this chapter. It was first described in individuals with HIV infection; although it has been reported in HIV-negative individuals, most cases are an oral manifestation of HIV infection. It almost always occurs on the lateral borders of the tongue and may extend onto the dorsal and ventral tongue (see Figure 4-27; **Figure 4-32**). On the lateral tongue, it appears as an irregular, white lesion that has a corrugated surface. The corrugations may not be present when the lesions extend onto the dorsal or ventral tongue. Histologically this lesion shows hyperkeratosis (often with hairlike projections), ep-

Figure 4-32 Hairy leukoplakia.

Figure 4-31 Herpes simplex ulceration of the hard palate in a patient with human immunodeficiency virus (HIV) infection. Arrows point to the periphery of the ulcer.

ithelial hyperplasia, vacuolated epithelial cells, and little or no inflammatory infiltrate in the underlying connective tissue.

Other white lesions, such as those resulting from chronic tongue chewing and hyperplastic candidiasis, can resemble hairy leukoplakia clinically. Biopsy of the lesions can reveal a histologic appearance that is consistent with hairy leukoplakia. However, the most reliable method of diagnosis is identification of the Epstein-Barr virus in the lesion.

Generally, hairy leukoplakia is not treated. Lesions may respond to antiviral medication such as acyclovir or zidovudine, but recur when treatment is discontinued. Studies have shown hairy leukoplakia to be predictive of the development of AIDS in HIV-infected persons.

Papillomavirus Infections

Lesions caused by papillomaviruses are described earlier in this chapter. Papillary oral lesions resulting from several different papillomaviruses have been described in persons with HIV infection. They have either normal color or slightly erythematous mucosa **(Figure 4-33)**. These lesions may be persistent and may occur in multiple oral mucosal locations. Results of studies have suggested that these lesions may be associated with antiretroviral treatment. Diagnosis of these lesions is made by biopsy and histologic examination with special tests to identify papillomavirus.

Kaposi Sarcoma

Kaposi sarcoma is one of the opportunistic neoplasms that occur in patients with HIV infection. HHV-8 has been associated with this neoplasm. Oral lesions appear as reddish-purple, flat or raised lesions and are seen anywhere in the oral cavity. The most common locations are the palate and gingiva **(Figure 4-34)**.

The diagnosis is made by biopsy. However, the clinical appearance of the lesion can be used when it is characteristic and the diagnosis of Kaposi sarcoma has been made at another site. At present, no effec-

A

Figure 4-33 Papillary lesion of the upper lip caused by human papillomavirus (HPV) in a patient with human immunodeficiency virus (HIV) infection.

B

Figure 4-34 Kaposi sarcoma in a patient with acquired immunodeficiency syndrome (AIDS). **A,** Skin. **B,** Gingiva. (Courtesy Dr. Fariba Younai.)

tive treatment for Kaposi sarcoma exists. Surgical excision to decrease the size of the lesion is sometimes attempted, as are radiation treatment and chemotherapy. Kaposi sarcoma is one of the intraoral lesions that may fulfill the criteria for the diagnosis of AIDS.

Lymphoma

Non-Hodgkin lymphoma is another of the malignant tumors that occur in association with HIV infection. It occasionally occurs in the oral cavity. These tumors have appeared as nonulcerated, necrotic, or ulcerated masses and have been surfaced by either ulcerated or normal-colored erythematous mucosa **(Figure 4-35).**

The diagnosis is made by biopsy and histologic examination. Treatment involves several different chemotherapeutic drugs. Oral lymphoma is another oral lesion that may meet the criteria for the diagnosis of AIDS.

Gingival and Periodontal Disease

In patients with HIV infection, unusual forms of gingival and periodontal disease can develop. These occur in HIV-infected individuals whose immune system has become deficient. These have been called **linear gingival erythema (LGE)** and **necrotizing ulcerative periodontitis (NUP).** A condition resembling NUG also occurs in individuals with HIV infection.

LGE has three characteristic features: (1) spontaneous bleeding, (2) punctate or petechiae-like lesions on the attached gingiva and alveolar mucosa, and (3) a bandlike erythema of the gingiva that does not respond to therapy. LGE is different from typical gingivitis in that gingivitis is generally not characterized by spontaneous bleeding, and the erythema of typical gingivitis responds within a few days to 1 week to scaling, root planing, and improvement of oral hygiene. LGE occurs independently of oral hygiene status.

Some patients experience gingivitis that resembles NUG, and it can be either generalized or localized to specific areas. NUP resembles NUG in that patients experience pain, spontaneous gingival bleeding, interproximal necrosis, and interproximal cratering **(Figure 4-36).** Patients also experience in-

A

B

Figure 4-35 Intraoral lymphoma in a patient with acquired immunodeficiency syndrome (AIDS).

Figure 4-36 **A** and **B,** Atypical periodontal disease in a patient with human immunodeficiency virus (HIV) infection.

tense erythema and, most characteristically, extremely rapid bone loss. **Necrotizing stomatitis** is characterized by extensive focal areas of bone loss along with the features of NUP.

The specific causes of these atypical gingival and periodontal diseases remain unclear. The microbiota associated with these diseases are being studied and have not been found to be distinctly different from those of inflammatory periodontal disease. These atypical gingival and periodontal conditions are not common in HIV-infected individuals and appear to occur in those patients whose immune systems have become severely compromised.

Treatment of HIV gingivitis and periodontitis involves scaling, root planing, and soft tissue curettage. In addition, intrasulcular lavage with povidone-iodine, use of chlorhexidine mouth rinse, and short-term systemic metronidazole administration have been helpful in the treatment of these conditions. Good oral hygiene, including the use of smaller toothbrushes and interproximal cleaning devices, has been a component of management.

Not all HIV-infected patients have periodontal problems. However, recognition of early lesions is essential to prevent extensive bone loss, and frequent recall is helpful in early identification of gingival and periodontal disease. Lack of response to periodontal treatment is a clue to the recognition of HIV-associated gingivitis and periodontitis.

Spontaneous Gingival Bleeding

A decrease in the number of platelets resulting from an autoimmune type of thrombocytopenic purpura is occasionally seen in patients with HIV infection. These patients can have bleeding gums or mucosal petechiae. Gingival bleeding not related to thrombocytopenia has also been described in LGE and NUP. A platelet count and bleeding time should be considered before deep scaling procedures are performed.

Aphthous Ulcers

Characteristic minor aphthous ulcers occur in patients with HIV infection and AIDS. Studies have suggested that an increase in the incidence of these ulcers occurs in patients with HIV infection. The clinical appearance and behavior of minor aphthous ulcers in HIV-infected patients is the same as in other individuals (see Chapter 3). Minor aph-

thous ulcers are diagnosed based on their clinical appearance.

Ulcers that resemble major aphthous ulcers also occur in patients with HIV infection **(Figure 4-37)**. They appear as deep, persistent, painful ulcers and must be differentiated from infectious ulcers. Biopsy and histologic examination of these ulcers does not show any evidence of an infectious cause. These ulcers respond to topical steroid application. Topical application of tetracycline and thalidomide have also been used in the management of these ulcers. Similar ulcers have been seen in the esophagus of patients with HIV infection.

Salivary Gland Disease

Bilateral parotid gland enlargement has been reported to occur in patients who are HIV positive **(Figure 4-38)**. The histologic appearance is reported to be that of a benign lymphoepithelial lesion, often with a prominent cystic component. Xerostomia has been reported to be associated with HIV infection. The cause is not clear. It may be related to medication administration or salivary gland disease.

Mucosal Melanin Pigmentation

Macular areas of melanin pigmentation of unknown cause also occur in patients with HIV infection. These do not require treatment, and the significance of these lesions is not known.

Figure 4-37 Persistent, nonspecific (major aphthouslike) ulcers in a patient with human immunodeficiency virus (HIV) infection. (Courtesy Dr. Sidney Eisig.)

Figure 4-38 Salivary gland enlargement was bilateral in this patient with human immunodeficiency virus (HIV) infection.

Selected References

Books

Kumar V: *Basic pathology,* ed 6, Philadelphia, 1997, WB Saunders.

Neville BW et al: *Oral and maxillofacial pathology,* ed 2, Philadelphia, 2002, WB Saunders.

New York State Department of Health AIDS Institute: *Oral health care for people with HIV infection,* December 2001, http://www.hivguidelines.org (clinical guidelines).

Regezi JA, Sciubba JJ: *Oral pathology. Clinical-pathologic correlations,* ed 4, Philadelphia, 2003, WB Saunders.

Rubin E, Farber JL: *Pathology,* ed 3, Philadelphia, 1999, Lippincott-Raven.

Journal Articles

Allen CM: Diagnosing and managing oral candidiasis, *J Am Dent Assoc* 123:77, 1992.

Barone R et al: Prevalence of oral lesions among HIV-infected intravenous drug abusers and other risk groups, *Oral Surg Oral Med Oral Pathol* 69:169, 1990.

Depaola LG: Human immunodeficiency virus disease: natural history and management, *Oral Surg Oral Med Oral Pathol Oral Radiol Endod* 90:266, 2000.

Centers for Disease Control and Prevention: 1993 revised classification system for HIV infection and expanded surveillance case definition for AIDS among adolescents and adults, *MMWR Recomm Rep* 41(RR-17):1, 1992.

Challacombe SJ: Immunologic aspects of oral candidiasis, *Oral Surg Oral Med Oral Pathol* 78:202, 1994.

Eisen D: The clinical characteristics of intraoral herpes simplex virus infection in 52 immunocompetent patients, *Oral Surg Oral Med Oral Pathol Oral Radiol Endod* 86:432, 1998.

Eisenberg E, Krutchkoff D, Yamase H: Incidental oral hairy leukoplakia in immunocompetent persons, *Oral Surg Oral Med Oral Pathol* 74:332, 1992.

Eng H-L et al: Oral tuberculosis, *Oral Surg Oral Med Oral Pathol Oral Radiol Endod* 81:415, 1996.

Fotos PG, Vincent SD, Hellstein JW: Oral candidiasis: clinical, historical, and therapeutic features of 100 cases, *Oral Surg Oral Med Oral Pathol* 74:41, 1992.

Glick M, Muzyka BC: Alternative therapies for major aphthous ulcers in AIDS patients, *J Am Dent Assoc* 123:61, 1992.

Green TL et al: Oral lesions mimicking hairy leukoplakia: a diagnostic dilemma, *Oral Surg Oral Med Oral Pathol* 67:422, 1989.

Greenspan JS: Sentinels and signposts: the epidemiology and significance of the oral manifestations of HIV disease, *Oral Dis* 3(suppl 1):S13, 1997.

Harris AM, Van Wyk CW: Heck's disease (focal epithelial hyperplasia): a longitudinal study, *Community Dent Oral Epidemiol* 21:82, 1993.

Hernandez YL, Daniels TE: Oral candidiasis in Sjögren's syndrome: prevalence, clinical correlations, and treatment, *Oral Surg Oral Med Oral Pathol* 68:324, 1989.

Holbrook WP, Gunnlaugur TG, Ragnarsson KT: Herpetic gingivostomatitis in otherwise healthy adolescents and young adults, *Acta Odontol Scand* 59:113, 2001.

Holmstrup P, Westergaard J: Periodontal diseases in HIV-infected patients, *J Clin Periodontol* 21:270, 1994.

Iacopino AM, Wathen WF: Oral candidal infection and denture stomatitis: a comprehensive review, *J Am Dent Assoc* 123:46, 1992.

Jones AC, Gulley ML, Freedman PD: Necrotizing ulcerative stomatitis in human immunodeficiency virus-seropositive individuals: a review of the histopathologic, immunohistochemical, and virologic characteristics of 18 cases, *Oral Surg Oral Med Oral Pathol Oral Radiol Endod* 89:323, 2000.

Kanas RJ et al: Oral hairy leukoplakia: a light microscopic and immunohistochemical study, *Oral Surg Oral Med Oral Pathol* 66:334, 1988.

Koorbusch GF, Fotos P, Terhark K: Retrospective assessment of osteomyelitis, *Oral Surg Oral Med Oral Pathol* 74:149, 1992.

Kulak-Ozkan Y, Kazazoglu E, Arikan A: Oral hygiene habits, denture cleanliness, presence of yeasts and stomatitis in elderly people, *J Oral Rehabil* 29:300, 2002.

Leggott PJ: Oral manifestations of HIV infection in children, *Oral Surg Oral Med Oral Pathol* 73:187, 1992.

Lynch DP: Oral candidiasis: history, classification and clinical presentation, *Oral Surg Oral Med Oral Pathol* 78:189, 1994.

MacPhail LA et al: Recurrent aphthous ulcers in association with HIV infection. Description of ulcer types and analysis of T-lymphocyte subsets, *Oral Surg Oral Med Oral Pathol* 71:678, 1991.

MacPhail LA et al: Differences in risk factors among clinical types of oral candidiasis in the Women's Interagency HIV Study, *Oral Sugr Oral Med Oral Pathol Oral Radiol Endod* 93:45, 2002.

McKenzie CD, Gobetti JP: Diagnosis and treatment of orofacial herpes zoster: report of cases, *J Am Dent Assoc* 120:679, 1990.

Miller RL: The differential diagnosis of white lesions resembling oral hairy leukoplakia, *J Tenn Dent Assoc* 73:20, 1993.

Morrow DJ, Sandhu HS, Daley TD: Focal epithelial hyperplasia (Heck's disease) with generalized lesions of the gingiva. A case report, *J Periodontol* 64:63, 1993.

Narana N, Epstein JB: Classifications of oral lesions in HIV infection, *J Clin Periodontol* 28:137, 2001.

Pindborg JJ: Classification of oral lesions associated with HIV infection, *Oral Surg Oral Med Oral Pathol* 67:292, 1989.

Praetorius F: HPV-associated diseases of the oral mucosa, *Clin Dermatol* 15:399, 1997.

Rams TE et al: Microbiological study of HIV-related periodontitis, *J Periodontol* 62:74, 1991.

Redding SW, Luce EB, Boren MW: Oral herpes simplex virus infection in patients receiving head and neck radiation, *Oral Surg Oral Med Oral Pathol* 69:578, 1990.

Ryder MI: An update on HIV and periodontal disease, *J Periodontol* 73:1071, 2002.

Samaranayake LP: Oral mycoses in HIV infection, *Oral Surg Oral Med Oral Pathol* 73:171, 1992.

Schiodt M: HIV-associated salivary gland disease, *Oral Surg Oral Med Oral Pathol* 37:164, 1992.

Sciubba J et al: Hairy leukoplakia: an AIDS-associated opportunistic infection, *Oral Surg Oral Med Oral Pathol* 67:404, 1989.

Siegel MA: Diagnosis and management of recurrent herpes simplex infections, *J Am Dent Assoc* 133:1245, 2002.

Swango PA, Kleinman D, Konzelman JL: HIV and periodontal health, *J Am Dent Assoc* 122:49, 1991.

Williams CA et al: HIV-associated periodontitis complicated by necrotizing stomatitis, *Oral Surg Oral Med Oral Pathol* 69:351, 1990.

Zhu WY et al: Human papillomavirus DNA in the dermis of condyloma acuminatum, *J Cutan Pathol* 20:447, 1993.

Review Questions

1. The most specific of the body's defense mechanisms against infection is:
   - A. Intact skin
   - B. Saliva
   - C. Skin secretions
   - D. The inflammatory response
   - E. The immune response

2. Which statement is *false*?
   - A. The primary lesion of syphilis is called a *chancre*.
   - B. The secondary lesion of syphilis occurs at the site of inoculation with the organism.
   - C. The tertiary lesion of syphilis is called a gumma.
   - D. Syphilis is caused by the spirochete *Treponema pallidum.*
   - E. The mucous patch is a lesion of secondary syphilis.

3. The lesions of impetigo may resemble:
   - A. Syphilis
   - B. Primary herpes simplex infection
   - C. Herpes zoster
   - D. Actinomycosis
   - E. Streptococcal sore throat

4. Which of the following are associated with group A, β hemolytic streptococcal infection?
   - A. Tonsillitis
   - B. Pharyngitis
   - C. Scarlet fever
   - D. Rheumatic fever
   - E. All of the above

5. Oral candidiasis is caused by a:
   - A. Bacterium
   - B. Virus
   - C. Spirochete
   - D. Protozoan
   - E. Yeastlike fungus

6. Which statement is *false*?
   A. Angular cheilitis may be caused by *Candida albicans.*
   B. White lesions resulting from candidiasis may not rub off the mucosal surface.
   C. Erythematous candidiasis is usually completely asymptomatic.
   D. Denture stomatitis may be a form of oral candidiasis.
   E. Chronic atrophic candidiasis is the most common type of candidiasis.

7. Which type of infection is involved when normal oral flora can cause disease?
   A. Chronic inflammatory
   B. Opportunistic
   C. Hyperplastic
   D. Granulomatous
   E. Subacute

8. The most characteristic clinical feature of herpes zoster is:
   A. Ulcer formation
   B. Pain
   C. Unilateral distribution of lesions
   D. White lesions
   E. Abscesses that drain through fistulas

9. A cytologic smear may be helpful in the diagnosis of:
   A. Coxsackievirus infection
   B. HPV infection
   C. Tuberculosis
   D. Candidiasis and herpes simplex infection
   E. Oral lesions of syphilis

10. Which condition is *not* associated with the Epstein-Barr virus?
    A. Hairy leukoplakia
    B. Herpangina
    C. Nasopharyngeal carcinoma
    D. Infectious mononucleosis
    E. Burkitt lymphoma

11. Which of the following stages of syphilis is or are infectious?
    A. Primary
    B. Secondary
    C. Tertiary
    D. All stages are infectious
    E. Both A and B

12. Which of the following is not associated with syphilis?
    A. Mucous patch
    B. VDRL and FTA
    C. Dark-field microscopy
    D. Hypodontia
    E. Chancre

13. Which of the following causes tuberculosis?
    A. *Mycobacterium israelii*
    B. *Actinomycosis tuberculum*
    C. *Mycobacterium tuberculosis*
    D. *Treponema pallidum*
    E. *Streptococcus pyogenes*

14. A positive skin reaction to PPD indicates:
    A. Active tuberculosis
    B. Contagious tuberculosis
    C. Has been infected with the tuberculosis bacteria
    D. Need for antibiotic therapy
    E. Need for hospitalization

15. A specific *clinical* characteristic found in actinomycosis is:
    A. Periapical radiolucency
    B. Filamentous bacteria
    C. Fungal infection
    D. Sulfur granules present in exudates
    E. Fever

16. Which of the following is or are clinical characteristics of NUG?
    A. Painful gingiva
    B. Punched out papillae
    C. Foul odor
    D. Metallic taste
    E. All of the above

17. Which of the following is or are associated with chronic osteomyelitis?
    A. Sickle cell anemia
    B. Paget disease
    C. Radiation treatment involving bone
    D. Inadequately treated acute osteomyelitis
    E. All of the above

18. Which of the following is *not* associated with the development of oral candidiasis?
    A. Antibiotic therapy
    B. HIV infection
    C. Xerostomia
    D. Dentures
    E. Herpangina

19. Verruca vulgaris:
    A. Clinically resembles an irritative fibroma
    B. Is caused by a HSV
    C. Is most commonly seen on the buccal mucosa
    D. Clinically resembles a pyogenic granuloma
    E. Is caused by HPV

20. Another name for a common wart is:
    A. Papilloma
    B. Verruca vulgaris
    C. Condyloma acumenatum
    D. Fibroma
    E. Pseudopapillomatosis

21. Which of the following is caused by a papillomavirus and is considered a sexually transmitted disease?
    A. Syphilis
    B. Tuberculosis
    C. Condyloma acuminatum
    D. Infectious mononucleosis
    E. Actinomycosis

22. Painful oral ulcers, gingivitis, fever, malaise, and cervical lymphadenopathy in a child younger than 6 years old would cause the hygienist to suspect which of the following diseases?
    A. Condyloma acuminatum
    B. Heck disease
    C. Primary herpes simplex infection
    D. Herpetic whitlow
    E. Infectious mononucleosis

23. The most common form of recurrent herpes simplex infection is:
    A. Herpes zoster
    B. Herpetic whitlow
    C. Herpangina
    D. Angular cheilitis
    E. Herpes labialis

24. The primary infection with the varicella zoster virus is called:
    A. Primary herpetic gingivostomatitis
    B. Herpes zoster
    C. Shingles
    D. Measles
    E. Chickenpox

25. Herpangina is caused by:
    A. Coxsackievirus
    B. Herpes simplex virus
    C. Varicella zoster virus
    D. Epstein-Barr virus
    E. HPV

26. Antibody testing to determine if a person has been infected with HIV includes which of the following tests?
    A. Schilling
    B. CBC
    C. PT and PTT
    D. ELISA and Western blot
    E. Immunohistochemistry

27. Which one of the following oral conditions is an early sign of a deficiency in the immune system and is commonly found in patients with HIV infection?
    A. Geographic tongue
    B. Advanced periodontitis
    C. Candidiasis
    D. Histoplasmosis
    E. Lichen planus

28. Hairy leukoplakia most commonly occurs on the:
    A. Buccal mucosa
    B. Dorsal tongue
    C. Lateral tongue
    D. Soft palate
    E. Labial mucosa

29. Which one of the following oral conditions is *not* a lesion associated with HIV or AIDS?
    A. Herpes simplex
    B. Hairy leukoplakia
    C. Kaposi sarcoma
    D. Leukoedema
    E. Candidiasis

30. LGE has specific characteristics that include spontaneous bleeding, petechiae on the attached gingiva and alveolar mucosa, and a band of erythema at the gingival margin. Which one of the following statements is *true*?
    A. These tissues respond well to scaling and root planing.
    B. Excellent oral hygiene and home care techniques will eliminate these gingival conditions.
    C. This condition will automatically develop into advanced periodontal disease in all HIV patients.
    D. LGE patients do not respond to scaling or oral hygiene techniques; the gingival condition exists independently of the patient's oral hygiene status.
    E. These are common conditions in HIV-infected individuals.

Chapter 4 Synopsis

Condition/ Disease	Cause	Age/Race/Sex	Location
Infectious Diseases			
Bacterial infections			
Impetigo			
Tonsillitis & Pharyngitis			
Tuberculosis	Infectious disease *Mycobacterium tuberculosis*	*	Primary infection of lung Bacteria can spread to other areas of the body
Actinomycosis	Infectious disease *Actinomyces israelii*	*	Skin/oral mucosa
Syphilis	Infectious disease *Treponema pallidum*	Usually seen in sexually active adults Congenital—infected mother to fetus (see Chapter 5)	Primary—site of inoculation Secondary—diffuse lesions of skin and mucous membranes Tertiary—cardiovascular system Central nervous system—oral lesions may occur
Necrotizing Ulcerative Gingivitis (NUG)	Infectious disease *Borrelia vincentii* + fusiform bacillus	†	Gingiva
Pericoronitis	Inflammatory process usually infection	More common in adolescents and young adults at the of eruption of third molars	Tissue around the crown of a partially erupted impacted tooth
Acute Osteomyelitis	Imflammation/infection	*	Bone
Chronic Osteomyelitis	Inflammation/infection	*	Bone

*No significant information.
†Not covered in this text.

Clinical Features	Radiographic Features	Microscopic Features	Treatment	Diagnostic Process
Oral lesions—rare Painful, nonhealing, slowly enlarging, deep or superficial ulcer Most common locations are tongue and palate	N/A	Granulomas containing the causative organism	Combination anti-tuberculosis agents	Laboratory Microscopic
Draining abscesses "Sulfur granules" in pus draining from abscess	N/A	Bacterial colonies in tissue from the lesion	Long term, high dose of antibiotic therapy	Clinical Microscopic
Oral lesions Primary—chancre Secondary—mucous patches Tertiary—gumma	N/A	Skin—dark-field identification of spirochetes	Antibiotic agents (usually penicillin)	Clinical Laboratory
Painful, erythematous gingivitis with necrosis and cratering of the interdental papillae, foul odor, metallic taste Fever, cervical lymphadenopathy	N/A	N/A	Antibiotic agents Débridement of necrotic tissue Oral hygiene care	Clinical
Erythematous, painful swollen tissue around the crown of the partially erupted tooth	Impacted tooth can be seen on radiograph	N/A	Débridement and irrigation Antibiotic therapy Extraction of impacted tooth	Clinical
	No radiographic change unless present for more than 1 week	Nonviable bone Necrotic debris Acute inflammation Bacterial colonies	Antibiotic therapy Drainage of area	Clinical Laboratory
Involved bone is painful with swelling	Irregular radio-lucency	Chronic inflammation of bone and bone marrow	Débridement Antibiotic therapy Hyperbaric oxygen	Clinical Radiographic Laboratory

Continued

Chapter 4 Synopsis—cont'd

Condition/ Disease	Cause	Age/Race/Sex	Location
Fungal Infections			
Oral Candidiasis	Opportunistic infectious disease *Candida albicans*	*	Oral mucosa
Deep Fungal Infections			
Histoplasmosis Coccidio- idomycosis Blastomycosis Cryptococcosis	*Histoplasma capsulatum* *Coccidioides immitis* *Blastomyces dermatitidis* *Cryptococcus neoformans*	*	Primary lung infection Secondary oral mucosal involvement
Mucormycosis	†	*	Nasal cavity Maxillary sinus Hard palate
Viral Infections			
Verruca Vulgaris	A human papillomavirus	†	Skin Lips—most common oral location
Condyloma Acuminatum	A human papillomavirus	†	Oral mucosa—any location
Focal Epithelial Hyperplasia	A human papillomavirus	Occurs in children	Oral mucosa

*No significant information.
†Not covered in this text.

Clinical Features	Radiographic Features	Microscopic Features	Treatment	Diagnostic Process
Appearance depends upon type Pseudomembranous Erythematous Chronic atrophic (denture stomatitis) Chronic hyperplastic Angular cheilitis Chronic mucocutaneous	N/A	Candida hyphae present on mucosal smear Candida hyphae in biopsy tissue	Antifungal therapy	Clinical Microscopic Therapeutic
Chronic nonhealing ulcers	Irregular radio-lucency if bone involvement	Identification of causative organism	Appropriate antifungal agents	Microscopic Laboratory
Proliferating mass with destruction of bone	Irregular radio-lucency if bone involvement	Identification of causative organism	Appropriate antifungal agent Management of underlying disease	Microscopic
White, papillary exophytic lesion resembling a papilloma	N/A	Fingerlike projections of keratotic squamous epithelium with central cores of well-vascularized fibrous connective tissue Cells with clear cytoplasm in the upper spinous layer	Surgical excision Immunologic staining to identify presence of papillomavirus May recur	Microscopic
Pink, papillary lesion usually more diffuse than papilloma or verruca vulgaris May be multiple lesions	N/A	Thickened epithelium with fingerlike projections covering cores of connective tissue Cells with clear cytoplasm seen throughout the epithelium	Surgical excision Recurrence is common	Microscopic
Multiple, whitish to pale pink nodules distributed throughout the oral mucosa	N/A	Thickened epithelium with broad, connected rete ridges Cells with clear cytoplasm seen in the epithelium	Self-limited disease	Clinical Microscopic

Continued

Chapter 4 Synopsis—cont'd

Condition/ Disease	Cause	Age/Race/Sex	Location
Viral Infections —cont'd			
Herpes Simplex Infection	Herpes simplex virus Most oral infections are type 1, some type 2		
Primary Herpetic Gingivo-stomatitis	Herpes simplex virus	Generally in children Less common in adolescents and adults	Lips, gingival, oral mucosa
Recurrent Herpes Simplex Infection	Herpes simplex virus	Usually seen in adolescents and adults	Herpes labialis—vermilion of lips Recurrent intraoral form keratinized mucosa (hard palate, gingiva)
Varicella-Zoster Virus Infection			
Chickenpox	Varicella-zoster virus	Usually seen in children Less common in adolescents and adults	Skin Mucous membranes
Herpes Zoster	Varicella-zoster virus	Occurs in adults	Skin Mucous membranes
Infectious Mononucleosis	Epstein-Barr virus	Usually occurs in adolescents and young adults	Systemic disease
Herpangina	A coxsackievirus	Usually young children and adults	Soft palate
Hand-Foot-Mouth Disease	A coxsackievirus	Affects children under 5 years old	Oral mucosa Skin—feet, hands, fingers

*No significant information.
†Not covered in this text.

Clinical Features	Radiographic Features	Microscopic Features	Treatment	Diagnostic Process
Multiple tiny vesicles that progress to form painful ulcers Painful, erythematous swollen gingiva Fever, malaise, cervical lymphadenopathy	N/A	Virally altered epithelial cells in mucosal smear or biopsy tissue	Self-limited disease	Clinical Microscopic
Focal crops of tiny vesicles that coalesce to form a single ulcer Prodromal symptoms	N/A	Virally altered epithelial cells in mucosal smear or biopsy tissue	Self-limited disease	Clinical Microscopic
Vesicular and pustular eruptions Oral lesions usually do not cause discomfort	N/A	Virally altered epithelial cells in mucosal smear or biopsy tissue	Self-limited disease	Clinical
Unilateral distribution of painful vesicles-ulcers along a sensory nerve Prodromal symptoms	N/A	Virally altered epithelial cells in mucosal smear or biopsy tissue	Antiviral agents Corticosteroids	Clinical
Palatal petechiae Sore throat Fever Generalized lymphadenopathy Enlarged spleen Malaise Fatigue	N/A	Mononucleosis cells in blood	Usually self-limited disease	Laboratory
Fever Malaise Vesicles on the soft palate	N/A	N/A	Self-limited disease	Clinical
Dysphagia Oral lesions—vesicles anywhere in the mouth	N/A	N/A	Self-limited disease	Clinical

Continued

Chapter 4 Synopsis—cont'd

Condition/ Disease	Cause	Age/Race/Sex	Location
Viral Infections —cont'd			
Acute Lympho-nodular Pharyngitis			
Measles	A paramyxovirus	Most commonly occurs in children	Primarily skin Oral mucosa—early lesions
Mumps	A paramyxovirus	Most commonly occurs in children	Salivary glands
HIV Infection/ AIDS	Immune deficiency resulting from infection with the human immunodeficiency virus	Newborn infants to adults	Systemic disease

*No significant information.
†Not covered in this text.

Clinical Features	Radiographic Features	Microscopic Features	Treatment	Diagnostic Process
Oral mucosa— Koplik spots— erythematous macules with white necrotic centers	N/A	N/A	Self-limited disease	Clinical
Painful, usually bilateral enlargement of salivary glands	N/A	N/A	Self-limited disease	Clinical
Opportunistic diseases Oral manifestations include oral candidiasis, herpes simplex infection, herpes zoster, hairy leukoplakia, papillomavirus lesions, Kaposi sarcoma, lymphoma and atypical periodontal disease, major aphthouslike ulcers, salivary gland disease and xerostomia, and mucosal pigmentation Autoimmune type thrombocytopenia may result in spontaneous gingival bleeding	Severe and rapid bone loss seen in atypical periodontal disease	Dependent upon opportunistic disease	Combination antiretroviral agents Management of specific opportunistic disease	Laboratory Microscopic

Developmental Disorders

Olga A.C. Ibsen
Joen Iannucci Haring

Objectives

After studying this chapter, the student will be able to:

1. Define each of the words in the vocabulary list for this chapter.
2. Define inherited disorders.
3. Recognize developmental disorders of the dentition.
4. Describe the embryonic development of the face, oral cavity, and teeth.
5. Define each of the developmental anomalies discussed in this chapter.
6. Identify (clinically, radiographically, or both) the developmental anomalies discussed in this chapter.
7. Distinguish between intraosseous cysts and extraosseous cysts.
8. Describe the differences between odontogenic and nonodontogenic cysts.
9. Name four odontogenic cysts that are intraosseous.
10. Name two odontogenic cysts that are extraosseous.
11. Name four nonodontogenic cysts that are intraosseous.
12. Name four nonodontogenic cysts that are found in the soft tissues of the head, neck, and oral region.
13. List and define three anomalies that affect the number of teeth.
14. List and define two anomalies that affect the size of teeth.
15. List and define five anomalies that affect the shape of teeth.
16. Define and identify each of the following anomalies affecting tooth eruption: impacted teeth, embedded teeth, and ankylosed teeth.
17. Identify the diagnostic process that contributes most significantly to the final diagnosis of each developmental anomaly discussed in this chapter.

Vocabulary

Ankyloglossia (ang″kĭ-lo-glos′e-ah) Extensive adhesion of the tongue to the floor of the mouth or the lingual aspect of the anterior portion of the mandible.

Ankylosed teeth (ang′kĭ-lōsd tēth) Teeth that are fused to the alveolar bone; a condition especially common with retained deciduous teeth.

Anodontia (an″o-don′she-ah) Congenital lack of teeth.

Anomaly (ah-nom′ah-le) Marked deviation from normal, especially as a result of congenital or hereditary defects.

Commissure (kom′ĭ-shūr) The site of union of corresponding parts; for example, the corners of the lips (labial commissure).

Concrescence (kon-kres′ens) In dentistry, a condition in which two adjacent teeth become united by cementum.

Congenital (kon-jen′ĭ-tal) Present at and existing from the time of birth.

Cyst (sist) An abnormal sac or cavity lined by epithelium and enclosed in a connective tissue capsule.

Dens in dente (dens in den′te) "A tooth within a tooth"; a developmental anomaly that results when the enamel organ invaginates into the crown of a tooth before mineralization.

Dentinogenesis (den″tĭ-no-jen′ĕ-sis) The formation of dentin.

Differentiation (dif′er-en″she-a′shun) The distinguishing of one thing from another.

Dilaceration (di-las″er-a′shun) An abnormal bend or curve, as in the root of a tooth.

Fusion (fu′zhun) The union of two adjacent tooth germs.

Gemination (jem-ĭ-na′shun) "Twinning"; a single tooth germ attempts to divide, resulting in the incomplete formation of two teeth; the tooth usually has a single root and root canal.

Hypodontia (hi″po-don′she-ah) Partial anodontia; the lack of one or more teeth.

Impacted teeth (im-pakt′ed tēth) Teeth that cannot erupt into the oral cavity because of a physical obstruction.

Macrodontia (mak″ro-don′she-ah) Abnormally large teeth.

Microdontia (mi″kro-don′she-ah) Abnormally small teeth.

Multilocular (mul-tĭ-lok′ū-ler) A radiographic appearance in which many circular radiolucencies exist; these can appear "soap bubble-like" or "honeycomb-like."

Nodule (nod′ūl) A small solid mass that can be detected through touch.

Predilection (prĕd-ĭ-lĕk′shun) A disposition in favor of something; preference.

Proliferation (pro-lif″ĕ-ra′shun) The multiplication of cells.

Stomodeum (sto″mo-de′um) The embryonic invagination that becomes the oral cavity.

Supernumerary (soo″per-nu′mer-ar″e) In excess of the normal or regular number, as in teeth.

The development of the human body is an extremely complex process that begins when an egg is fertilized by a sperm. It continues with a series of cell divisions, multiplications, and differentiation into various tissues and structures. A failure or disturbance that occurs during these processes may result in a lack, excess, or deformity of a body part. These disorders are called **developmental disorders,** or **developmental anomalies.**

Inherited disorders are different from developmental disorders in that they are caused by an abnormality in the genetic makeup (genes and chromosomes) of an individual and are transmitted from parent to offspring through the egg or sperm (see Chapter 6).

A **congenital disorder** is one that is present at birth. It can be either inherited or developmental; however, the cause of most congenital abnormalities is unknown.

The complex process of proliferation and differentiation that takes place in the human body provides numerous possibilities for errors or defects in development. The head and neck region is a common location for such errors because of its intricate sequence and pattern of development. This chapter includes descriptions of developmental disorders of the face, oral cavity, and teeth with which the dental hygienist should be familiar.

Some of the developmental disturbances discussed in this chapter can be identified clinically, whereas others are identified by radiographic examination; still others require biopsy and histologic examinations. A thorough clinical examination, including examination of extraoral and intraoral structures, is an essential component. Dental radiographs are an important part of the examination. Any developmental anomalies observed either clinically or radiographically are documented in the patient's record even if no treatment is indicated. The patient is informed of all dental anomalies, their possible implications, and the treatment necessary, if any. In some instances, referral to a specialist is indicated. To better understand these developmental disorders, a brief review of the embryonic development of the face, oral cavity, and teeth is included in this chapter.

Embryonic Development of the Face, Oral Cavity, and Teeth

FACE

Development of the face is a process of selective growth or proliferation and differentiation (**Figures 5-1** and **5-2**). During the third week of embryonic life, an invagination or infolding of the ectoderm

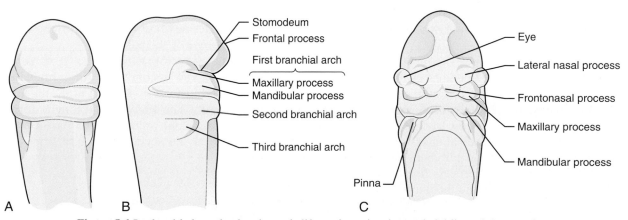

Figure 5-1 In the third week of embryonic life, an invagination or infolding of the ectoderm forms the primitive oral cavity called the stomodeum. **A** and **B,** As facial development continues, the first branchial arch divides into two maxillary processes. **C,** The fourth week of development.

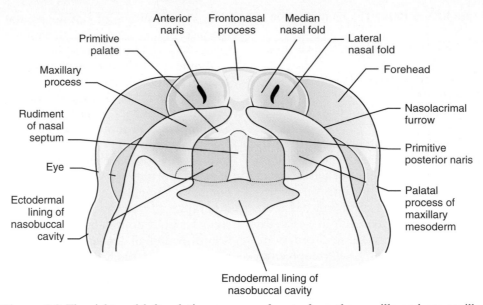

Figure 5-2 The right and left palatine processes fuse to form the maxilla and premaxilla. A Y-shaped pattern results.

forms the primitive oral cavity, which is called the **stomodeum.** Just above the stomodeum is a process called the **frontal process,** and just below it is a structure called the first branchial arch. Additional branchial arches form below the first branchial arch. All of the face and most of the structures of the oral cavity develop from either the frontal process or the first branchial arch. The first branchial arch divides into two **maxillary processes** and the **mandibular process.** The maxillary processes give rise to the upper part of the cheeks, the lateral portions of the upper lip, and part of the palate. The mandibular arch forms the lower part of the cheeks, the mandible, and part of the tongue.

As development continues, two pits (called **olfactory pits**) mark the future openings of the nose that develop on the surface of the frontal process. They divide the frontal process into three parts: (1) the **median nasal process,** (2) the **right lateral nasal process,** and (3) the **left lateral nasal process.** The lateral nasal processes form the sides of the nose, whereas the median nasal process forms the center and tip of the nose. Later, the median nasal process grows downward between the maxillary processes to form a pair of bulges called the **globular process.** This continues to grow downward, forming the portion of the upper lip called the **philtrum.** Most of

these developments are completed by the end of the eighth week of embryonic life.

ORAL AND NASAL CAVITIES

The area of the palate called the **premaxilla** develops from the globular process. The **lateral palatine processes** (left and right) are formed from the maxillary processes. These lateral palatine processes then fuse with the premaxilla. The fusion creates a Y-shaped pattern (see Figure 5-2). The nasal septum arises from the median nasal process. The right and left maxillary processes fuse together with the nasal septum at the center of the palate.

The tongue develops from the first three branchial arches. The second and third branchial arches are located just below the first branchial arch (see Figure 5-1, *B*). The body of the tongue forms from the first branchial arch, and the base of the tongue forms from the second and third branchial arches.

TEETH

Tooth development, or **odontogenesis,** in the human embryo takes place at about the fifth week of embryonic life and involves both ectoderm and

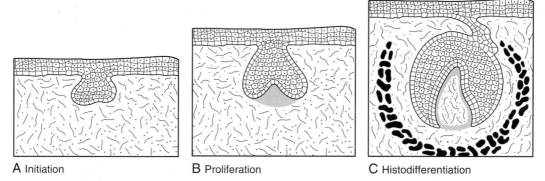

A Initiation   B Proliferation   C Histodifferentiation

Figure 5-3 Development of a tooth germ showing initiation of dental lamina **(A)**, proliferation of dental lamina **(B)**, and differentiation of the components of the tooth germ **(C).**

ectomesenchyme. The ectomesenchyme is derived from neural crest cells.

Odontogenesis begins with the formation of a band of ectoderm in each jaw called the **primary dental lamina.** Ten small knoblike proliferations of epithelial cells develop on the primary dental lamina in each jaw **(Figure 5-3, *A*).** Each of these proliferations extends into the underlying mesenchyme, becoming the early enamel organ for each of the primary teeth **(Figure 5-3, *B*).**

The tooth germ is composed of three parts: (1) the enamel organ, (2) the dental papilla, and (3) the dental sac or follicle **(Figure 5-3, *C*).** The enamel organ develops from ectoderm, and the dental papilla and dental sac or follicle develop from mesenchyme. Cell differentiation in the enamel organ progresses to produce ameloblasts, which form enamel. In the dental papilla, odontoblasts are produced to form dentin. The permanent or **succedaneous** enamel organs form at the same time.

Formation of dental hard tissues occurs during the fifth month of gestation **(Figure 5-4). Dentinogenesis** is the formation of dentin. Dentin is the first mineralized tooth tissue to appear. When it begins to form, the mesenchymal tissue within the tooth germ is called the **dental papilla.** After dentin is produced, the dental papilla is called the dental pulp. Enamel is the product of the enamel organ. Enamel matrix begins to form shortly after dentin, and mineralization and maturation of enamel follow the formation of the matrix. **Amelogenesis** refers to the formation of enamel.

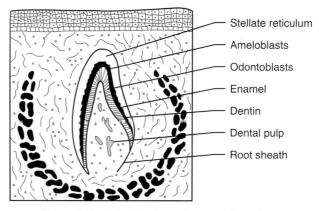

Stellate reticulum
Ameloblasts
Odontoblasts
Enamel
Dentin
Dental pulp
Root sheath

Figure 5-4 Deposition of enamel and dentin.

The dental sac or follicle that surrounds the developing tooth germ provides cells that form cementum, the periodontal ligament, and alveolar bone. **Cementogenesis** (the formation of cementum) occurs after crown formation is complete. An epithelial structure called the ***Hertwig's epithelial root sheath*** proliferates to shape the root of the tooth and induces the formation of the root dentin. The cells of the Hertwig's epithelial root sheath must break up and pull away from the root surface before cementum can be produced. Very little cementum is produced until the tooth has erupted and is in occlusion and functioning. Root length is not completed until 1 to 4 years after the tooth erupts into the oral cavity.

Developmental Soft Tissue Abnormalities

ANKYLOGLOSSIA

Ankyloglossia is an extensive adhesion of the tongue to the floor of the mouth, which is often referred to as "tongue-tied." Ankyloglossia is derived from the Greek words "ankylos," meaning adhesion, and "glossa," meaning tongue. This adhesion results from the complete or partial fusion of the lingual frenum to the floor of the mouth. Total ankyloglossia is rare. Partial ankyloglossia appears clinically as a very short lingual frenum connecting the anteroventral portion of the tongue to the floor of the mouth **(Figure 5-5)**. Patients with a short lingual frenum may exhibit no adverse effects, but some may have problems with speech. Gingival recession and bone loss can occur if the frenum is attached high on the lingual alveolar ridge. Surgical removal of a portion of the lingual frenum, known as **frenectomy**, is the usual treatment for ankyloglossia.

COMMISSURAL LIP PITS

Commissural lip pits are epithelium-lined blind tracts located at the corners of the mouth **(Figure 5-6)**. These tracts may be shallow, or they may be several millimeters deep. They are a relatively common developmental anomaly. The cause of commissural lip pits is not clear; both the incomplete fusion of the maxillary and mandibular processes and the defec-

tive development of the horizontal facial cleft have been suggested. The commissural lip pit may be observed during examination.

Another lip pit that occasionally may be seen is the **congenital lip pit**. It occurs near the midline of the vermilion border of the lip and may appear as either a unilateral or a bilateral depression. No treatment is indicated for lip pits.

LINGUAL THYROID

Lingual thyroid, or **ectopic lingual thyroid nodule**, is a small mass of thyroid tissue located on the tongue away from the normal anatomic location of the thyroid gland. It is an uncommon developmental anomaly that results from the failure of the primitive thyroid tissue to migrate from its developmental location in the area of the foramen cecum on the posterior portion of the tongue to its normal position in the neck.

Clinically the lingual thyroid nodule appears as a smooth nodular mass at the base of the tongue posterior to the circumvallate papillae on or near the midline. It can be asymptomatic or can cause a feeling of fullness in the throat or difficulty in swallowing. Histologically the lingual thyroid is composed of immature or mature thyroid tissue.

Figure 5-6 Commissural lip pit. A deep depression is seen at the labial commissure.

Figure 5-5 Ankyloglossia. The short lingual frenum is attached near the tip of the tongue. (Courtesy Dr. George Blozis.)

On occasion, the size of the lingual thyroid necessitates its removal. However, this nodule may be the patient's only functioning thyroid tissue. Therefore it is necessary to establish the presence of functioning thyroid tissue elsewhere before any nodular lesion located in the posterior aspect of the tongue is removed. If a normally located thyroid gland is lacking or nonfunctional, the lingual thyroid is not removed.

Developmental Cysts

A **cyst** is an abnormal, pathologic sac or cavity lined by epithelium and enclosed in a connective tissue capsule. Cysts occur throughout the body, including the oral region.

The cysts discussed in this chapter are all related to the development of the face, jaws, and teeth. Some have a distinctive histologic appearance, and a definitive diagnosis is based on microscopic examination of the tissue. Other cysts are lined by less distinctive epithelium. The diagnosis of these cysts is based on both the histologic appearance of the tissue and the location of the cyst.

The most common cyst observed in the oral cavity is caused by pulpal inflammation and is called the radicular cyst (see Chapter 2). The **residual cyst** is a radicular cyst that remains after extraction of the offending tooth. Because cysts are commonly observed in the jaws and surrounding soft tissues, the dental hygienist should understand their diagnostic criteria, pathogenesis, and prognosis. The preliminary identification of a cystic lesion is within the scope of dental hygiene practice.

Developmental cysts are classified as **odontogenic** (related to tooth development) and **nonodontogenic** (not related to tooth development). Cysts are also classified according to location, cause, origin of the epithelial cells, and histologic appearance **(Table 5-1)**. Developmental cysts can vary in size from small, asymptomatic lesions to large lesions that can cause expansion of bone. Very large and long-standing lesions can resorb tooth structure or move teeth. Oral cysts that occur within bone are called **intraosseous cysts**, and cysts that occur in soft tissue are called **extraosseous cysts**.

Radiographically, cysts within bone generally appear as well-circumscribed radiolucencies. All cysts may appear **unilocular**, but some are more likely to appear as **multilocular** radiolucencies. When cysts are found within soft tissue, no radiographic change usually occurs.

ODONTOGENIC CYSTS

Dentigerous Cyst

A **dentigerous cyst**, also called a **follicular cyst**, forms around the crown of an unerupted or developing tooth **(Figure 5-7)**. The epithelial lining originates from the reduced enamel epithelium after the crown has completely formed and calcified. Fluid accumulates between the crown and the reduced enamel epithelium. The reduced enamel epithelium results from remnants of the enamel organ. The most common location for the dentigerous cyst is around the crown of an unerupted or impacted third molar. However, a dentigerous cyst may form around the crowns of other unerupted or impacted teeth, such as the maxillary cuspid or a supernumerary tooth. This cyst is most often seen in young adults and can range from small and asymptomatic to very large. When

---

Table 5-1 Classification of Developmental Cysts

Odontogenic		Nonodontogenic	
Intraosseous	*Extraosseous*	*Intraosseous*	*Extraosseous*
Dentigerous cyst	Eruption cyst	Nasopalatine duct cyst	Nasolabial cyst
Primordial cyst		Median palatal cyst	Lymphoepithelial
Odontogenic keratocyst		Globulomaxillary cyst	(branchial cleft) cyst
Lateral periodontal cyst	Gingival cyst	Median mandibular cyst	Epidermal cyst
			Thyroglossal duct cyst

DENTIGEROUS CYST

A

Figure 5-7 Schematic of a dentigerous cyst located around the crown of an unerupted or impacted tooth.

B

large, it is capable of displacing teeth or causing a fracture of the mandible.

Radiographically, the dentigerous cyst appears as a well-defined, unilocular radiolucency around the crown of an unerupted or impacted tooth (**Figure 5-8**, *A* and *B*). Histologically, the lumen is most characteristically lined with cuboidal epithelium surrounded by a wall of connective tissue (**Figure 5-8**, *C*). It may also be lined with stratified squamous epithelium. The lumen may be filled with a watery or serous fluid.

Treatment of a dentigerous cyst involves the complete removal of the cystic lesion and usually the tooth involved. If it is not removed, the cyst wall continues to enlarge. In addition, a risk exists that a neoplasm (tumor) may develop.

Eruption Cyst

An **eruption cyst** is similar to a dentigerous cyst. It is found in the soft tissue around the crown of an erupting tooth.

Because the tooth erupts through the cyst, this condition usually does not require treatment. Occasionally the dome of the eruption cyst is removed to expose the crown. The tooth is allowed to erupt naturally.

C

Figure 5-8 Radiographs of dentigerous cysts around the crown of an unerupted bicuspid **(A)** and an impacted third molar **(B). C,** Microscopic appearance of a dentigerous cyst.

Primordial Cyst

A **primordial cyst** develops in place of a tooth and is most commonly found in place of the third molar or posterior to an erupted third molar **(Figure 5-9)**. It originates from remnants and degeneration of the enamel organ. A history that the tooth was never present is an essential component of the diagnostic process.

Primordial cysts are most often seen in the young adult; no sex predilection has been reported. Clinically the cyst usually is asymptomatic and is discovered on radiographic examination. Radiographically it is a well-defined, radiolucent lesion that can be either unilocular or multilocular. The histologic appearance and diagnosis of the primordial cyst may vary. Histologically the lumen is lined by stratified squamous epithelium surrounded by parallel bundles of collagen fibers. A layer of orthokeratin or parakeratin can cover the epithelium. The term *primordial cyst* simply refers to its development in place of a tooth. For this reason, biopsy and histologic examination of primordial cysts are essential. Histologically a primordial cyst can be an odontogenic keratocyst or a lateral periodontal cyst.

Treatment of a primordial cyst involves surgical removal of the entire lesion. The prognosis depends on the histology; the risk of recurrence depends on the histologic diagnosis. For example, if the cyst is histologically an odontogenic keratocyst, the risk of recurrence is greater than if the cyst is lined by nonkeratinized stratified squamous epithelium.

PRIMORDIAL CYST

Figure 5-9 Schematic of a primordial cyst occurring in place of a tooth: the third molar, in this instance.

Odontogenic Keratocyst

An **odontogenic keratocyst** is an odontogenic cyst that is characterized by its unique histologic appearance and frequent recurrence. The lumen is lined by epithelium that is 8 to 10 cell layers thick and surfaced by parakeratin. The basal cell layer is palisaded and prominent; the interface between the epithelium and the connective tissue is flat (**Figure 5-10,** *A* and *B*).

These cysts are most often seen in the mandibular third molar region. Radiographically the odontogenic keratocyst frequently appears as a well-defined, multilocular, radiolucent lesion (**Figure 5-10,** *C*). Unilocular lesions may also occur. The radiographic appearance of an odontogenic keratocyst can be identical to that of an odontogenic tumor. The odontogenic keratocyst is an expansive lesion that can move teeth and resorb tooth structure.

Treatment of an odontogenic keratocyst is rather aggressive because of the high recurrence rate (**Figure 5-10,** *D* and *E*). The cyst generally extends beyond the borders that are seen on the radiograph because it extends between the trabeculae of bone. Therefore thorough surgical excision and osseous curettage are recommended. Careful follow-up and evaluation are essential.

Calcifying Odontogenic Cyst

The **calcifying odontogenic cyst** is a nonaggressive cystic lesion lined by odontogenic epithelium that closely resembles the epithelium of the odontogenic tumor called an ameloblastoma; in addition, it has a characteristic feature called ghost cells. Generally the cyst is treated conservatively and does not recur. A solid variant of the calcifying odontogenic cyst has been reported; it has been suggested that this solid variant represents a neoplasm rather than a cyst. Because of its histologic resemblance to the ameloblastoma, the calcifying odontogenic cyst is described in detail in Chapter 7.

Lateral Periodontal Cyst and Gingival Cyst

The **lateral periodontal cyst** is named for its location. It is most often seen in the mandibular cuspid and premolar area. It presents as an asymptomatic, unilocular or multilocular radiolucent lesion located

Figure 5-10 A, Microscopic appearance of an odontogenic keratocyst (OKC) showing a thin uniform epithelial lining (low power). *Lu,* Lumen; *E,* epithelium; *CT,* connective tissue. **B,** Microscopic appearance of an OKC showing a corrugated parakeratotic surface *(P)* and a prominent basal cell layer *(B)* (high power). **C,** Radiograph of an OKC showing a multilocular radiolucency. **D,** Radiograph of an OKC extending to the third molar. **E,** Same patient in **D,** 2 years later, showing recurrence of OKC. The reader should note the third molar has been removed.

on the lateral aspect of a tooth root (**Figure 5-11,** *A*). Histologically a thin band of stratified squamous epithelium that exhibits focal epithelial thickenings lines the cyst (**Figure 5-11,** *B*). The **gingival cyst** exhibits the same type of epithelial lining as the lateral periodontal cyst and is located in the soft tissue of the same area. The gingival cyst appears as a small bulge or swelling of the attached gingiva or interdental papillae (**Figure 5-11,** *C*).

The lateral periodontal cyst is found most often in males. No sex predilection has been reported for gingival cysts. Both the lateral periodontal cyst and the gingival cyst are treated by surgical excision. A few cases of recurrence of lateral periodontal cysts have been reported.

NONODONTOGENIC CYSTS

Nasopalatine Canal Cyst

A **nasopalatine canal cyst (incisive canal cyst)** is located within the nasopalatine canal or the incisive papilla. When found in the papilla, it is referred to as a **cyst of the palatine papilla.** This cyst arises from epithelial remnants of the embryonal nasopalatine ducts. The lesion is most commonly seen in adults between 40 and 60 years of age, and a strong predilection exists for males. The cyst is usually asymptomatic. There may be a small pink bulge near the apices and between the roots of the maxillary central incisors on the lingual surface. The adjacent teeth are usually vital.

Figure 5-11 A, Radiograph of a lateral periodontal cyst. This biloculated, well-defined radiolucency is located lateral to the tooth root. **B,** Microscopic appearance of a lateral periodontal cyst showing a thin epithelial lining with focal epithelial thickenings. **C,** Gingival cyst. (**C** courtesy Drs. Paul Freedman and Stanley Kerpel.)

Radiographically the nasopalatine canal cyst is a well-defined, radiolucent lesion that is often heart shaped (**Figure 5-12,** *A*), resulting from the anatomic Y shape of the canal. When it is heart shaped, it is evenly distributed to the right and left of the midline.

Histologically the cyst is lined by epithelium that varies from stratified squamous to pseudostratified ciliated columnar epithelium (**Figure 5-12,** *B*). The connective tissue wall contains nerves and blood vessels that are normally found in the area and may also contain inflammatory cells.

Treatment of a nasopalatine canal cyst is surgical excision. It is especially important that surgery take place in the edentulous patient before the fabrication of a prosthesis. Recurrence is not expected.

Median Palatine Cyst

A **median palatine cyst** appears as a well-defined unilocular radiolucency and is located in the midline of the hard palate (**Figure 5-13**). The cyst is thought to be a more posterior form of a nasopalatine canal cyst. Histologically the median palatine cyst is lined with stratified squamous epithelium that is sur-

rounded by dense fibrous connective tissue. The median palatine cyst is treated by surgical enucleation. The prognosis is good, and recurrence is rare.

Globulomaxillary Cyst

Radiographically a **globulomaxillary cyst** is a well-defined, pear-shaped radiolucency found between the roots of the maxillary lateral incisor and cuspid (**Figure 5-14**). Although it was once thought to be a fissural cyst, it is now believed to be of odontogenic epithelial origin. The size of the lesion can vary; however, when it is large enough, a divergence of the roots can result. The adjacent teeth are usually vital. Surgical enucleation of the globulomaxillary cyst is recommended. The prognosis is good, and recurrence is rare.

Median Mandibular Cyst

A **median mandibular cyst** is a rare lesion. It is located, as its name indicates, in the midline of the mandible. The origin of the median mandibular cyst is also unclear. Some believe it to be of odontogenic

A

B

Figure 5-12 A, An incisive canal cyst may be located in the anterior maxilla in either bone, soft tissue, or both. This radiograph of an incisive canal cyst shows a well-circumscribed radiolucency between the maxillary central incisors. **B,** Microscopic appearance of an incisive canal cyst showing a pseudostratified, ciliated, columnar epithelial lining.

origin, possibly a primordial cyst. Because no midline fusion occurs between the bony processes, there can be no epithelial entrapment. The cyst is lined with squamous epithelium, and the surrounding teeth are vital. Radiographically a well-defined radiolucency is seen below the apices of the mandibular incisors. A median mandibular cyst is treated by surgical removal, and prognosis is good. Recurrence is not expected.

Nasolabial Cyst

A **nasolabial cyst** is a soft tissue cyst with no alveolar bone involvement. The origin of this cyst is uncertain. At present it is thought to originate from the lower anterior portion of the nasolacrimal duct. The cyst is observed in adults 40 to 50 years of age; a strong predilection (4:1) exists for females.

Clinically there may be an expansion or swelling in the mucolabial fold in the area of the maxillary canine and the floor of the nose. Usually no radiographic change is associated with this cyst. However, when the lesion is large enough, expansive pressure can cause the resorption of bone **(Figure 5-15)**. Histologically the cyst is lined with pseudostratified, ciliated columnar epithelium and multiple goblet cells. Treatment of a nasolabial cyst is surgical excision, prognosis is good, and recurrence is rare.

Lymphoepithelial Cyst

A **lymphoepithelial cyst (branchial cleft cyst)** is most commonly found in the major salivary glands. It is composed of a stratified squamous epithelial lining surrounded by a well-circumscribed component of lymphoid tissue **(Figure 5-16)**. It appears to arise from epithelium trapped in a lymph node during

Figure 5-13 Radiograph of a median palatine cyst showing a well-defined radiolucency located in the midline of the maxilla.

Figure 5-14 Radiograph of a globulomaxillary cyst showing a characteristic pear-shaped radiolucency between the roots of the maxillary lateral incisor and cuspid.

development. When found intraorally, the floor of the mouth and the lateral borders of the tongue are the most common locations. When occurring intraorally, the lymphoepithelial cyst appears as a pinkish yellow, raised nodule. Treatment of a lymphoepithelial cyst consists of surgical excision, and prognosis is good.

Epidermal Cyst

An **epidermal cyst** presents as a raised nodule in the skin of the face or neck. Histologically the cyst is lined by keratinizing epithelium that resembles the epithelium of skin (epidermis). The cyst lumen is usually filled with keratin scales. Most epidermal cysts are thought to originate from the epithelium of the hair follicle. Occasionally when located in the skin of the cheek, the nodule may be noted intraorally from the buccal mucosal aspect and the skin. An epidermoid cyst is treated by surgical excision, and prognosis is good.

Dermoid Cyst and Benign Cystic Teratoma

A **dermoid cyst** is a developmental cyst that is often present at birth or noted in young children. It is more common in other parts of the body than in the head and neck. When the dermoid cyst occurs in the oral cavity, it is usually found in the anterior floor of the mouth. The cyst may cause displacement of the tongue and may have a doughlike consistency when palpated.

Histologically the dermoid cyst is lined by ortho-keratinized, stratified squamous epithelium surrounded by a connective tissue wall. The lumen is usually filled with keratin. Hair follicles, sebaceous glands, and sweat glands may be seen in the cyst wall. A **benign cystic teratoma** has a cystic component that resembles the dermoid cyst. In addition, teeth, bone, muscles, and nerve tissue may be found in the wall of this lesion. Teeth are usually not found in the malignant form of the teratoma. Treatment of the dermoid cyst is surgical excision; prognosis is good, and malignant transformation is rare.

Thyroglossal Tract Cyst

A **thyroglossal tract (duct) cyst** forms along the same tract that the thyroid gland follows in development, from the area of the foramen cecum to its permanent location in the neck (**Figure 5-17**, *A* and *B*). Most of these cysts occur below the hyoid bone. The epithelial lining varies from stratified squamous to ciliated columnar epithelium. Cysts above the hyoid bone are usually lined with squamous epithelium, and those below the hyoid bone with ciliated columnar epithelium. Thyroid tissue may also be found within the connective tissue wall.

Figure 5-15 Nasolabial cyst causing a swelling in the nasolabial fold area.

Figure 5-16 Microscopic appearance of a lymphoepithelial cyst showing lumen *(Lu)*, epithelial lining *(E)*, surrounding lymphocytes *(L)*, and connective tissue *(CT)* (low power).

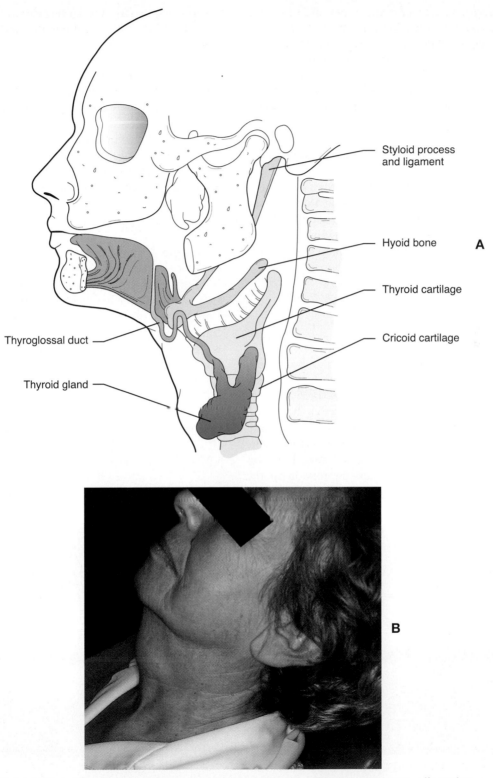

Styloid process
and ligament

Hyoid bone

Thyroid cartilage

Cricoid cartilage

Thyroglossal duct

Thyroid gland

A

B

Figure 5-17 A, The thyroglossal tract extends from the area of the foramen cecum lingual to the lower part of the neck. **B,** A thyroglossal tract cyst is the cause of this enlargement at the midline of the neck.

The thyroglossal tract cyst is most often found in young individuals under 20 years of age. There is no sex predilection. Clinically if this cyst is located below the hyoid bone, it presents as a smooth bulge or swelling in the area of the midline of the neck. If located on the posterior aspect of the tongue, a smooth, rather firm mass of tissue is present, which can vary in size from a few millimeters to several centimeters. The patient may complain of dysphagia (difficulty in swallowing) or difficulty when extending the tongue.

Treatment of a thyroglossal tract cyst consists of complete excision of the cyst and the tract, usually including a portion of the hyoid bone and muscle tissue along the thyroglossal tract. Prognosis is generally good, but a few cases of malignant transformation have been reported.

PSEUDOCYSTS

Static Bone Cyst

A **static bone cyst (lingual mandibular bone concavity** or **Stafne bone cyst)** is not a true cyst because it is not a pathologic cavity and is not lined with epithelium. It is therefore often referred to as a *pseudocyst.* Radiographically a well-defined cystlike radiolucency is observed in the posterior region of the mandible inferior to the mandibular canal. The radiolucency is caused by a lingual depression in the mandible, which surrounds normal salivary gland tissue **(Figure 5-18).** The salivary gland tissue may be an extension of the sublingual gland. The lesion is usually asymptomatic. Occasionally the depression can be palpated.

This variant of normal requires no treatment. If any question exists about the diagnosis, the patient is followed until it is determined that no enlargement of the radiolucency has occurred. If the radiolucency occurs above the mandibular canal, a biopsy may be indicated to establish the diagnosis and differentiate this variant of normal from cysts and tumors having a predilection for that location.

Simple Bone Cyst

A **simple bone cyst (traumatic bone cyst)** is a pathologic cavity in bone that is not lined with epithelium. The cause is uncertain, although an association with trauma has been suggested. The lesion is found most often in young individuals, and at one time it was reported to be more commonly found in males; more recently, an equal distribution among males and females has been reported. The lesion is observed radiographically as a well-defined unilocular or multilocular radiolucent lesion that characteristically shows scalloping around the roots of teeth **(Figure 5-19).** The lesion is usually asymptomatic

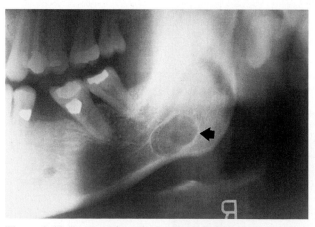

Figure 5-18 Panoramic radiograph of a lingual mandibular bone concavity (Stafne bone cyst). Arrow points to a well-circumscribed radiolucency inferior to the mandibular canal.

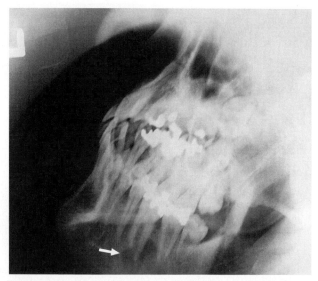

Figure 5-19 Extraoral radiograph showing a simple (traumatic) bone cyst in the mandible with its unique radiolucent characteristic, scalloping around the roots. (Courtesy Dr. Edward V. Zegarelli.)

and is discovered on routine radiographs. Surgical intervention reveals a void within the bone. A curettage is performed on the wall lining the void, which fills up with bone 6 months to 1 year after the surgical procedure. Prognosis is excellent, and recurrence is unusual.

Aneurysmal Bone Cyst

An **aneurysmal bone cyst** is a pseudocyst that consists of blood-filled spaces surrounded by multinucleated giant cells and fibrous connective tissue (similar to the giant cell granuloma). The radiolucent lesion has a multilocular appearance that is often described as a "honeycomb" or "soap bubble." It is usually seen in individuals less than 30 years of age, and a slight predilection is reported for females. The clinical presentation may be that of expansion of the involved bone.

A previous history of trauma to the area has been reported in some cases, but no direct correlation exists. Other reports have noted an association between the aneurysmal bone cyst and other bone lesions. It has frequently been associated with fibrous dysplasia. Surgical excision is the recommended treatment of an aneurysmal bone cyst, and there may be excessive bleeding from the lesion during the procedure.

Developmental Abnormalities of Teeth

ABNORMALITIES IN THE NUMBER OF TEETH

Anodontia

Anodontia is the congenital lack of teeth. Total anodontia (lack of all teeth) is a rare condition that may affect either the deciduous or the permanent dentition. Because development of both deciduous and permanent teeth begins before birth, their failure to develop is congenital. However, teeth may not be identified as missing until the time of normal eruption or initial radiographic examination. Total anodontia is often associated with the hereditary disturbance ectodermal dysplasia, which is described in Chapter 6. Missing teeth require prosthetic replacement.

Hypodontia

Hypodontia is the lack of one or more teeth. This developmental anomaly is rather common and may affect either deciduous or permanent teeth (**Figure 5-20**, *A* and *B*). Any tooth in either dentition may be missing. The permanent dentition is most commonly affected. The teeth most often missing are the maxillary and mandibular third molars, the maxillary lateral incisors, and the mandibular second premolars. Teeth are often missing bilaterally. The mandibular incisor is the tooth most commonly missing in the deciduous dentition. Teeth are identified as congenitally lacking by careful clinical and radiographic examination along with a thorough patient history.

Missing teeth tend to be **familial**, that is, affecting more members of a family than would be expected by chance. In addition, factors such as jaw lesions in infancy and radiation therapy during tooth formation may result in the destruction of tooth germs and the subsequent lack of affected teeth.

Figure 5-20 A and **B,** Hypodontia. Teeth missing have not been extracted; they never developed. (**A** courtesy Dr. George Blozis; **B** courtesy Dr. Margot Van Dis.)

Missing teeth may require prosthetic replacement. Their absence can also result in problems in occlusion caused by drifting or tipping of teeth. Orthodontic evaluation and treatment may be necessary. In addition, congenitally missing teeth may be a component of a **syndrome.** A syndrome is a group of findings that occur together. Patients with congenitally missing teeth should be evaluated for other abnormalities.

Supernumerary Teeth

Supernumerary teeth are extra teeth found in the dental arches **(Figure 5-21).** *Supernumerary* means more than the normal or regular number. Supernumerary teeth result either from the formation of extra tooth buds in the dental lamina or from the cleavage of already existing tooth buds and may occur in either the deciduous or the permanent dentition. Extra teeth are most often seen in the maxilla and may occur singly or in multiples and unilaterally or bilaterally.

Typically the supernumerary tooth is smaller than a normal-sized tooth and often does not erupt. Most are discovered on radiographs as incidental findings. A supernumerary tooth may or may not resemble a normal tooth in shape and position.

The most common supernumerary tooth is called the **mesiodens,** which is located between the maxillary central incisors at or near the midline. It is usually a small tooth with a conical crown and short roots **(Figure 5-22).** It may occur singly or in pairs and may be inverted when seen on a radiograph. The mesiodens can erupt or remain embedded or impacted.

The second most common supernumerary tooth is the maxillary fourth molar, which is also called a **distomolar** because it is located distal to the third molar **(Figure 5-23,** *A* and *B*). The distomolar can look like a miniature third molar or can be of normal third molar size and shape. It rarely erupts into the oral cavity and is usually discovered on a radiograph.

Other supernumerary teeth include mandibular and maxillary premolars, maxillary lateral incisors, and the maxillary paramolar, a small rudimentary tooth that occurs buccal to the third molar. Erupted supernumerary teeth can cause crowding, malpositioning of adjacent teeth, or noneruption of normal teeth; therefore removal is often necessary. Nonerupted supernumerary teeth should be extracted because a risk exists for cyst development around the crown. Multiple supernumerary teeth may be a component of a syndrome such as cleidocranial dysplasia

Figure 5-21 A, Supernumerary teeth. This patient has four maxillary lateral incisors. **B,** Radiograph showing unerupted supernumerary teeth. **C,** Supernumerary mandibular incisor. (**A** courtesy Dr. Margot Van Dis; **B** courtesy Dr. George Blozis.)

or Gardner syndrome. These syndromes are described in Chapter 6.

ABNORMALITIES IN THE SIZE OF TEETH

Microdontia

Microdontia is a developmental anomaly in which one or more teeth in a dentition are smaller than normal. The term is derived from the Greek words "mikros," meaning small, and "odontos," meaning

Figure 5-22   **A,** Mesiodens seen between the maxillary central incisors. **B,** Radiograph of an erupted mesiodens. **C,** Radiograph showing a pair of inverted impacted mesiodens. (**A** and **B** courtesy Dr. George Blozis.)

tooth. Microdontia is classified as true generalized microdontia, generalized relative microdontia, or microdontia involving a single tooth.

True generalized microdontia is seen in the pituitary dwarf and is extremely rare. All the teeth are smaller than normal. In **generalized relative microdontia,** normal-sized teeth appear small in large

jaws. Heredity plays a role in generalized relative microdontia. For example, a child may inherit large jaws from one parent and normal-sized teeth from the other, resulting in the illusion of small teeth. **Microdontia involving a single tooth** is far more common than true generalized microdontia or generalized relative microdontia. The maxillary lateral

Figure 5-23 **A,** Small erupted microdont distal to the maxillary second molar. **B,** Radiograph of a pair of distomolars, located distal to the second molar. (**A** courtesy Dr. Margot Van Dis; **B** courtesy Dr. George Blozis.)

incisor and the maxillary third molar are the teeth most often affected **(Figure 5-24).** The maxillary lateral incisors often appear peg shaped, with the mesial and distal tooth surfaces converging toward the incisal edge. This "peg lateral" is smaller than normal, tends to occur bilaterally, has short roots, and is thought to be familial. The maxillary third molar microdont typically appears small but normally shaped. Microdonts are identified clinically if erupted or radiographically if unerupted. For cosmetic reasons, erupted microdonts may be restored to resemble teeth of normal size and shape. Impacted microdonts should be surgically removed to prevent cyst formation.

Macrodontia

Macrodontia is an uncommon developmental anomaly in which one or more teeth in a dentition are larger than normal. The term is derived from the Greek words "makros," meaning large, and "odontos," meaning tooth. Macrodontia is classified in the same manner as microdontia: true generalized macrodontia, relative generalized macrodontia, and macrodontia involving a single tooth.

True generalized macrodontia is rare and is occasionally seen in cases of pituitary gigantism. **Relative generalized macrodontia** is seen in individuals with normal or slightly larger than normal teeth in small jaws and is generally caused by the patient's inheriting tooth size from one parent and jaw size from the other. **Macrodontia affecting a single tooth** is uncommon. Localized macrodontia affecting

Figure 5-24 Peg-shaped lateral incisor. (Courtesy Dr. George Blozis.)

one side of the dental arches may be seen in a condition called **facial hemihypertrophy,** which involves the enlargement of half of the head with enlarged teeth on the involved side. No treatment is indicated for macrodontia.

ABNORMALITIES IN THE SHAPE OF TEETH

Gemination

Gemination is a developmental anomaly that occurs when a single tooth germ attempts to divide and results in the incomplete formation of two

Figure 5-25 **A,** Clinical picture of gemination in a mandibular cuspid. **B,** Gemination seen in a maxillary central incisor. **C,** Radiograph of the same maxillary central incisor. (**A** courtesy Dr. George Blozis.)

teeth. **Geminate** means paired or occurring in twos. The cause of this aborted twinning of a single tooth germ is unknown. Gemination is uncommon and is more frequently seen in the deciduous dentition, but occasionally it occurs in the permanent dentition. Gemination most often affects anterior teeth and is most often seen in the deciduous mandibular incisors and the permanent maxillary incisors.

Clinically, gemination appears as two crowns joined together by a notched incisal area (**Figure 5-25,** *A* and *B*). Radiographically, usually one single root and one common pulp canal exist (**Figure**

5-25, *C*). The patient has a full complement of teeth.

A geminated tooth poses an aesthetic problem, particularly when it occurs in the maxillary anterior region. It also poses a prosthetic challenge. Treatment therefore usually involves alteration of the tooth so that it resembles a normal tooth in size and shape.

Fusion

Fusion results from the union of two normally separated adjacent tooth germs. The cause of fusion is uncertain; heredity, external pressure, and crowding have all been suggested. Fusion of adjacent teeth can be complete or incomplete, depending on the stage of tooth development at the time of contact. Early contact of developing tooth germs can result in a single, large tooth; later contact can result in the union of crowns only or the union of roots only. True fusion always involves confluence of dentin. Fusion tends to occur in the anterior region, and the incisors are the teeth most often affected. Fusion of deciduous teeth occurs more often than fusion of permanent teeth.

Clinically, fused teeth appear as a single large crown that occurs in place of two normal teeth and may exhibit an observable separation **(Figure 5-26)**. Radiographically either separate or fused roots and root canals are seen. To differentiate fusion from gemination, the teeth must be counted. If the neighboring teeth of the tooth in question are present, the tooth is geminated; if a neighboring tooth is lacking, the tooth in question is fused. Fusion can occur between two adjacent normal teeth or between a normal tooth and a supernumerary tooth. It may be difficult to distinguish between a geminated tooth and the fusion of a normal tooth to a supernumerary tooth.

As with geminated teeth, fused teeth may present aesthetic and occlusal problems; they also pose a restorative challenge. Treatment involves alteration of the size and shape of the tooth and may involve replacement of one of the fused teeth.

Concrescence

In dentistry, **concrescence** is a condition in which two adjacent teeth are united by cementum only. It is actually a form of fusion that takes place after tooth formation is complete and is usually discovered as an incidental radiographic finding **(Figure 5-27)**. The cause of concrescence is thought to be crowding or trauma that results in the close approximation of adjacent tooth roots. Subsequent cementum deposition acts to fuse the two adjacent roots. Concrescence is most often seen in adjacent maxillary molars and adjacent supernumerary teeth and may involve erupted, unerupted, or impacted teeth.

Concrescence generally does not require treatment. If one of the teeth joined by cementum requires extraction, extraction of the fused neighbor is inevitable. However, the extraction of involved teeth is difficult, and excessive fracture of the associated alveolar bone may result.

Dilaceration

In dentistry, **dilaceration** refers to an abnormal curve or angle in the root or, less frequently, the crown of a tooth (**Figure 5-28,** *A* to *C*). This dental anomaly is thought to be caused by trauma to the tooth germ during root development. The position of the calcified portion of the tooth is changed, and the

Figure 5-26 A, Clinical picture of fusion involving a permanent mandibular lateral incisor. **B,** Fusion of mandibular molars. (**A** courtesy Dr. George Blozis; **B** courtesy Dr. Rudy Melfi.)

remainder of the tooth forms at an angle. A dilaceration can appear anywhere along the root portion of a tooth and can occur in any tooth in either the deciduous or the permanent dentition. A root dilaceration is usually discovered as an incidental radiographic finding.

Dilacerations do not require treatment. However, they may cause problems if extraction or endodontic therapy becomes necessary. The importance of a preoperative radiograph is obvious.

Enamel Pearl

An **enamel pearl**, or **enameloma**, is a small, spherical enamel projection located on a root surface **(Figure 5-29)**. This developmental anomaly is thought to occur as a result of the abnormal displacement of ameloblasts during tooth formation. The enamel pearl is usually found on maxillary molars. It is attached to cementum near the root bifurcation or trifurcation area. Occasionally it is located near the cementoenamel junction. The enamel pearl may consist of enamel only or enamel, dentin, and pulp.

The enamel pearl is an uncommon finding. It appears radiographically as a small, spherical radiopacity. Clinically the enamel pearl may be mistaken for calculus. Generally no treatment is necessary for this anomaly. Removal may be necessary if periodontal problems occur in the furcation area when an enamel pearl is present.

Talon Cusp

A **talon cusp** is an accessory cusp located in the area of the cingulum of a maxillary or mandibular permanent incisor **(Figure 5-30)**. A talon is a claw of a predatory animal. The talon cusp is said to resemble an eagle's talon. The talon cusp often projects lingually to the height of the incisal edge of the involved tooth. The talon cusp is composed of normal enamel and dentin and contains a pulp horn. Frequently, a caries-susceptible fissure is present between the cusps. Removal of the talon cusp is often indicated because it interferes with occlusion. Because of the presence of the pulp horn, endodontic therapy is necessary.

A   **B**

Figure 5-27 Concrescence illustrated in a photograph **(A)** of extracted teeth and in a corresponding radiograph **(B).** (Courtesy Dr. George Blozis.)

Figure 5-28 **A,** Dilaceration on the distal root of an extracted tooth. **B,** Mesial root dilaceration on a mandibular second molar. **C,** Radiograph of root dilaceration in maxillary lateral and cuspid. (**A** courtesy Dr. Rudy Melfi.)

Taurodontism

Taurodontism is a term used to describe a developmental dental anomaly in which the teeth exhibit elongated, large pulp chambers and short roots **(Figure 5-31).** Taurodontism means "bull-like" teeth. The term was first used to describe teeth that resembled those of cud-chewing animals. Although the cause of taurodontism is uncertain, a variety of causes have been suggested, ranging from a primitive pattern of tooth development to the developmental failure of the Hertwig epithelial root sheath to invaginate at the proper level.

Taurodontism is uncommon and seen in both the deciduous and the permanent dentitions and usually affects a single molar tooth or several molars in the same quadrant. Taurodontism can occur unilaterally or bilaterally. The crown of the tooth appears clinically normal. A taurodont is identified by its characteristic radiographic appearance. The tooth tends to have a stretched appearance, and the pulp chamber is greatly enlarged and elongated without a constriction at the cementoenamel junction. The roots appear short, with the furcation located near the apices. No treatment is indicated for taurodontism.

Figure 5-29 Enamel pearl in the furcation area. (Courtesy Dr. Rudy Melfi.)

A

B

Figure 5-31 **A,** Taurodont in the mandibular third molar. **B,** Taurodont in the mandibular second molar. (**A** courtesy Dr. Margot Van Dis; **B** courtesy Dr. George Blozis.)

Figure 5-30 Talon cusp on the lingual aspect of the maxillary right lateral permanent incisor.

Dens in Dente

Dens in dente, also called **dens invaginatus,** is a developmental anomaly that results when the enamel organ invaginates into the crown of a tooth before mineralization **(Figure 5-32). Invaginate** means that one portion infolds into another portion of a struc-

ture. Radiographically a toothlike structure appears within the involved tooth. An elongated bulb or pear-shaped mass of enamel is seen in dentin surrounding a radiolucent area; hence, the name *dens in dente,* or "tooth within a tooth." This defect is typically confined to the coronal third of the tooth, but in some cases it extends to include the entire root length. Clinically the dens in dente may appear as either a normally shaped or malformed crown that exhibits a deep pit or crevice in the area of the cingulum. The invaginated toothlike structure retains a communication with the outside of the tooth via the pit or crevice visible on the crown surface.

Dens in dente customarily affects a single tooth. Anterior teeth, particularly the maxillary and mandibular incisors, are more commonly affected

A

Figure 5-33 Dens evaginatus of maxillary premolar. (Courtesy Dr. Margot Van Dis.)

B

Figure 5-32 A, Clinical illustration of dens in dente in maxillary lateral incisor. **B,** Radiograph of dens in dente in maxillary lateral incisor. (**A** courtesy Dr. George Blozis.)

than the posterior teeth. The maxillary lateral incisor is the most frequently affected tooth, and when affected it is often peg shaped.

The dens in dente is vulnerable to caries, pulpal infection, and necrosis as a result of the communication between the oral cavity and the invaginated area of the tooth. Consequently the dens in dente is often nonvital and is seen in association with a periapical lesion (periapical cyst, periapical granuloma, periapical abscess). If the dens in dente is detected shortly after eruption, a prophylactic restoration can be placed in the deep pit or crevice to prevent caries and subsequent pulpal necrosis. A nonvital dens in dente

may be treated endodontically. A malformed crown can be restored with composite materials or a full-coverage crown.

Dens Evaginatus

Dens evaginatus is an accessory enamel cusp found on the occlusal tooth surface **(Figure 5-33)**. This is a rare developmental anomaly that occurs most often on the mandibular premolars. When affected, they are called **tuberculated premolars.** Molars, cuspids, and incisors can also be affected. Dens evaginatus is thought to result from the proliferation and outpouching of enamel epithelium during tooth development.

Clinically the dens evaginatus appears as a small, rounded nodule on the occlusal surface of a mandibular premolar between the buccal and lingual cusps. A pulp horn may extend into this extra cusp. The dens evaginatus may not require treatment. However, it can cause occlusal problems, and removal may be necessary. Occlusal wear or fracture of this accessory cusp may result in pulp exposure, and endodontic treatment may be necessary.

Supernumerary Roots

Supernumerary or extra roots can involve any tooth **(Figure 5-34)**. No cause for this developmental anomaly has been identified. External pressure, trauma, and metabolic dysfunction during root development have been suggested. Supernumerary roots are not uncommon and tend to occur in teeth that exhibit root formation after birth. The multirooted teeth most often affected are the maxillary

Figure 5-34 Supernumerary roots in mandibular premolars.

Figure 5-35 Enamel hypoplasia. In this patient the enamel hypoplasia follows a pattern that is suggestive of a systemic problem such as a high fever.

and mandibular third molars. The single-rooted teeth most often affected are the mandibular bicuspids and cuspids. Supernumerary roots may exhibit dilaceration and are diagnosed radiographically.

Generally no treatment is indicated for supernumerary roots. However, they become clinically significant if extraction of the involved tooth or endodontic therapy becomes necessary.

ABNORMALITIES OF TOOTH STRUCTURE

Enamel Hypoplasia

Enamel hypoplasia is the incomplete or defective formation of enamel, resulting in the alteration of tooth form or color. **Hypoplasia** is defined as the incomplete development of an organ or tissue. Enamel hypoplasia results from a disturbance of or damage to ameloblasts during enamel matrix formation. Enamel hypoplasia can affect either the deciduous or the permanent dentition.

Numerous factors can cause enamel hypoplasia:
- Amelogenesis imperfecta
- Febrile illness (measles, chickenpox, scarlet fever)
- Vitamin deficiency (vitamins A, C, D)
- Local infection of a deciduous tooth
- Ingestion of fluoride
- Congenital syphilis
- Birth injury, premature birth
- Idiopathic factors

Enamel hypoplasia that is inherited is called **amelogenesis imperfecta** (see Chapter 6). The factors that cause enamel hypoplasia by injuring the sensitive ameloblasts during enamel formation are discussed in this chapter.

Enamel Hypoplasia Caused by Febrile Illness or Vitamin Deficiency.   Ameloblasts
are one of the most sensitive cell groups in the body. It is believed that any serious systemic disease or severe nutritional deficiency is capable of producing enamel hypoplasia. Febrile illnesses (measles, chickenpox, and scarlet fever) and vitamin deficiencies (vitamins A, C, and D) that occur during the time of tooth formation can result in a type of enamel hypoplasia characterized by pitting of the enamel. Only the crowns of teeth that are developing at the time of the febrile illness or vitamin deficiency are affected.

This type of hypoplasia usually involves the permanent central incisors, laterals, cuspids, and first molars, which are the teeth that form during the first year of life. One or more horizontal rows of tiny, deep pits are seen traversing the affected tooth surface. The number of pits and rows of pits may vary, depending on the extent and severity of injury to the ameloblasts. These enamel pits tend to stain and appear unsightly **(Figure 5-35)**.

Teeth affected with enamel hypoplasia of the pitting type may be restored with composites during childhood and later with porcelain veneers or full-crown coverage.

Enamel Hypoplasia Resulting from Local Infection or Trauma.

Enamel hypoplasia of a permanent tooth may result from infection of a deciduous tooth. A single tooth is usually affected and is referred to as a **Turner tooth**. A carious deciduous tooth with periapical involvement can disturb the ameloblasts of the underlying permanent tooth. The severity of the defect depends on the severity of the deciduous tooth infection, the degree of periapical tissue involvement, and the stage of development of the underlying permanent tooth.

The teeth most often affected are the permanent maxillary incisors and the permanent mandibular premolars. The clinical appearance of the affected tooth depends on the extent of the injury. The color of the enamel of these teeth may range from yellow to brown, or severe pitting and deformity may be involved. These enamel defects can frequently be identified radiographically before the eruption of the involved tooth. An anterior Turner tooth may be restored to provide an improved aesthetic appearance; a posterior Turner tooth may require a restoration to provide improved function.

Enamel Hypoplasia Resulting from Fluoride Ingestion.

Enamel hypoplasia resulting from **fluoride ingestion**, or **dental fluorosis**, occurs as a result of the patient ingesting high concentrations of fluoride during tooth formation, usually in drinking water. Affected teeth exhibit a mottled discoloration of enamel **(Figure 5-36)**. **Mottling** refers to irregular areas of discoloration. The more fluoride ingested, the more severe the mottling. The optimum range of fluoride is 0.7 to 1.2 parts fluoride/million gallons of water. Ingestion of water with a fluoride concentration two to three times the recommended amount results in mild fluorosis that appears as white flecks and chalky opaque areas of enamel.

Ingestion of water containing four times the recommended amount of fluoride causes brown or black staining and a pitted or overall corroded enamel appearance.

All permanent teeth are involved in this type of enamel hypoplasia. The teeth affected by fluorosis are generally decay resistant. To improve the aesthetic appearance of these teeth, bleaching, bonding, composites, porcelain veneers, or full-coverage crowns can be used.

Enamel Hypoplasia Resulting from Congenital Syphilis.

Syphilis is a contagious sexually transmitted disease caused by the spirochete *Treponema pallidum*. It is described in detail in Chapter 4. Congenital syphilis is transmitted from an infected mother to her fetus via the placenta. Children with congenital syphilis have numerous developmental anomalies and may be blind, deaf, or paralyzed. In utero infection by *Treponema pallidum* results in enamel hypoplasia of the permanent incisors and first molars. This is so rare that a lengthy discussion is not warranted.

The affected incisors are shaped like screwdrivers: broad cervically and narrow incisally, with a notched incisal edge **(Figure 5-37, A)**. They are called **Hutchinson incisors**. First molars appear as irregularly shaped crowns made up of multiple tiny globules of enamel instead of cusps **(Figure 5-37, B)**. Because of their berrylike appearance, these molars are called **mulberry molars.** Not every case of congenital syphilis exhibits these dental findings, and similarly shaped teeth may be seen in individuals without congenital syphilis.

Treatment to improve the aesthetic appearance of these teeth includes full-coverage crowns.

Enamel Hypoplasia Resulting from Birth Injury, Premature Birth, or Idiopathic Factors.

Enamel hypoplasia can occur as a result of trauma or change of environment at the time of birth or in premature infants. In addition, many cases of enamel hypoplasia do not have an identifiable cause despite careful and thorough history taking. The ameloblast is a

Figure 5-36 Mottled enamel. The discoloration of the enamel in this patient occurred as a result of high fluoride intake.

sensitive cell that is easily damaged. For this reason, even a mild illness or systemic problem can result in enamel hypoplasia. Such illnesses may be so insignificant that they are not known to the patient or remembered by the patient's parents. To improve the aesthetic appearance of these teeth, composites, porcelain veneers, or full-coverage crowns can be used.

Enamel Hypocalcification

Enamel hypocalcification is a developmental anomaly that results in a disturbance of the maturation of the enamel matrix. It usually appears as a localized, chalky white spot on the middle third of smooth crowns. The underlying enamel may be soft and susceptible to caries. The cause of enamel hypocalcification is uncertain; however, trauma during the maturation of enamel matrix has been suggested. Bleaching, composites, porcelain veneers, or full-coverage crowns can be used to improve the aesthetic appearance of these teeth.

Endogenous Staining of Teeth

Endogenous or **intrinsic staining of teeth** occurs as a result of the deposition of substances circulating systemically during tooth development. For example, ingestion of tetracycline during tooth development causes a yellowish-green discoloration of dentin that is visible through the enamel. At the time of eruption, the teeth fluoresce under ultraviolet light. Later the tetracycline is oxidized, the color changes from yellowish to brown, and the teeth no longer fluoresce. Other conditions, such as Rhesus (Rh) incompatibility (erythroblastosis fetalis), neonatal liver disease, and congenital porphyria (an inherited metabolic disease) also cause endogenous staining of teeth.

Regional Odontodysplasia

Regional odontodysplasia, or **ghost teeth**, is an unusual developmental problem in which one or several teeth in the same quadrant radiographically exhibit a marked reduction in radiodensity and a characteristic ghostlike appearance **(Figure 5-38)**. Very thin enamel and dentin are present. Occasionally the enamel is not visible on the radiograph. The pulp chambers of these teeth are extremely large. Either the teeth do not erupt, or eruption is incomplete. If ghost teeth erupt into the oral cavity, they are typically nonfunctional and malformed.

A

B

Figure 5-37 **A,** Hutchinson incisors. **B,** Mulberry molars. (Courtesy Dr. George Blozis.)

Figure 5-38 Regional odontodysplasia.

Regional odontodysplasia can affect either the deciduous or the permanent dentition. The maxilla, especially the anterior maxilla, is more often involved than the mandible. The cause of regional odontodysplasia is unknown. A vascular phenomenon has been suggested. Extraction usually is the treatment of choice for ghost teeth.

ABNORMALITIES OF TOOTH ERUPTION

Impacted and Embedded Teeth

Impacted teeth are teeth that cannot erupt because of a physical obstruction. **Embedded teeth** are those that do not erupt because of a lack of eruptive force. An impacted tooth is one of the most common developmental defects occurring in humans. Any tooth can be impacted. The most commonly impacted teeth are the maxillary and mandibular third molars, the maxillary cuspids, the maxillary and mandibular premolars, and supernumerary teeth. Impacted teeth are identified radiographically **(Figure 5-39)**.

Third molar impactions are classified according to the position of the tooth: mesioangular, distoangular, vertical, and horizontal. The most common position of an impacted third molar is mesioangular. The crown of the third molar points in a mesial direction and is in contact with the second molar, which is preventing its eruption. In a distoangular impaction, the crown of the third molar points in a distal direction toward the ramus, and the roots of the impacted tooth are adjacent to the distal root of the second molar. In a vertical impaction, the crown of the third molar is in a normal position for eruption, but eruption is prevented by the distal aspect of the second molar or by the anterior border of the ramus. In a horizontal impaction, the crown of the third molar is seen in a horizontal position relative to the inferior border of the mandible.

Teeth can be completely impacted in bone with no communication with the oral cavity, or they can be partially impacted. In a partial impaction, the tooth lies partly in soft tissue and partly in bone. Partially impacted teeth often have a communication with the oral cavity and are susceptible to infections (see Pericoronitis, Chapter 4). For unknown reasons, some completely impacted teeth undergo resorption. This resorption usually begins in the crown portion of the tooth, and the tooth is slowly replaced by bone. Radiographically this resorption should not be confused with caries. Caries of an impacted tooth is impossible, unless communication with the oral cavity occurs.

Impacted teeth are surgically removed to prevent odontogenic cyst and tumor formation, dam-

A

B

Figure 5-39 **A,** Horizontal impaction of the third molar. **B,** Mesioangular impaction of the third molar.

Figure 5-40 Ankylosis of deciduous molar. (Courtesy Dr. Margot Van Dis.)

age (resorption) to adjacent teeth, or because the bone (in some cases) may be more susceptible to fracture. Partially impacted third molars are removed to prevent infections. Studies have shown that the optimal time to extract impacted third molars is between the ages of 12 and 24 years. With increased age, a greater incidence of nerve paresthesia exists.

Ankylosed Teeth

Ankylosed or **submerged teeth** are deciduous teeth in which bone has fused to cementum and dentin, preventing exfoliation of the deciduous tooth and eruption of the underlying permanent tooth **(Figure 5-40).** Deciduous molars are most often affected by ankylosis. The cause is unknown; trauma and infection of the periodontal ligament have been suggested.

Initially the tooth erupts into the oral cavity into normal occlusion. The ankylosed tooth is not exfoliated. When the permanent teeth erupt, the permanent teeth adjacent to the ankylosed tooth have taller occlusocervical heights. Compared with the adjacent teeth, the ankylosed tooth appears submerged and has a different, more solid sound when percussed.

The presence of an ankylosed tooth is usually suspected based on the clinical appearance and is confirmed radiographically. The periodontal ligament space is lacking or indistinct because of the union of bone and cementum, and the tooth usually exhibits root resorption. Ankylosis may be seen in permanent teeth that have been avulsed and reimplanted.

Extraction of ankylosed deciduous teeth is necessary to allow eruption of the underlying permanent tooth. Extraction of ankylosed permanent teeth is often necessary to prevent malocclusion, caries, and periodontal disease.

Selected References

Books

Alley KE, Melfi RC: *Permar's oral embryology and microscopic anatomy: a textbook for students in dental hygiene,* ed 10, Baltimore, 2000, Lippincott, Williams & Wilkins.

Langlais RP, Miller CS: *Color atlas of common oral diseases,* ed 2, Baltimore, 1998, Lippincott, Williams & Wilkins.

Miller BF: *Miller-Keane encyclopedia and dictionary of medicine, nursing, and allied health,* ed 6, Philadelphia, 1997, WB Saunders.

Neville BW et al: *Oral and maxillofacial pathology,* ed 2, Philadelphia, 2002, WB Saunders.

Regezi JA, Sciubba JJ: *Oral pathology: clinical-pathologic correlations,* ed 4, Philadelphia, 2003, WB Saunders.

Regezi JA, Sciubba JJ, Posrel MA: *Atlas of oral and maxillofacial pathology,* Philadelphia, 2000, WB Saunders.

Woelfel JB, Scheid RC: *Dental anatomy: its relevance to dentistry,* ed 5, Baltimore, 1997, Lippincott, Williams & Wilkins.

Wood NK, Goaz PW: *Differential diagnosis of oral lesions,* ed 5, St Louis, 1997, Mosby.

Journal Articles

Alexander WN, Lilly GE, Irby WB: Odontodysplasia, *Oral Surg* 22:814, 1966.

Alfors E, Larson A, Sjögren S: The odontogenic keratocyst: a benign cystic tumor? *J Oral Maxillofac Surg* 42:10, 1984.

Al-Talabani NG, Smith CJ: Experimental dentigerous cysts and enamel hypoplasia: their possible significance in explaining the pathogenesis of dentigerous cysts, *J Oral Pathol* 9:82, 1980.

Baker BR: Pits of the lip commissures in Caucasoid males, *Oral Surg* 21:56, 1966.

Barker GR: A radiolucency of the ascending ramus of the mandible associated with invested parotid salivary gland material and analogous with a Stafne bone cavity, *Br J Oral Maxillofac Surg* 26:81, 1988.

Baum BJ, Cohen MM: Patterns of size reduction in hypodontia, *J Dent Res* 50:779, 1971.

Bodin I, Julin P, Thomsson M: Hyperdontia III. Supernumerary anterior teeth, *Dentomaxillofac Radiol* 10:35, 1981.

Bodin I, Julin P, Thomsson M: Hyperdontia IV. Supernumerary premolars, *Dentomaxillofac Radiol* 19:99, 1981.

Brannon RB: The odontogenic keratocyst—a clinicopathologic study of 312 cases. I. Clinical features, *Oral Surg* 42:54, 1976.

Brannon RB: The odontogenic keratocyst—a clinicopathologic study of 312 cases. II. Histologic features, *Oral Surg* 43: 233, 1977.

Buchner A, Hansen LS: Lymphoepithelial cysts of the oral cavity. A clinicopathologic study of 38 cases, *Oral Surg* 50:441, 1980.

Burton DJ, Saffos RO, Scheffer RB: Multiple bilateral dens in dente as a factor in the etiology of multiple periapical lesions, *Oral Surg* 49:496, 1980.

Carter L, Carney Y, Perez-Pudlewski D: Lateral periodontal cyst: multifactorial analysis of a previously unreported series, *Oral Surg Oral Med Oral Pathol Oral Radiol Endod* 81:210, 1996.

Cavanha AO: Enamel pearls, *Oral Surg* 19:373, 1965.

Christ TF: The globulomaxillary cyst—an embryologic misconception, *Oral Surg Oral Med Oral Pathol* 30:515, 1970.

Conklin WW: Bilateral dens invaginatus in the mandibular incisor region, *Oral Surg* 45:905, 1978.

Dachi SF, Howell FV: A survey of 3874 routine full-mouth radiographs. II. A study of impacted teeth, *Oral Surg* 14:1165, 1961.

Darling AI, Levers BGH: Submerged human deciduous molars and ankylosis, *Arch Oral Biol* 18:1021, 1973.

Dean HT, Arnold FA: Endemic dental fluorosis or mottled teeth, *J Am Dent Assoc* 30:1278, 1943.

Dehlers FAC, Lee KW, Lee EC: Dens evaginatus (evaginated odontoma), *Dent Pract* 17:239, 1967.

Delany GM, Goldblatt LI: Fused teeth: a multidisciplinary approach to treatment, *J Am Dent Assoc* 103:732, 1981.

DiFiore PM, Hartwell GR: Median mandibular lateral periodontal cysts, *Oral Surg Oral Med Oral Pathol* 63:545, 1987.

Eisenbud LE et al: Aneurysmal bone cyst of the mandible, *Oral Surg Oral Med Oral Pathol* 64:202, 1987.

el-Mofty SK, Shannon MT, Mustoe TA: Lymph node metastasis in spindle cell carcinoma arising in an odontogenic cyst, *Oral Surg Oral Med Oral Pathol* 71:209, 1991.

Everett FG, Wescott WB: Commissural lip pits, *Oral Surg* 14:202, 1961.

Fantasia JE: Lateral periodontal cyst. An analysis of 46 cases, *Oral Surg* 48:237, 1979.

Freedman PD, Lumerman H, Gee JK: Calcifying odontogenic cyst, *Oral Surg* 40:93, 1975.

Gardner DG: An evaluation of reported cases of median mandibular cysts, *Oral Surg Oral Med Oral Pathol* 65:208, 1988.

Gardner DG: The dentinal changes in regional odontodysplasia, *Oral Surg* 38:887, 1974.

Gardner DG, Girgis SS: Taurodontism, shovel-shaped incisors and the Klinefelter syndrome, *J Can Dent Assoc* 8:372, 1978.

Gardner DG, Sapp JP: Regional odontodysplasia, *Oral Surg* 35:351, 1973.

Grahnen H, Granath LE: Numerical variations in primary dentition, *Odontol Revy* 12:342, 1961.

Grahnen H, Larsson PG: Enamel defects in deciduous dentition of prematurely born children, *Odontol Rev* 9:143, 1958.

Hamner JE III, Witko CJ, Metro PS: Taurodontism. Report of a case, *Oral Surg* 18:409, 1964.

Henderson HZ: Ankylosis of primary molars: a clinical, radiographic, and histologic study, *J Dent Child* 46:117, 1979.

Hernandez GA et al: Aneurysmal bone cyst versus hemangioma of the mandible, *Oral Surg Oral Med Oral Pathol* 76:790, 1993.

Holt RD, Brook AH: Taurodontism: a criterion for diagnosis and its prevalence in mandibular first molars in a sample of 1115 British school children, *J Int Assoc Dent Child* 10:41, 1979.

Howell RE et al: CEA immunoreactivity in odontogenic tumors and keratocysts, *Oral Surg Oral Med Oral Pathol* 66:576, 1988.

Jasmin J, Ionesco-Benaiche N, Muller M: Latent fluorides: report of a case, *J Dent Child* 62:220, 1995.

Keith A: Problems relating to the teeth of the earlier forms of prehistoric man, *Proc R Soc Med* 6(part 3):103, 1913.

Kelly JR: Gemination, fusion, or both? *Oral Surg* 45:326, 1978.

King RC, Smith BR, Burk JL: Dermoid cyst in the floor of the mouth, *Oral Surg Oral Med Oral Pathol* 78:567, 1994.

Kitchin PC: Dens in dente, *J Dent Res* 15:1176, 1935.

Krolls SO, Donalhue AH: Double-rooted maxillary primary canines, *Oral Surg* 49:379, 1980.

Leamas R, Jimenez-Planas A: Taurodontism in premolars, *Oral Surg Oral Med Oral Pathol* 75:501, 1993.

Mathewson RJ, Siegel MJ, McCanna DL: Ankyloglossia: a review of the literature and a case report, *J Dent Child* 33:238, 1966.

Mellor JK, Ripa LW: Talon cusp: a clinically significant anomaly, *Oral Surg* 29:224, 1970.

Milazzo A, Alexander SA: Fusion, gemination, oligodontia and taurodontism, *J Pedodontics* 6:194, 1982.

Mlynarczyk G: Enamel pitting: a common symptom of tuberous sclerosis, *Oral Surg Oral Med Oral Pathol* 71:63, 1991.

Morningstar CH: Effect of infection of deciduous molar on the permanent tooth germ, *J Am Dent Assoc* 24:786, 1937.

Partridge M, Towers JF: The primordial cyst (odontogenic keratocyst): its tumor-like characteristics and behavior, *Br J Oral Maxillofac Surg* 25:271, 1987.

Pendrys DG: Dental fluorosis in perspective, *J Am Dent Assoc* 122:63, 1991.

Ray GE: Congenital absence of permanent teeth, *Br Dent J* 90:213, 1951.

Reaume CE, Sofie VL: Lingual thyroid: review of the literature and a report of a case, *Oral Surg* 45:841, 1978.

Redman RS: Respiratory epithelium in an apical periodontal cyst of the mandible, *Oral Surg Oral Med Oral Pathol* 67:77, 1989.

Rushton MA: Invaginated teeth (dens in dente): contents of the invagination, *Oral Surg* 11:1378, 1958.

Rushton MA: Odontodysplasia: "ghost teeth," *Br Dent J* 119:109, 1965.

Sapp PJ, Stark M: Self-healing traumatic bone cysts, *Oral Surg Oral Med Oral Pathol* 69:597, 1990.

Shafer WG: Dens in dente, *NY Dent J* 19:220, 1953.

Suchina JA, Ludington JR Jr, Madden RM: Dens invaginatus of a maxillary lateral incisor: endodontic treatment, *Oral Surg Oral Med Oral Pathol* 68:467, 1989.

Tolson G et al: Report of a lateral periodontal cyst and gingival cyst in the same patient, *J Periodontol* 67:541, 1996.

Trope M: Root resorption of dental and traumatic origin: classification based on etiology, *Pract Periodontics Anesthet Dent* 10(4):515, 1998.

van Gool AV: Injury to the permanent tooth germ after trauma to the deciduous predecessor, *Oral Surg* 35:2, 1973.

Vorheis JM, Gregory GT, McDonald RE: Ankylosed deciduous molars, *J Am Dent Assoc* 44:68, 1952.

Weinmann JP, Svoboda JF, Woods RW: Hereditary disturbances of enamel formation and calcification, *J Am Dent Assoc* 32:397, 1945.

Yip WK: The prevalence of dens evaginatus, *Oral Surg* 38:80, 1974.

Yoshikazu S, Tanimoto K, Wada T: Simple bone cyst: evaluation of contents with conventional radiography and computed tomography, *Oral Surg Oral Med Oral Pathol* 77:296, 1994.

Zegarelli DJ, Zegarelli EV: Radiolucent lesions in the globulomaxillary region, *J Oral Surg* 31:767, 1973.

Review Questions

1. Which term refers to a defect present at birth?
   A. Anomaly
   B. Inherited defect
   C. Congenital defect
   D. Developmental defect
   E. Embryonic defect

2. Which term refers to the origin and tissue formation of teeth?
   A. Odontogenesis
   B. Dentinogenesis
   C. Amelogenesis
   D. Cementogenesis
   E. Stomatogenesis

3. Which term refers to the joining of teeth by cementum *only*?
   A. Fusion
   B. Gemination
   C. Twinning
   D. Concrescence
   E. Hypodontia

4. Which teeth are most often missing?
   A. Canines
   B. Deciduous second molars
   C. Lateral incisors
   D. Premolars
   E. Third molars

5. Which tooth is the most common supernumerary tooth?
   A. Mandibular lateral incisors
   B. Distomolar
   C. Paramolar
   D. Hutchinson incisor
   E. Mesiodens

6. Which teeth most often appear smaller than normal?
   A. Mandibular premolars
   B. Maxillary premolars
   C. Mandibular lateral incisors
   D. Mandibular third molars
   E. Maxillary lateral incisors

7. Which term refers to the developmental anomaly that arises when a single tooth germ attempts to divide and results in the incomplete formation of two teeth?
   A. Fusion
   B. Gemination
   C. Concrescence
   D. Dilaceration
   E. Osteogenesis

8. Which term refers to the developmental anomaly that arises from the union of two normally separated adjacent tooth germs?
   A. Twinning
   B. Gemination
   C. Concrescence
   D. Dilaceration
   E. Fusion

9. Which term refers to an abnormal angulation or curve in the root or crown of a tooth?
   A. Fusion
   B. Gemination
   C. Concrescence
   D. Dilaceration
   E. Twinning

10. Which term refers to a developmental anomaly in which teeth exhibit elongated, large pulp chambers and short roots?
    A. Dens in dente
    B. Dens evaginatus
    C. Taurodontism
    D. Dilaceration
    E. Concrescence

11. Which *developmental* anomaly is often associated with a nonvital tooth and periapical lesions?
    A. Dens in dente
    B. Dens evaginatus
    C. Taurodontism
    D. Talon cusp
    E. Radicular cyst

12. Which of the following teeth most often exhibit supernumerary roots?
    A. Maxillary first premolars
    B. Maxillary third molars
    C. Mandibular first molars
    D. Maxillary first molars
    E. Maxillary second molars

13. Which one of the following describes the appearance of enamel hypoplasia resulting from a febrile illness or vitamin deficiency?
    A. Pitting defects
    B. Yellowish-brown discoloration
    C. Blackish-brown staining
    D. Chalky white spots
    E. Opalescent dentin

14. Which one of the following is associated with enamel hypoplasia resulting from congenital syphilis?
    A. Turner tooth
    B. Hutchinson incisors
    C. Taurodont
    D. Dens evaginatus
    E. Dens invaginatus

15. Which one of the following describes the appearance of enamel hypocalcification?
    A. Pitting defects
    B. Yellowish-brown discoloration
    C. Blackish-brown stains
    D. Chalky white spots
    E. No clinical change

16. Which term describes a tooth that has not erupted because of the lack of eruptive force?
    A. Ankylosed
    B. Impacted
    C. Embedded
    D. Fused
    E. Congenital defect

17. Which teeth are most often impacted?
    A. Distomolars
    B. Maxillary and mandibular first molars
    C. Mandibular cuspids
    D. Mandibular bicuspids
    E. Mandibular third molars

18. Which term describes a tooth in which bone has fused to cementum and dentin and prevents the eruption of an underlying permanent tooth?
    A. Concrescence
    B. Embedded
    C. Impacted
    D. Fused
    E. Ankylosed

19. Which cyst is *not* an odontogenic cyst?
    A. Dentigerous cyst
    B. Primordial cyst
    C. Median palatal cyst
    D. Lateral periodontal cyst
    E. Follicular cyst

20. The most common cause of the radicular cyst is:
    A. Caries
    B. Trauma
    C. Malignant infiltration
    D. Food impaction
    E. Open contact

21. Which cyst is an odontogenic intraosseous cyst that forms around the crown of a developing tooth?
    A. Coronal cyst
    B. Dentigerous cyst
    C. Lateral periodontal cyst
    D. Eruption cyst
    E. Primordial cyst

22. Which cyst develops in place of a tooth?
    A. Dentigerous cyst
    B. Primordial cyst
    C. Follicular cyst
    D. Odontogenic keratocyst
    E. Fissural cyst

23. Which cyst is characterized by its unique histologic appearance and frequent recurrence?
    A. Residual cyst
    B. Stafne bone cyst
    C. Odontogenic keratocyst
    D. Eruption cyst
    E. Primordial cyst

24. The lateral periodontal cyst is defined by its location. In which area is the lateral periodontal cyst most commonly found?
    A. Mandibular third molar area
    B. Maxillary tuberosity area
    C. Between the maxillary premolars
    D. Between the mandibular cuspid and first premolar
    E. Between the maxillary cuspid and first premolar

25. The teeth are vital with all of the following cysts except:
    A. Nasopalatine canal cyst
    B. Cyst of the palatine papilla
    C. Dentigerous cyst
    D. Median mandibular cyst
    E. Radicular cyst

26. Which cyst is characteristically pear shaped?
    A. Globulomaxillary cyst
    B. Median palatal cyst
    C. Incisal canal cyst
    D. Median mandibular cyst
    E. Nasopalatine cyst

27. Which cyst was probably a radicular cyst left behind after the extraction of the offending tooth?
    A. Periodontal cyst
    B. Gingival cyst
    C. Odontogenic cyst
    D. Residual cyst
    E. Eruption cyst

28. With which cyst may the patient complain of dysphagia?
    A. Thyroglossal tract cyst
    B. Median palatal cyst
    C. Static bone cyst
    D. Traumatic bone cyst
    E. Stafne bone cyst

29. Which cyst is considered a pseudocyst?
    A. Odontogenic keratocyst
    B. Dentigerous cyst
    C. Lymphoepithelial cyst
    D. Primordial cyst
    E. Traumatic bone cyst

30. In addition to the odontogenic keratocyst, which lesion would the hygienist suspect if a radiograph revealed a multilocular radiolucency?
    A. Globulomaxillary cyst
    B. Aneurysmal bone cyst
    C. Stafne bone cyst
    D. Radicular cyst
    E. Dentigerous cyst

31. Which term refers to the adhesion of the tongue to the floor of the mouth?
    A. Ankylosis
    B. Ankyloglossia
    C. Anodontia
    D. Amelogenesis
    E. Glossodynia

32. Which location is the most common for lip pits?
    A. Commissure
    B. Philtrum
    C. Nasolabial groove
    D. Labiomental groove
    E. Midline of lower lip

33. Which term refers to an ectopic mass of thyroid tissue located on the dorsal tongue?
    A. Thyroid cyst
    B. Thyroid tumor
    C. Lingual tonsil
    D. Lingual thyroid
    E. Thyroglossal cyst

34. Which term refers to the total absence of all teeth?
    A. Anodontia
    B. Hypodontia
    C. Hyperdontia
    D. Microdontia
    E. Odontodysplasia

35. Which term refers to the lack of one or more teeth?
    A. Anodontia
    B. Hypodontia
    C. Hyperdontia
    D. Microdontia
    E. Partial anodontia

36. Which tooth is the second most common supernumerary tooth?
    A. Taurodont
    B. Mesiodens
    C. Paramolar
    D. Distomolar
    E. Maxillary lateral incisor

37. Which term refers to abnormally small teeth?
    A. Taurodontia
    B. Macrodontia
    C. Microdontia
    D. Hypodontia
    E. Dens invaginatus

38. Which term refers to abnormally large teeth?
    A. Taurodontia
    B. Acromegaly
    C. Microdontia
    D. Hypodontia
    E. Macrodontia

39. Which location is the most likely for an enamel pearl?
    A. Maxillary molars
    B. Maxillary second premolar
    C. Mandibular premolars
    D. Mandibular molars
    E. Maxillary first premolar

40. Which location is the most likely for a talon cusp?
    A. Canines
    B. Incisors
    C. Molars
    D. Premolars
    E. Mandibular incisors

41. Which term refers to an accessory cusp located on the occlusal surface of a tooth?
    A. Mulberry cusp
    B. Talon cusp
    C. Dens invaginatus
    D. Dens evaginatus
    E. Supernumerary cusp

42. Which term refers to the enamel hypoplasia of a permanent tooth that results from infection of a deciduous tooth?
    A. Hutchinson tooth
    B. Talon tooth
    C. Turner tooth
    D. Gorlin tooth
    E. Ghost tooth

43. Which term refers to the irregular areas of discoloration that result from fluoride ingestion?
    A. Pitting defects
    B. Developmental defect
    C. Endogenous staining
    D. Extrinsic staining
    E. Mottling defect

44. Which term refers to teeth that appear ghostlike on a dental radiograph?
    A. Taurodontism
    B. Enamel hypocalcification
    C. Regional odontodysplasia
    D. Enamel hypoplasia
    E. Supernumerary teeth

45. Which term refers to teeth that cannot erupt because of physical obstruction?
    A. Fused
    B. Ankylosed
    C. Embedded
    D. Impacted
    E. Occlusal trauma

Chapter 5 Synopsis

Condition/ Disease	Cause	Age/Race/Sex	Location
Ankyloglossia	Developmental	*	Tongue/floor of mouth
Commisural Lip Pits	Developmental	*	Commisures of the lip (corners of the mouth)
Lingual Thyroid	Developmental	*	Posterior, dorsal tongue
Dentigerous Cyst	Developmental	Young adults	Around the crown of an unerupted, impacted, or developing tooth
Eruption Cyst	Developmental	Children	Soft tissue around the crown of an erupting tooth
Primordial Cyst	Developmental	Young adults	Develops in place of a tooth Mandibular third molar area most common site
Odontogenic Keratocyst	Developmental (dental lamina)	Age: most common 20–30	Posterior mandible most common site
Lateral Periodontal Cyst	Developmental (dental lamina)	M > F Median age 50–60	Lateral aspect of tooth root Mandibular cuspid—premolar area
Gingival Cyst	Developmental (dental lamina)	Median age 50–60	Soft tissue of mandibular cuspid—premolar area

*Specific information not included in text.

Clinical Features	Radiographic Features	Microscopic Features	Treatment	Diagnostic Process
Complete or partial fusion of the lingual frenum of the tongue to the floor of the mouth	N/A	N/A	Surgical removal of a portion of the lingual frenum	Clinical
Tiny blind tracts are present in the corners of the lips	N/A	N/A	None	Clinical
A mass of tissue at the midline posterior to the circumvallate papillae	N/A	Normal thyroid tissue	Usually none, may be the individual's only functioning thyroid tissue Removal may be indicated if the mass is large	Clinical Laboratory (to identify thyroid tissue)
When large, can displace teeth	Well-defined unilocular radiolucency	Cyst lined by cuboidal to squamous epithelium	Removal of cyst and associated tooth	Radiographic Microscopic
Swelling at site of erupting tooth	N/A	Cyst lined by cuboidal to squamous epithelium	Usually none Tooth erupts through cyst	Clinical Radiographic (erupting tooth)
Asymptomatic	Well-defined radiolucency	Cyst lined by cuboidal to squamous epithelium	Surgical removal of the cyst	Radiographic Microscopic
When large, may cause buccal expansion	Well-defined, usually multilocular radiolucency	Cyst lined by thin corrugated parakeratotic squamous epithelium 8-10 cell layers thick Prominent, palisaded basal cell layer with flat interface between the epithelium and connective tissue	Surgical removal of the cyst with peripheral osseous curettage (recurrence high)	Microscopic
Asymptomatic	Unilocular or multilocular radiolucency	Cyst lined by thin nonkeratinized squamous epithelium with focal thickenings	Surgical removal	Microscopic Radiographic
Bulge or swelling of gingival papilla or alveolar mucosa	N/A	Cyst lined by thin nonkeratinized squamous epithelium that may have focal thickenings	Surgical removal	Clinical Microscopic

Continued

Chapter 5 Synopsis—cont'd

Condition/ Disease	Cause	Age/Race/Sex	Location
Nasopalatine Canal Cyst (Nasopalatine Duct Cyst)	Developmental	M > F Age: most 40–60	Anterior maxilla Nasopalatine canal– incisive papillae area
Median Palatine Cyst	Developmental	*	Midline of hard palate posterior to the palatine papilla
Globulomaxillary Cyst	Unclear	*	Between maxillary lateral and cuspid
Median Mandibular Cyst	Unknown	*	Midline of mandible

Nasolabial Cyst	Developmental	F:M 4:1
		Age: adults
		  40–50 years
			Soft tissue of face
			Nasolabial fold area (maxillary canine-floor
			  of the nose area)

Lymphoepithelial Cyst	Developmental (epithelium
	  trapped in lymph node)
		*	Major salivary glands
			Soft tissue of neck
			Intraoral: lateral border of tongue and floor
			  of the mouth

Epidermal Cyst	Epithelium of hair follicle	*	Skin of the face and neck
Dermoid Cyst	Developmental	Present at birth or young child	Anterior floor of mouth

Thyroglossal Tract Cyst (Thyroglossal Duct Cyst)	Developmental	Under 20 years
		  of age
			Along the thyroglossal tract from the foramen
			  cecum to the normal location of the
			  thyroid gland below the hyoid bone

*Specific information not included in text.

Clinical Features	Radiographic Features	Microscopic Features	Treatment	Diagnostic Process
Asymptomatic Pink bulge at the incisive papillae area	Well-circumscribed radiolucency between the maxillary central incisors Open heart shaped	Cyst lined by squamous or respiratory epithelium Blood vessels and small nerves in cyst wall	Surgical removal	Radiographic Microscopic
If large—swelling at midline of hard palate	Unilocular radiolucency	Cyst lined by stratified squamous epithelium surrounded by dense fibrous connective tissue	Surgical removal	Radiographic Microscopic
Asymptomatic	Pear-shaped radiolucency	Cyst lining varies from squamous to cuboidal to respiratory epithelium	Surgical removal	Radiographic Microscopic
Asymptomatic If very large, may cause expansion of lingual aspect of mandible	Well-circumscribed radiolucency below the apices of the mandibular incisors	Cyst lined by squamous epithelium	Surgical removal	Radiographic Microscopic
Expansion or swelling in nasolabial fold area or in mucolabial fold area	N/A	Cyst lined by respiratory epithelium (Pseudostratified ciliated columnar epithelium with goblet cells)	Surgical removal	Clinical Microscopic
Intraoral: pink-yellow, well-delineated, raised nodule	N/A	Cyst lined by stratified squamous epithelium surrounded by lymphoid tissue	Surgical removal	Microscopic
Localized, firm movable swelling	N/A	Cyst lined by keratinized stratified squamous epithelium Lumen filled with keratin scales	Surgical removal	Microscopic
If large, can displace tongue Doughlike consistency	N/A	Cyst lined by stratified squamous epithelium surrounded by a connective tissue wall Hair follicles and glands seen in cyst wall	Surgical removal	Microscopic
If below the hyoid bone—bulge or swelling in the midline of the neck	N/A	Cyst lined by epithelium Thyroid tissue in connective tissue wall of cyst	Surgical removal Complete excision of cyst and tract	Microscopic

Continued

Chapter 5 Synopsis—cont'd

Condition/ Disease	Cause	Age/Race/Sex	Location
Static Bone Cyst (Developmental Salivary Gland Inclusion)	Developmental depression in mandible	*	Anterior to angle of ramus Inferior to the mandibular canal
Simple Bone Cyst (Traumatic Bone Cyst) (Hemorrhagic Bone Cyst)	Unclear Trauma suggested as possible cause	Age: teenage and young adults	Mandible
Aneurysmal Bone Cyst	Unclear Often associated with other bone lesions	Age: < 30 yr F > M	Posterior maxilla or mandible
Anodontia	Developmental	*	Throughout arches
Hypodontia	Developmental	*	Maxillary third molars Mandibular third molars Maxillary lateral incisors Mandibular second premolars
Supernumerary Teeth	Developmental	*	Maxilla > mandible
Mesiodens	Developmental	*	Near/at midline between maxillary central incisors
Distomolar	Developmental	*	Distal to third molars
Microdontia	Developmental	*	Maxillary lateral incisors *Peg lateral* is most common Maxillary third molars

*Specific information not included in text.

Clinical Features	Radiographic Features	Microscopic Features	Treatment	Diagnostic Process
Asymptomatic	Well-circumscribed radiolucency in the mandible below the inferior alveolar canal	Not a true cyst (pseudocyst) Normal salivary gland tissue found within depression	No treatment	Radiographic
Usually asymptomatic Occasionally— enlargement of bone	Radiolucency Characteristic scalloping around the roots of teeth	Not a true cyst (pseudocyst) Space in bone not lined by epithelium	Surgical intervention	Surgical
Expansion of involved bone	Multilocular radiolucency "Honeycomb/soap bubble" appearance	Not a true cyst (pseudocyst) Blood-filled spaces surrounded by multinucleated giant cells and cellular connective tissue	Surgical removal Curettage Cryotherapy	Microscopic
Absence of all primary or permanent teeth	All teeth absent	N/A	Prosthetic replacement of missing teeth	Clinical Radiographic
Absence of one or more teeth	Absence of one or more teeth	N/A	Prosthetic replacement of missing teeth	Clinical Radiographic
Presence of one or more extra teeth; usually smaller than normal; may be erupted or unerupted	One or more extra teeth	N/A	Extraction may be necessary	Clinical Radiographic
Most common extra tooth; may be erupted or unerupted/impacted Usually appear conical and small	Extra tooth seen at the midline of the anterior maxilla	N/A	Extraction No treatment	Clinical Radiographic
Second most common supernumerary tooth May be erupted (appears small) or impacted	Extra tooth distal to third molar	N/A	No treatment Extraction	Clinical Radiographic
Affected tooth appears smaller than normal One or more teeth may be affected	Tooth smaller than normal	N/A	If erupted, restore to resemble a normal-sized tooth	Clinical Radiographic

Continued

Chapter 5 Synopsis—cont'd

Condition/ Disease	Cause	Age/Race/Sex	Location
Macrodontia	Developmental	*	Any tooth
Gemination	Developmental	*	Primary > permanent Anterior > posterior
Fusion	Developmental	*	Primary > permanent Anterior > posterior Incisors
Concrescence	Developmental	*	Maxillary molars
Dilaceration	Developmental	*	Any tooth
Enamel Pearl	Developmental	*	Maxillary molars (furcation area)
Talon Cusp	Developmental	*	Cingulum of incisors
Taurodontism	Developmental	*	Molars
Dens in Dente	Developmental	*	Anterior > posterior Maxillary and mandibular incisors Maxillary lateral incisor
Dens Evaginatus	Developmental	*	Mandibular premolars, molars, cuspids, incisors

*Specific information not included in text.

Clinical Features	Radiographic Features	Microscopic Features	Treatment	Diagnostic Process
Affected tooth appears larger than normal One or more teeth may be affected	Tooth larger than normal	N/A	No treatment	Clinical Radiographic
Tooth appears larger than normal Large crown (appears bifid) Normal number of teeth present	Appears as a single tooth with a bifid crown and one common root canal	N/A	If esthetic problem, restore to resemble normal tooth	Clinical Radiographic
Adjacent teeth appear fused together Large crown seen	Appears as a single large crown with separate or fused roots and root canals	N/A	If esthetic problem, alteration of tooth to resemble normal-sized tooth	Clinical Radiographic
Cannot observe clinically	Appears as though the roots of adjacent teeth are connected	N/A	No treatment	Radiographic
Cannot observe clinically	Appears as a sharp bend in a tooth root	N/A	No treatment	Radiographic
Cannot observe clinically	Appears as a small sphere of enamel on a tooth root	N/A	No treatment	Radiographic
Cusp that resembles the talon of an eagle is seen on the cingulum	Appears as an area of increased radiopacity	N/A	Removal of cusp and restoration of tooth if cusp interferes with occlusion	Clinical
Crown appears normal	Appears as a tooth with abnormally short roots and low furcation area Pulp chamber is abnormally large	N/A	No treatment	Radiographic
Tooth may appear normal or peg shaped	Enamel invagination noted with crown of involved tooth	N/A	If tooth is vital, placement of a prophylactic restoration If nonvital, root canal therapy	Clinical Radiographic
Accessory enamel cusp seen on occlusal surface	May see pulp horn extending into accessory cusp	N/A	No treatment	Clinical

Continued

Chapter 5 Synopsis—cont'd

Condition/Disease	Cause	Age/Race/Sex	Location
Supernumerary Roots	Developmental	*	Maxillary and mandibular third molars, mandibular premolars and cuspids
Enamel Hypoplasia	Febrile illness or vitamin deficiency during tooth development	*	Permanent central and lateral incisors, cuspids, first molars
	Local infection or trauma during tooth development	*	Permanent maxillary incisor and mandibular premolars
	Fluoride ingestion during tooth development	*	All permanent teeth
	Congenital syphilis	*	Permanent incisors and molars
	Birth injury, premature birth, and idiopathic factors	*	Any teeth
Enamel Hypocalcification	Trauma to enamel during maturational phase	*	Any teeth
Endogenous Staining of Teeth	Ingestion of tetracycline or systemic disturbance during tooth development	*	Any teeth
Regional Odontodysplasia	Developmental	*	Several teeth in the same quadrant Primary or permanent teeth Maxilla > mandible
Impacted Teeth	Developmental	*	Maxillary and mandibular third molars Maxillary cuspids
Ankylosed Teeth	Developmental	*	Most common in deciduous molars

*Specific information not included in text.

Clinical Features	Radiographic Features	Microscopic Features	Treatment	Diagnostic Process
Cannot observe clinically	Visible extra root(s)	N/A	No treatment	Radiographic
Crowns have one or more rows of tiny deep pits and stains	N/A	N/A	If necessary, restoration can be placed to improve appearance	Clinical
Crowns have a yellowish-brown color; pitting and enamel deformity may be present	N/A	N/A	If necessary, restoration can be placed to improve appearance	Clinical
Crowns have a mottled discoloration ranging from chalky white spots to brown-black staining	N/A	N/A	Restoration or bleaching can be used to produce a more aesthetic appearance	Clinical
Hutchinson incisors are screwdriver shaped Mulberry molars resemble berries	N/A	N/A	Full-coverage crowns	Clinical
Crowns may have pitting, grooves, or staining	N/A	N/A	If necessary, restoration can be placed to improve appearance	Clinical
Crowns have chalky white spots on the middle third			If necessary, restoration can be placed to improve appearance	
With tetracycline staining, crowns appear yellowish green or brownish gray	N/A	N/A	If necessary, restoration can be used to improve appearance	Clinical
Affected teeth do not erupt or eruption is incomplete	Reduced radiodensity of involved teeth Teeth appear "ghostlike" with large pulp chambers and thin enamel	*	Extraction	Clinical Radiographic
Teeth do not erupt	Impacted teeth are surrounded by bone	N/A	Surgical removal	Clinical Radiographic
A primary ankylosed tooth prevents the eruption of the permanent tooth	Ankylosed teeth do not exhibit a periodontal ligament space	N/A	Extraction	Clinical Radiographic

Chapter 6

Genetics

Heddie O. Sedano

Objectives

After studying this chapter, the student will be able to:

1. Define each of the words listed in the vocabulary for this chapter.
2. State the purpose of mitosis.
3. State the purpose of meiosis.
4. Explain what is meant by the Lyon hypothesis and give an example of its clinical significance.
5. Explain what is meant by a gross chromosomal abnormality and give three examples of syndromes that result from gross chromosomal abnormalities.
6. List the four inheritance patterns.
7. Explain what is meant by X-linked inheritance.
8. State the inheritance pattern and describe the oral manifestations and, if appropriate, the characteristic facies for each of the following: cyclic neutropenia, Papillon-Lefèvre syndrome (PLS), cherubism, chondroectodermal dysplasia (Ellis-van Creveld syndrome), mandibulofacial dysostosis (Treacher Collins syndrome), osteogenesis imperfecta, hereditary hemorrhagic telangiectasia (Osler-Rendu-Parkes Weber syndrome), Peutz-Jeghers syndrome, white sponge nevus (Cannon disease), hypohidrotic ectodermal dysplasia, hypophosphatasia, and hypophosphatemic vitamin D–resistant rickets.
9. State the inheritance pattern, the oral or facial manifestations, and the type and location of the malignancy associated with each of the following syndromes: Gardner syndrome; nevoid basal cell carcinoma syndrome (Gorlin syndrome); multiple mucosal neuromas, medullary carcinoma of the thyroid gland, and pheochromocytoma syndrome (multiple endocrine neoplasia type 2B [MEN 2B]); and neurofibromatosis of von Recklinghausen.
10. State the location and malignant potential of the intestinal polyps in Peutz-Jeghers syndrome and Gardner syndrome.
11. List the four types of amelogenesis imperfecta.
12. Briefly compare and contrast dentinogenesis imperfecta, amelogenesis imperfecta, and dentin dysplasia, including the inheritance patterns, the clinical manifestations, and the radiographic appearance of each.

Vocabulary

Alleles (ah-lēlz′) Genes that are located at the same level or locus in the two chromosomes of a pair and that determine the same functions or characteristics.

Amino acid (ah-me′no as′id) Organic compound containing the amino group NH_2; amino acids are the main component of proteins.

Autosomes (aw′to-sōmz) (adjective, autosomal) Nonsex chromosomes, which are identical for men and women.

Barr body (bahr bod′e) Condensed chromatin of the inactivated X chromosome, which is found at the periphery of the nucleus of cells in women.

Carrier (kar′e-er) In genetics, a heterozygous individual who is clinically normal but who can transmit a recessive trait or characteristic; also, a person who is homozygous for an autosomal dominant condition with low penetrance.

Centromere (sen′tro-mēr) Constricted portion of the chromosome that divides the short arms from the long arms.

Chromatid (kro′mah-tid) Either of the two vertical halves of a chromosome that are joined at the centromere.

Chromatin (kro′mah-tin) General term used to refer to the material (deoxyribonucleic acid [DNA]) that forms the chromosomes.

Codon (ko′don) Vertical sequence of three bases in DNA that codes for an amino acid.

Consanguinity (kon″san-gwin′ĭ-te) Blood relationship; in genetics the term is generally used to describe a mating or marriage between close relatives.

DNA; deoxyribonucleic acid (de-ok″se-ri″bo-nu-kle′ik as′id) A substance composed of a double chain of polynucleotides; both chains coiled around a central axis form a double helix; it is the basic genetic code or template for amino acid formation.

Diploid (dip′loid) Having two sets of chromosomes; the normal constitution of somatic cells.

Dominant (dom′ĭ-nant) In genetics a trait or characteristic that is manifested when it is carried by only one of a pair of homologous chromosomes.

Expressivity (eks″pres-siv′ĭ-te) Degree of clinical manifestation of a trait or characteristic.

Facies (fa′she-ēz) Appearance of the face.

Gamete (gam′ēt) Spermatozoon or ovum.

Genetic heterogeneity (je-net′ik het″er-o-jĕ-ne′ĭ-te) Having more than one inheritance pattern.

Haploid (hap′loid) Cell with a single set of chromosomes; a gamete is haploid.

Heterozygote (het″er-o-zi′gōt) (adjective, heterozygous) Individual with two different genes at the allele loci.

Homozygote (ho″mo-zi′gōt) (adjective, homozygous) Individual having identical genes at the allele loci.

Hypohidrosis (hi′po-hǐ-dro′sis) Abnormally diminished secretion of sweat.

Hypotrichosis (hi′po-trǐ-ko′sis) Presence of less than the normal amount of hair.

Karyotype (kar′e-o-tīp) Photomicrographic representation of a person's chromosomal constitution arranged according to the Denver classification.

Locus (lo′kus) (plural, loci) Position occupied by a gene on a chromosome.

Meiosis (mi-o′sis) Two-step cellular division of the original germ cells, which reduces the chromosomes from 4nDNA to 1nDNA.

Metaphase (met′ah-fāz) Phase of cellular division in which the chromosomes are lined up evenly along the equatorial plane of the cell and in which the chromosomes are most visible.

Mitochondria (mi″to kon′dre-ĕ) Cytoplasmic organelles that have their own DNA in a circular chromosome.

Mitochondrial DNA (mi″to kon′dre-ĕl DNA) Unique DNA that is maternally inherited.

Mitosis (mi-to′sis) Way in which somatic cells divide so that the two daughter cells receive the same number of identical chromosomes.

Mutation (mū-ta′shun) Permanent change in the arrangement of genetic material.

Oogenesis (o″o-jen′ĕ-sis) Process of formation of female germ cells (ova).

Ovum (o′vum) (plural, ova) Egg; mature feminine germ cell.

Penetrance (pen′ĕ-trans) Frequency with which a heritable trait is exhibited by individuals carrying the gene or genes that determine that trait.

Phenotype (fe′noh-tīp) Entire physical, biochemical, and physiologic makeup of an individual; genotype is the genetic composition, and phenotype is its observable appearance.

Recessive (re-ses′iv) Trait or characteristic that shows clinically when a double-gene dose (homozygous) exists in autosomic chromosomes or a single-gene dose exists in males if the trait is X linked.

RNA; ribonucleic acid (ri″bo-noo-kle′ik as′id) Single strands of polynucleotides found in all cells; different types of RNA have different functions in the production of proteins by the cell.

Ribosome (ri′bo-sōm) Cytoplasmic organelles in which proteins are formed based on the genetic code provided by RNA.

Spermatogenesis (sper″mah-to-jen′ĕ-sis) Process of formation of spermatozoa (sperm).

Spermatozoon (sper″mah-to-zo′on) (plural, spermatozoa) Mature male germ cell.

Syndrome (sin′drōm) Set of signs or symptoms (or both) occurring together.

Translocation (trans″lo-ka′shun) Portion of a chromosome attached to another chromosome.

Trisomy (tri′so-me) Pair of chromosomes with an identical extra chromosome.

Genetics is the science that studies inheritance and the expression of inherited traits. The main objectives of this chapter are to introduce some of the basic concepts of genetics and present the clinical manifestations of some inherited oral disorders of interest to the dental hygienist. The descriptions of many syndromes are included. As explained in previous chapters, a **syndrome** is a distinctive association of signs and symptoms occurring together in the same patient. The syndromes included in this chapter are inherited. However, other syndromes, such as acquired immunodeficiency syndrome (AIDS), are acquired, not inherited. In addition, the fact that an alteration is found as part of a syndrome does not mean that it cannot also occur independently. For example, cleft lip and palate occur as components of several syndromes and can also occur independently. The classification of syndromes is difficult because they are composed of several associated anomalies and because the anomalies that compose the syndrome may not be present consistently in all patients with the same syndrome.

The term **phenotype** is used often in this chapter. It refers to the physical, biochemical, and physiologic traits of an individual. A phenotype can occur as a result of genetic factors or from a combination of genetic factors and environmental influences.

In this chapter, as in previous chapters, basic concepts are discussed first. These concepts are followed by descriptions of specific inherited disorders.

Chromosomes

The hereditary units that are transmitted from one generation to another are called **genes**. They are found on **chromosomes**, which are located in the

Figure 6-1 High-power photomicrograph shows a dividing cell with visible chromosomes and nuclei of cells with scattered chromatin.

nucleus of the cell. Using a microscope, one can see chromosomes clearly only when the nucleus and cell are dividing **(Figure 6-1).** At other times the genetic material is dispersed in the nucleus (see Figure 6-1). Each cell of the human body, with the exception of mature germ cells (ova and spermatozoa), has 46 chromosomes. Half of these chromosomes are derived from the father and the other half from the mother. Chromosomes contain **DNA,** which directs the production of amino acids, polypeptides, and proteins by the cell. In addition, DNA has the ability to duplicate itself (self-replication). It creates exact copies of itself, and through the process of cell division, cells identical to the original cell are formed.

Normal Cell Division

MITOSIS

All cells in the body, with the exception of ova and spermatozoa, are called **somatic cells.** Cellular division is achieved by **mitosis** during a part of the somatic cell's life span, called the **mitotic cycle.** The function of mitosis is to create an exact copy of each chromosome and, through division of the original cell, distribute an identical set of chromosomes to each daughter cell. After each cell division is completed and before the next division can occur, the cell enters the **gap 1 (G₁)** phase, which is followed by the **S phase,** in which replication of the DNA takes place. The **gap 2 (G₂)** phase follows the S phase and ends when mitotic division begins. The cell cycle is illustrated in **Figure 6-2.**

Stages of Mitosis

Mitosis is composed of four stages: (1) metaphase, (2) prophase, (3) anaphase, and (4) telophase. In each of these four stages, the chromosomes are distributed in a specific arrangement. In **metaphase,** the chromosomes stain intensely and are arranged almost symmetrically at both sides of the center, or **equatorial plane,** of the cell. The appearance of a metaphase chromosome resembles the letter *X* **(Figure 6-3),** having a pair of "long arms" also known as *q arms* (see Figure 6-3, *3*) and a pair of "short arms" also known as *p arms* (see Figure 6-3, *1*). The size of the chromosome at metaphase and the length of the long and short arms vary from chromosome to chromosome. The constriction present in all chromosomes, which joins the short and long arms, is called the **centromere** (see Figure 6-3, *2*). During metaphase, chromosomes are actually formed by two identical vertical halves, each composed of either left or right short and long arms and half of the centromere. Each of these identical halves is called a **chromatid** (see Figure 6-3, *4*). At metaphase, each chromatid contains one molecule of DNA, and therefore the DNA content of each chromosome is doubled **(Figure 6-4).** When cell division takes place, each chromosome splits vertically at the centromere; 46 chromatids (which now become chromosomes) form one daughter cell, and the other 46 chromatids form a second daughter cell. During **prophase** the chromosomes are lining up toward metaphase; in **anaphase** and **telophase** the chromatids are in the process of splitting.

MEIOSIS

Primitive germ cells (oogonia, spermatogonia) have 46 chromosomes. Mature germ cells (ova, spermatozoa) have 23 chromosomes. **Meiosis** is a two-step special type of cell division in which the primitive germ cells reduce their chromosome number by half and become mature germ cells. The primitive germ cells have two chromosomes for each pair and are

Mitotic   G1   S (replication)   G2   Mitotic
division   division

Figure 6-2 Schematic representation of the mitotic cycle shows the end of mitosis, followed by the G_1, S, and G_2 phases and the next mitosis.

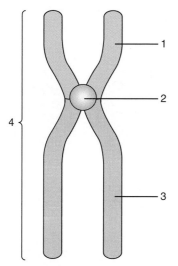

Figure 6-3 Autosomal chromosome at metaphase shows **(1)** short arm, **(2)** centromere, **(3)** long arm, and **(4)** chromatid.

1nDNA + 1nDNA + 1nDNA + 1nDNA

4nDNA

Figure 6-4 Pair of autosomal chromosomes at metaphase. Each chromatid represents 1nDNA.

called **diploid.** The suffix *ploid* refers to the number of sets of chromosomes, and its prefix refers to the degree of ploidy. In diploid, *di* indicates two. The mature germ cells (or gametes) have half the number of chromosomes and are called **haploid.** During the period in which the cell is not in division, the DNA content of diploid cells is designated 2nDNA, and in metaphase it is double or 4nDNA. After the two stages of meiosis have been completed, the 4nDNA is reduced to 1nDNA. The two steps are called **first meiosis** and **second meiosis.** This reduction is necessary to maintain the normal number of human chromosomes. A new embryo must have 46 chromosomes per cell as did its parents. Therefore the union of germ cells needs to result in 46 chromosomes. If two cells with 46 chromosomes were combined, the resulting cell would have 92 chromosomes.

First Meiosis

Before the first meiosis in the primitive germ cells, a replication of DNA occurs that is similar to that observed in the S phase of somatic cells. After replication the members of each pair of chromosomes line up next to each other in an intimate point-by-point relationship (**Figure 6-5,** *A*). This pairing does not occur in mitosis. After pairing, the two chromosomes establish actual contact at different locations. These contacts are known as **chiasmata** (meaning X shaped) and determine points of crossing over (**Figure 6-5,** *B*). This crossing over achieves the exchange of chromosome segments between a chromatid of one chromosome and a chromatid of the other chromosome of a pair (between homologous chromosomes) (**Figure 6-5,** *C*). This special aspect of

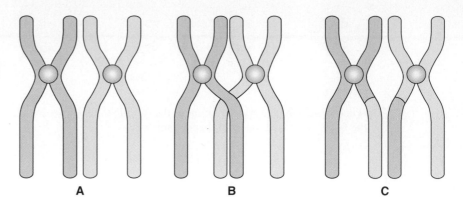

Figure 6-5 Homologous autosomal chromosomes line up in first meiosis **(A)**, cross over during metaphase of first meiosis **(B)**, and exchange segments after crossing over **(C)**.

the first meiosis takes place at metaphase. After metaphase of the first meiotic division, the chromosomes separate from each other but no splitting of the centromere occurs. The chromosomes remain intact, and each member of the pair migrates to one of the new cells, each of which contains 23 chromosomes but twice the final amount of DNA. During this migration, chromosomes of the paternal and maternal lines segregate at random, thus ensuring diversity of the species by creating a new combination of chromosomes.

Occasionally the chromosomes that were crossing over do not separate, and both migrate to the same cell. This is known as nondisjunction and results in the formation of a germ cell with an extra chromosome. If this occurs and that cell (either an ovum or a spermatozoon) participates in the formation of an embryo, three chromosomes **(trisomy)** instead of two result. An example of this type of abnormality is **Down syndrome,** also called **trisomy 21,** in which three of chromosome 21 are found instead of two. Trisomy has been reported for several different chromosomes.

In a female embryo, **oogenesis (ovum development)** starts around the third month of prenatal life, and the future ova remain in suspended crossing over from about the time of birth until the time ovulation starts. At the beginning of ovulation, the first meiosis is completed. Nondisjunction is more prevalent in female oogenesis than in male spermatogenesis. This is probably because of the period of prolonged crossing over; therefore the older the woman, the greater the chance of shedding a trisomic ovum and of bearing a child with Down syndrome or other trisomy.

Figure 6-6 Two haploid cells after second meiosis, each having 1nDNA.

Second Meiosis

The second stage of meiosis is essentially a mitotic division in which each chromosome splits longitudinally. No replication of DNA occurs before the second meiosis. After the splitting, two cells are formed, each containing the right amount of DNA (1nDNA) **(Figure 6-6).** Nondisjunction can occur during the first and second meiosis. If it occurs in second meiosis, a chromosome does not split, and one daughter cell has a full chromosome and the other has none.

Immediately after fertilization, the chromosomes of the ovum and spermatozoon, each having 1nDNA, condense independently and form round structures, each known as a pronucleus. The DNA in these

— Cytoplasm

— Nucleus

Barr body —

Figure 6-7 Buccal smear shows Barr body (*arrow* points to small dark dot on nuclear membrane) at the periphery of the nucleus of a desquamated epithelial cell from a woman's buccal mucosa. (Courtesy Dr. Carl J. Witkop.)

pronuclei replicates, forming a set of 23 full chromosomes for each, the maternal and paternal pronuclei. When the membranes of these pronuclei break, the 46 chromosomes mix at random, initiating the first cellular division (mitosis) that starts the development of the new embryo.

Lyon Hypothesis

The sex chromosomes are designated XX in women and XY in men. During the early period of embryonic development (possibly by the end of the second week), the genetic activity of one of the X chromosomes in each cell of a female embryo is inactivated. The inactivation is a random process affecting either the X chromosome derived from the mother or the X chromosome derived from the father. Activated chromosomes are dispersed in the nucleus. The inactivated chromosome remains contracted when the cell is not dividing and forms a structure known as the **Barr body.**

In female cells the Barr body can easily be seen under the light microscope, especially in cytologic smears, including those obtained from the oral mucosa. The Barr body appears as a dark dot at the periphery of the nucleus **(Figure 6-7)**.

This inactivation of one of the X chromosomes in a female embryo was postulated by Mary Lyon and is known as the **Lyon hypothesis.** This hypothesis has interesting clinical implications for female carriers of conditions caused by genes located on the X chromosome, which are explained later in this chapter.

Molecular Composition of Chromosomes

DEOXYRIBONUCLEIC ACID (DNA)

Chromosomes contain DNA. DNA contains the basic code or template that carries all genetic information. The basic unit of DNA is called a

nucleotide, which is formed by a nitrogen-containing base, a five-carbon sugar (deoxyribose), and a phosphate. Four bases are found in DNA: adenine (A), guanine (G), thymine (T), and cytosine (C). These chains of polynucleotides are coiled to form a structure called a *double helix* **(Figure 6-8)**. In DNA the base adenine is always bound to the base thymine, and guanine is always bound to cytosine. This is a constant arrangement and is identical in all species from bacteria to humans, with just a few exceptions. Therefore the ratio of adenine to thymine (A/T) is always equal, and the same is true for the ratio of guanine to cytosine (G/C). In humans, G/C pairs are about four times greater than A/T pairs. The polynucleotide chains run vertically in opposite directions. Therefore a sequence of adenine, guanine, and cytosine (AGC) is always matched by the sequence of thymine, cytosine, and guanine (TCG).

In the linear representation shown, the number 1 indicates the nucleotide of one chain and the number 2 indicates the nucleotide of the other chain. A molecule of hydrogen (H) binds both nucleotides. This arrangement is repeated horizontally to form the polynucleotide double spiral staircase (or helix) appearance of DNA (Figure 6-8).

The vertical sequence of three bases is called a codon. It codes for an amino acid. Several amino acids form a polypeptide, and one or more polypeptides form a protein. A gene is often equated with the unit that forms a polypeptide.

DNA has the unique capability of self-replication, which is achieved by unwinding its double chain like the plaits of a braid. Each separated chain serves as a blueprint for another chain.

Mitochondrial DNA is found in the circular chromosome of the mitochondria, and it is maternally inherited. This is the DNA present in the cytoplasmic mitochondrial organelles of the ovum. Mitochondrial DNA is passed from the mother to all her offspring regardless of sex.

RIBONUCLEIC ACID (RNA)

To produce amino acids, polypeptides, and proteins, the genetic code contained in the DNA is transcribed into **RNA**, which differs from DNA in that it is a single strand (in its simplest form), its sugar is a ribose (the sugar in DNA is deoxyribose), and the base uracil (U) replaces the thymine (T) in DNA.

Figure 6-8 Schematic representation of the DNA double helix.

Types of RNA

The four types of RNA are (1) messenger RNA (mRNA), (2) transfer RNA (tRNA), (3) ribosomal RNA (rRNA), and (4) heterogeneous RNA (hnRNA). RNA can be found in both the nucleus and the cytoplasm of a cell.

The first type of RNA, **mRNA**, is a blueprint of the genetic DNA for the coding of proteins. It carries the message for the DNA to ribosomes in the cytoplasm, in which proteins are produced. The second type of RNA, **tRNA**, transfers amino acids from the cytoplasm to the mRNA, positioning amino acids in the proper sequence to form polypeptides and hence proteins. The third type of RNA, **rRNA**, combines with several polypeptides to form ribosomes. The fourth type of RNA, **hnRNA**, is found within the nucleus and is the precursor of mRNA.

In the production of a protein **(Figure 6-9)**, the mRNA carries the genetic code for the formation of that protein to the ribosomes. The tRNA brings amino acids to the ribosomes from the cellular cytoplasm. The amino acid sequence forms proteins according to the genetic code, and these proteins exit the ribosomes as they are formed.

NUCLEUS   **CYTOPLASM**

Figure 6-9 Production (synthesis) of protein from DNA.

Genes and Chromosomes

Genes in a chromosome are located in a vertical linear manner. The genes in both members of a pair of chromosomes (homologous chromosomes) govern the same functions or dictate the same characteristics. The genes that are located at the same level (or **locus**) in homologous chromosomes and that dictate the same functions or characteristics are called **alleles.**

The manifestations **(phenotype)** of a gene action are not necessarily the same from one individual to another. This is best explained with the ABO blood group system. The locus can be occupied by either the factor that determines the blood group A or the factor that determines the blood group B. If it is empty, it results in the blood group O. The locus is always the same, and the three genes govern the same function; however, the clinical result is different. In this situation the trait or condition is said to have multiple alleles. For example, if both loci are AA, or if they are AO, the person is said to have blood group A. If both loci are BB or BO, the person is said to have blood group B. If the loci are AB or BA, the person is said to have blood group AB. Only if both the loci are empty does the person have blood group O. The locus always controls blood group, but the group is dependent on the alleles that are present or lacking in each person.

When the allelic genes are identical, the person is said to be homozygous for that gene, or a homozygote. Using the ABO blood group system again, for example, a person with AA, BB, and OO would be homozygous. When the genes are different (for example, AB, AO, or BO) the person is said to be heterozygous for that gene, or a heterozygote. If a gene can express its effect clinically with a single dose (heterozygous), as in the combination AO = blood group A, the characteristic is said to be dominant. If the gene needs a double dose to exhibit its action (homozygous), the resulting characteristic or function is said to be recessive. For example, only the combination OO results in the blood group O.

CHROMOSOMAL ABNORMALITIES

Abnormalities of chromosomes can be divided into two categories: (1) molecular abnormalities and (2) gross abnormalities. Molecular alterations occur at the DNA level and are not detectable microscopically. Most inherited disorders represent examples of molecular changes (mutations) at the level of one or both allelic genes. Examples of these conditions are presented later in this chapter.

Gross chromosomal alterations can be observed in a karyotype. A **karyotype (Figures 6-10 and 6-11)** is a photographic representation of a person's chromosomal constitution. Clinicians can create a karyotype by culturing cells from blood, skin, or other tissues. One method uses peripheral blood by placing it in a test tube with heparin to avoid coagulation and centrifuging it. After centrifugation, the white blood cells (leukocytes) are deposited at the bottom of the tube. The leukocytes are removed and are placed in a culture medium containing phytohemagglutinin, which is a substance that enhances mitosis. Because chromosomes are best observed when cell division is arrested at metaphase, colchicine is added to the culture after 72 hours of culture at 37° C to stop mitosis at metaphase. This also prevents the centromere from dividing. A hypotonic solution is then added to the culture to make the cells swell. The cells are then fixed (preserved) and stained and observed under the microscope. Examples of well-defined mitoses are chosen and photographed. The photograph is enlarged, and each chromosome is cut out of the photographic print. When stained, the chromosomes have a bandlike appearance that allows an accurate identification of each. These cutouts are then pasted on a special chart to construct the karyotype.

Figure 6-10 Karyotype from a female shows the 22 pairs of autosomal chromosomes and the pair of X chromosomes. (Courtesy Dr. Jaroslav Cervenka.)

Figure 6-11 Karyotype from a male shows the 22 pairs of autosomal chromosomes and the X and Y chromosomes. (Courtesy Dr. Jaroslav Cervenka.)

GROSS CHROMOSOMAL ABNORMALITIES

Alterations in Number and Structure of Chromosomes

Gross chromosomal abnormalities are caused by either alterations in chromosome number, which are almost always a result of nondisjunction (explained earlier), or alterations in structure, which develop because of chromosomal breaks or abnormal rearrangements. The following illustrate alterations in number:

- Euploid: A complete second set of chromosomes, the total number being 92. This is incompatible with life.
- Polyploid: Three (triploid) or four (tetraploid) complete sets of chromosomes. This has been occasionally described in humans and is incompatible with life.
- Aneuploid: Any extra number of chromosomes that do not represent an exact multiple of the total chromosome complement, for example, trisomy (a pair with an identical extra chromosome) and monosomy (a missing chromosome from a pair).

Examples of structural abnormalities include the following:

- Deletion: The loss of part of a chromosome.
- Translocation: A portion of a chromosome attached to another chromosome.
- Inversion: A portion of a chromosome is upside-down.
- Duplication: A chromosome is larger than normal, the extra segment being identical to a segment of the normal chromosome.

Clinical Syndromes Resulting from Gross Chromosomal Abnormalities

Trisomy 21

This condition, also known as **Down syndrome,** is the most frequent of the trisomies. Ninety-five percent of cases of Down syndrome are the result of nondisjunction, mostly associated with late maternal age at the time of conception.

Slanted eyes characterize the **facies** (the appearance of the face). Patients are generally shorter than normal, and heart abnormalities are present in more than 30% of individuals with trisomy 21. The

Figure 6-12 Newborn with trisomy 13. Cleft lip, frontal hemangioma, and abnormal position of fingers should be noted.

intelligence level varies from near normal to marked retardation.

Fissured tongue is frequently seen in patients with trisomy 21. Premature loss of teeth, especially the mandibular central incisors, caused by alveolar bone loss is frequently seen. Gingival and periodontal disease has been reported in 90% of affected individuals. Hypodontia (fewer teeth than normal), abnormally shaped teeth, and anomalies in eruption with malposition and crowding of teeth are common findings. Dental hygienists play an important role in the maintenance of oral health in these patients.

Trisomy 13

This disorder is characterized by multiple abnormalities in various organs. Seventy percent of live-born infants die within the first 7 months of life. Characteristic clinical findings include bilateral cleft lip and palate, microphthalmia or anophthalmia (small eyes or no eyes), superficial hemangioma of the forehead or nape of the neck, growth retardation, severe mental retardation, polydactyly of hands and feet (supernumerary digits), clenching of the fist with the thumb under the fingers, rocker-bottom feet, heart malformations, and several anomalies of the external genitals. The facial appearance is quite striking because of the cleft lip, cleft palate, and ocular abnormalities **(Figure 6-12).**

Turner syndrome

Patients with Turner syndrome have a female phenotype, and in the majority of cases the karyotype has the normal 44 autosomic chromosomes and only one

X chromosome. A normal female would have two X chromosomes: one from the mother and one from the father. Most cases of Turner syndrome are due to nondisjunction of the X chromosome in the paternal gamete. Clinically these women are of short stature and have webbing of the neck and edema of the hands and feet **(Figure 6-13)**. They frequently exhibit a low hairline on the nape of the neck. The chest is broad with wide-spaced nipples. The aorta is frequently abnormal, and body hair is sparse. The external genitals appear infantile, and generally the ovaries are not developed; therefore these individuals have primary amenorrhea (abnormal temporary or permanent cessation of the menstrual cycle). Smears taken from the oral mucosa demonstrate the lack of Barr bodies.

Klinefelter syndrome

This condition occurs when an ovum carrying two X chromosomes is fertilized by a spermatozoon with a Y chromosome, and therefore the fertilized ovum will have two X chromosomes plus a Y chromosome. The majority of cases result from nondisjunction of the X chromosome, generally in the ova of older women. Affected individuals have a male phenotype, and the condition cannot be detected until after puberty. These patients are taller than normal and have wide hips and a female pubic hair distribution. About 50% have gynecomastia (development of female breasts), and intelligence levels are lower than normal in 10% of affected individuals. The penis appears normal, but the testes are smaller and harder than normal and lack seminiferous tubules.

The maxilla is slightly hypoplastic (underdeveloped). Buccal smears reveal the presence of one Barr body.

Variations of Klinefelter syndrome also occur, and they are represented by karyotypes containing XXXY or XXXXY. The greater the number of X chromosomes, the more pronounced the clinical manifestations and the lower the level of intelligence. The maxilla becomes increasingly hypoplastic with increasing number of X chromosomes. Buccal smears show one Barr body for each extra X chromosome.

Cri du chat (cat cry) syndrome and Wolf-Hirschhorn syndrome

These syndromes are examples of abnormalities caused by deletions. The cri du chat syndrome results

Figure 6-13 Patient with Turner syndrome. Note the webbing of the neck.

from a deletion on the short arm of chromosome 5, and the Wolf-Hirschhorn syndrome results from a deletion on the short arm of chromosome 4. Newborns with a chromosome 5 deletion exhibit a catlike cry at birth and are mentally retarded. No oral abnormalities occur. Most newborns with the deletion in the short arm of chromosome 4 have a cleft palate and intelligence quotients of less than 30.

PATTERNS OF INHERITANCE

Because loci are present in both autosomal and X chromosomes and because of a double- and single-dose effect, four possible inheritance patterns exist. Dominant genes need only a single dose, and recessive genes need a double dose. The inheritance patterns are autosomal dominant, autosomal recessive, X-linked dominant, and X-linked recessive. Autosomal chromosomes include all chromosomes except those that determine sex (X and Y). The Y chromosome participates only in the differentiation of the masculine gonads.

Autosomal Dominant Inheritance

A condition having autosomal dominant inheritance is transmitted vertically from one generation to the next. Males and females are equally affected. When a person has a gene for the condition, the risk of having an affected offspring is 50% for each pregnancy.

Genetic risk is always a mathematical estimate of probability governed by chance. Therefore none, less than half, half, more than half, or all of the offspring could be affected by a condition that is transmitted by autosomal dominant inheritance.

An individual can carry a gene with a dominant effect without presenting any clinical manifestations. This is referred to as **lack of penetrance**. This situation can be partially explained by the presence of modifying genes in the same or other chromosomes. The clinical manifestations in autosomal dominant disorders frequently vary among affected individuals. This is known as variable expressivity. **Penetrance** refers to the number of individuals affected, and **expressivity** pertains to the degree to which an individual is affected.

Autosomal Recessive Inheritance

As stated earlier, individuals exhibiting an autosomal recessive trait must be homozygous for the gene. Clinically normal parents of affected children are heterozygous and are both carriers of the trait. They are not generally recognized as carriers until after the birth of an affected child. If the enzymatic defect is known, carriers can be recognized before the birth of a child by assessing levels of the responsible enzyme in clinically normal members of a family with the trait. For parents who are carriers of the same recessive trait, the risk of having an affected child is 25%; the risk of having a homozygotic normal child is 25%; and the chance of having a heterozygotic carrier is 50% for each pregnancy. As in other inheritance patterns, risk is a mathematical estimate of the probability of an event occurring. If both parents are homozygous (have two of the genes of the trait) for a recessive trait, they would be expected to be affected and all their children would be equally affected because they would also be homozygous (have two of the same genes) for the trait. In humans this type of situation is quite rare because individuals affected by the same recessive trait usually do not mate.

In genetics, **consanguinity** means a familial relationship and is generally used to describe matings or marriages among close relatives, usually including first cousins. In the United States, marriage or mating among very close relatives (parent-offspring, brother-sister, uncle-niece, aunt-nephew) is illegal, and in most states, marriage of first cousins is also illegal. However, consanguineous matings occur sporadically. The chances of having deleterious genes in common increases among close relatives. When consanguinity exists among the members of a family, the chance of the offspring being homozygous for a deleterious gene increases. The closer the degree of consanguinity, the greater the risk.

X-Linked Inheritance

Women have two X chromosomes and therefore can be either heterozygous or homozygous for a gene that is located on the X chromosome. Therefore in women, X-linked traits can be dominant or recessive. Men have only one X and one Y chromosome. If a deleterious gene occurs on the X chromosome in a male, the condition or trait will be seen clinically regardless of the dominant or recessive behavior of the same gene in women. The man's X chromosome is transmitted to all of his daughters and to none of his sons. The X chromosome in his sons comes from the mother. Consequently, no male-to-male (from father to son) transmission of X-linked traits occurs. Some X-linked dominant traits are lethal in males. Females probably survive because of the action of the allelic normal gene on the second X chromosome. All offspring, male and female, of a woman homozygotic for a dominant X-linked condition will be affected with the condition. This is because all her X chromosomes contain that gene (and all offspring receive an X chromosome). Because the gene is dominant, only one of the genes is necessary for that condition to occur. A mother who is a carrier of an X-linked recessive trait has a 50% risk of having an affected son and a 50% risk of having a carrier daughter. This is because both daughters and sons have a 50% risk of getting the X chromosome with the gene for that condition. Again, the reader should remember that risk is a mathematic prediction. A male affected with an X-linked trait will have no affected sons because he does not give the X chromosome to his sons. All his daughters will be carriers or affected, depending on the recessive or dominant nature of the trait, because all daughters will receive his X chromosome.

Lyon hypothesis and X-linked recessive traits

As discussed previously, according to the Lyon hypothesis, one of the X chromosomes in the female is genetically cancelled at an early stage of embryonic development. This cancellation affects X chromosomes from both maternal and paternal lines. If a female embryo is a carrier of an X-linked recessive trait, half of the X chromosomes have the normal gene and the other half have the abnormal gene (allele) for the given trait before cancellation occurs. Classic hemophilia (hemophilia A) is a good example. Hemophilia A is inherited as an X-linked recessive condition. In this disorder, blood does not coagulate because of the low or almost nonexistent levels of Factor VIII (antihemophilic globulin) in circulating blood. Males with the abnormal gene have a severe coagulation defect. In the female carrier, some of the cancelled X chromosomes have the abnormal gene and others have the normal one. The female carrier is a **mosaic,** that is, she has both normal and abnormal X chromosomes. Because cancellation is random, the number of X chromosomes that remain genetically active and contain the normal or abnormal gene will vary. The female carrier's levels of Factor VIII are often reduced; however, this reduction and the length of coagulation time will vary, depending on the number of X chromosomes that contain the abnormal gene and remain genetically active. Although female carriers of the gene for hemophilia do not have as severe a problem as males, they tend to bleed more than usual after extraction of teeth or scaling and curettage. The variation in the bleeding problem in female carriers of the gene for hemophilia reflects the Lyon hypothesis. Other inherited disorders that reflect this hypothesis are described in detail later in this chapter. They include the X-linked type of amelogenesis imperfecta and hypohidrotic ectodermal dysplasia.

Genetic Heterogeneity

The term genetic heterogeneity is used when a condition has more than one inheritance pattern as well as differences in the degree of clinical manifestations for each of the inherited varieties. Amelogenesis imperfecta (described later in the chapter) is a condition that illustrates genetic heterogeneity.

In general, alterations in structural proteins (complex substances formed by one or more polypeptide) are inherited as a dominant trait, whereas alterations in enzymatic proteins (a protein inducing changes in other body substances) are inherited in a recessive manner; however, exceptions to this rule are seen.

Physical characteristics can be inherited either as dominant or as recessive traits. The term **recessive**

does not mean deleterious or abnormal. It means instead that the individual must be homozygous for the trait for it to be seen. For example, in the ABO blood group system, blood group O is recessive, whereas groups A and B are dominant. However, no blood group is abnormal.

Genes can be codominant. Again, a good example is the ABO blood group. A and B are dominant over O, but when A and B are allelic, the result is blood group AB in which both genes are exhibited. This is called codominance.

The four inheritance patterns refer to those characteristics that are governed by the action of one gene. This is called single-gene inheritance. **Oligogenic inheritance** refers to those characteristics or traits that are inherited by the participation of several genes. These conditions show greater clinical variation than do those inherited through single-gene action. Characteristics such as tooth shape and form, as well as eye color, are determined by oligogenic inheritance. Most physical characteristics are oligogenic. The various genes that participate in determining a trait or condition can be located in the same chromosome or in different chromosomes.

Examples of Inherited Abnormalities

All the inherited disorders in this section include oral and dental alterations and are discussed by location—gingiva and periodontium, jawbones and facies, oral mucosa, and teeth. Patients affected with these genetic abnormalities should receive routine dental hygiene care to maintain oral health. Specific dental hygiene management considerations are included only if they are unique to the disorder described.

Inherited Disorders Affecting the Gingiva and Periodontium

Most of the disorders included here are rare. However, they exhibit severe gingival or periodontal alterations (or both); therefore the dental hygienist should be aware of the disorders and their clinical manifestations.

Cyclic neutropenia

The inheritance pattern of **cyclic neutropenia** is autosomal dominant. The disorder is characterized by a cyclic decrease in the number of circulating neutrophilic leukocytes (neutrophils); a decrease in the number of circulating neutrophils is called *neutropenia*. The cycles usually occur in intervals of 21 to 27 days, but in some patients the interval may be extended to several months. These episodes of neutropenia generally persist for 2 to 3 days.

The clinical manifestations are related to the decrease in neutrophils. Systemic manifestations of cyclic neutropenia include fever, malaise, sore throat, and occasional cutaneous infections. Oral manifestations consist of severe ulcerative gingivitis or gingivostomatitis **(Figure 6-14)**. In addition to the gingiva, areas of ulceration can also occur on the tongue and surfaces of the oral mucosa. The ulcers are of variable size and have a craterlike appearance. They are very painful and have a bleeding base. Generally the oral lesions are secondarily infected. When neutrophils return to normal, the oral lesions tend to improve.

Patients with cyclic neutropenia are usually managed by first determining the frequency of the cycles through periodic neutrophil counts and then by instituting preventive antibiotic therapy to protect against secondary opportunistic infections. Over time, episodes of neutropenia and associated ulcerative gingivitis lead to severe periodontal disease, with loss of alveolar bone, tooth mobility, and exfoliation of teeth. Treatment should be done when the circulating neutrophil count is normal to reduce the risk of complications such as gingival hemorrhage and secondary infection. Dental hygiene care, including frequent appointments for removal of local irritants and maintenance of optimal oral hygiene, reduces the risk of opportunistic infections in patients with cyclic neutropenia.

Recently, patients with cyclic neutropenia treated with periodic granulocyte colony-stimulating factor (G-CSF) have a reduced symptomatology and show a substantial clinical improvement.

Papillon-Lefèvre syndrome

Papillon-Lefèvre syndrome has an autosomal recessive inheritance pattern and is composed of marked destruction of the periodontal tissues (periodontoclasia) of both dentitions with premature loss of teeth and hyperkeratosis of the palms of the hands and soles of the feet (palmar and plantar hyperkeratosis).

The gene for this syndrome has been mapped to the long arm of chromosome 11 regions 14-21 (11q14-21). These patients are normal at birth except for a reddening of the palms of the hands and soles of the feet. Teeth erupt in normal sequence, position, and time. At about 1½ to 2 years of age, a marked

Figure 6-14 Hypertrophic gingivitis with areas of gingival recession is exhibited in a patient with cyclic neutropenia.

gingivoperiodontal inflammatory process develops marked by edema, bleeding, alveolar bone resorption, and mobility of teeth with consequent exfoliation. A red, scaly keratosis develops on the palms and soles concurrent with these oral lesions and occasionally extends to the dorsal surfaces of the hands and feet. The oral lesions are complicated by superimposed inflammation, and radiographs reveal marked alveolar bone resorption with vertical pockets. Teeth are lost in the same sequence in which they erupted. When the last tooth is lost, the gingiva regains a normal appearance.

The lesions on the hands and feet remain as reddish-white, scaly, thick areas of hyperkeratinization **(Figure 6-15)**. The permanent dentition begins to erupt at the proper time. At about 8 or 9 years of age, the gingivoperiodontal destruction is repeated in the same manner as occurred in the primary dentition **(Figure 6-16)**. All permanent teeth are lost before 14 years of age. The gingiva again resumes a normal appearance.

Peripheral blood neutrophil is depressed in all patients with Papillon-Lefèvre syndrome. This suggests that the neutrophils may be an important factor in the pathogenesis of severe periodontal disease in these patients. Retinoid therapy markedly improves the skin condition but has no effect on the periodontal disease in patients with this syndrome. To date, all therapeutic attempts at preventing the gingival and periodontal destruction and subsequent loss of teeth have been unsuccessful. The basic defect that causes the condition is unknown. Peripheral blood neutrophil chemotaxis has been reported to be depressed in patients with Papillon-Lefèvre syndrome. This decreased chemotaxis suggests that neutrophils may play a role in periodontal destruction in patients

Figure 6-15 Areas of hyperkeratinization of the palms are exhibited in a patient with Papillon-Lefèvre syndrome (PLS). (From Sedano HO, Sauk JJ, Gorlin RJ: *Oral manifestations of inherited disorders,* Boston, 1977, Butterworth. Used with permission.)

with this syndrome. Current research suggests bacterial and viral involvement as the initiating factors for the periodontal destruction. It has been suggested that the genetic component of Papillon-Lefèvre syndrome is a predisposition rather than the main determinant of periodontal disease.

The skin manifestations remain for life, but treatment with retinol (oral etretinate) has proved somewhat effective in controlling the hyperkeratinization. These patients do not have any other abnormalities.

Focal palmoplantar and gingival hyperkeratosis

Areas of hyperkeratinization of the palms and soles and marked hyperkeratinization of the labial and lingual gingiva characterize **focal palmoplantar** and **gingival hyperkeratosis.** This syndrome has an autosomal dominant inheritance pattern. The palmar and plantar hyperkeratosis starts at the tips of the fingers and toes and extends to the surface of the palms and soles. This process increases with age and also becomes localized, with calluses forming on the weight-bearing areas.

The oral hyperkeratinization is bandlike and a few millimeters in width **(Figure 6-17).** It follows the normal festooned contour of the gingiva. The free gingiva is not affected. Palatal and lingual mucosa can occasionally be affected with areas of hyperkeratinization. These changes start in childhood and increase with age. The rest of the oral cavity is normal.

Figure 6-16 Panoramic radiograph shows marked periodontal destruction with alveolar bone resorption in the patient in Figure 6-15. (From Sedano HO, Sauk JJ, Gorlin RJ: *Oral manifestations of inherited disorders,* Boston, 1977, Butterworth. Used with permission.)

Gingival fibromatosis

Gingival fibromatosis is a component of several inherited syndromes. The gingival hypertrophy generally develops early in life, and within a few years the teeth are completely covered. The fibromatosis is composed of very firm tissue with a granular corrugated surface. The color is generally paler than that of the normal gingiva and results from the marked collagenization of the fibrous connective tissue. The extensive gingival enlargement leads to protrusion of the lips.

In addition to isolated gingival fibromatosis **(Figure 6-18)**, which has an autosomal dominant inheritance pattern and has no other associated abnormalities, gingival fibromatosis is a component of a number of syndromes. Because of the gingival involvement, several of these syndromes, though rare, are described here. However, only those that are well known and occur most frequently are included.

In patients with gingival fibromatosis, dental hygiene care can reduce the risk of secondary inflammation and infection.

Laband syndrome

The inheritance pattern of **Laband syndrome** is autosomal dominant. In addition to gingival fibromatosis, patients have dysplastic or absent nails and malformed nose and ears because of soft and pliable cartilage formation, hepatosplenomegaly (enlarged liver and spleen), and hypoplasia of terminal phalanges of the fingers and toes with a resultant frog-like appearance.

Gingival fibromatosis with hypertrichosis, epilepsy, and mental retardation syndrome

This syndrome has an autosomal dominant inheritance pattern. Hypertrichosis (excessive growth of hair), especially of the eyebrows, extremities, genitals, and sacral region, characterize gingival fibromatosis with hypertrichosis, epilepsy, and mental retardation. Epilepsy and mental retardation can also occur in this syndrome but are inconsistent features.

Gingival fibromatosis with multiple hyaline fibromas

Gingival fibromatosis with multiple hyaline fibromas has an autosomal dominant inheritance pattern and is also known as the **Murray-Puretic Drescher syndrome.** In addition to gingival fibromatosis, it is characterized by hypertrophy of the nail beds and multiple hyaline fibrous tumors developing on the nose, chin, head, back, fingers, thighs, and legs. These tumors on the extremities can produce contractures of various joints, including hips, knees, shoulders, and elbows.

Inherited Disorders Affecting the Jaw Bones and Facies

Cherubism

The inheritance pattern of **cherubism** is autosomal dominant with marked penetrance (when the gene is present, the clinical manifestations are usually seen) in males and variable expressivity and incomplete penetrance in females. The gene for cherubism has been mapped to the short arm of chromosome 4 region 16 (4p16). The first clinical manifestation is a progressive bilateral facial swelling that appears when the patient is between 1½ and 4 years of age. This change can affect either the mandible or the maxilla, but involvement of the mandible is most common. Displacement of the eyes is evident when the maxilla is affected. This, added to the bilateral deformity, produces the

Figure 6-17 Marked hyperkeratosis follows the normal contour of the gingiva in focal palmoplantar and gingival hyperkeratosis. (From Sedano HO, Sauk JJ, Gorlin RJ: *Oral manifestations of inherited disorders,* Boston, 1977, Butterworth. Used with permission.)

Figure 6-18 Gingival hypertrophy is shown in a patient with isolated gingival fibromatosis.

characteristic cherubic facial appearance that is responsible for the name of the syndrome. Increased distance between the eyes (ocular hypertelorism) is always present in affected patients. Radiographs of the jaws show a typical "soap-bubble" or multilocular appearance **(Figure 6-19)**, which usually occupies the ascending ramus of the mandible and extends into the molar and premolar areas. Severe cases can involve the full mandible, but the condyle is always spared. When the maxilla is affected, the changes are observed at the level of the tuberosity and involve the antrum.

These areas of bone radiolucency are occupied by fibrous connective tissue containing multinucleated giant cells. The microscopic appearance resembles the central giant cell granuloma (described in Chapter 2). The bone lesions interfere with tooth development and eruption. Most of these patients have **pseudoanodontia** (teeth falsely appear to be lacking), especially of molars and premolars, because of delayed eruption.

The size of the jaws tends to increase rapidly until about puberty and then generally remains stable. After the individual reaches age 20 or 30 years, radiographs show an almost normal bone appearance, with a few areas of increased bone density. The facial deformity remains for life, and in some patients it can be quite striking.

Chondroectodermal dysplasia

Chondroectodermal dysplasia, also known as the **Ellis-van Creveld syndrome,** has an autosomal recessive inheritance pattern. The gene for this syn-drome has been mapped to the short arm of chromosome 4 region 16 (4p16). Affected individuals are dwarfs because of distal shortening of the extremities. One third of these patients are mildly retarded. The hands show polydactyly (supernumerary digits) on the ulnar side, and fingernails and toenails are hypoplastic and deformed. Other skeletal anomalies include curvature of the legs and feet. Fifty percent of affected individuals have congenital heart defects. Anomalies of the external genitals, especially in males, are also observed.

The oral manifestations are constant and characteristic and include fusion of the anterior portion of the maxillary gingiva to the upper lip from canine to canine. Thus the anterior maxillary vestibular sulcus is lacking **(Figure 6-20)**. This anomaly induces a V-notch appearance in the midline of the upper lip. The anterior lower alveolar ridge presents a serrated appearance caused by thick frenula, which start at the vestibular sulcus and traverse the alveolar ridge. The central incisors of both maxilla and mandible are generally lacking and are replaced by a centrally located abnormal tooth. Most of the teeth have a conical shape and exhibit enamel hypoplasia. More than 50% of newborns with this syndrome have natal teeth.

Cleidocranial dysplasia

The inheritance pattern of **cleidocranial dysplasia** is autosomal dominant; however, about half the cases are isolated examples caused by either spontaneous mutation or a gene with poor penetrance. The gene for this syndrome has been mapped to the short arm

Figure 6-19 Panoramic radiograph of the jaws shows typical bilateral soap-bubble image in a patient with cherubism. (From Young WG, Sedano HO: *Atlas of oral pathology,* Minneapolis, 1981, University of Minnesota Press. Used with permission.)

of chromosome 6 region 21 (6p21). The cranium develops a mushroom shape because the fontanelles remain open. This makes the face appear small. Frontal, parietal, and occipital enlargement is quite noticeable. Skull radiographs reveal the open fontanelles, which are often open for life. The paranasal sinuses are lacking or hypoplastic. The neck is long and narrow because of unilateral or bilateral aplasia (lack of development) or hypoplasia of the clavicles. Affected individuals are able to approximate their shoulders to the midline because of this clavicular alteration. Various other bone anomalies can also be present.

The premaxilla is generally underdeveloped, resulting in pseudoprognathism. These patients have many supernumerary teeth, sometimes even simulating a third dentition **(Figure 6-21)**. These teeth are crowded in the jaws and do not erupt. They also interfere with the eruption of normal teeth, resulting in pseudoanodontia. A lack of cellular cementum has been reported in patients with this syndrome. Multiple cysts can develop in association with the impacted teeth. About 1% of affected patients have cleft lip, cleft palate, or both.

Gardner syndrome

Gardner syndrome, also known as **familial colorectal polyposis,** has an autosomal dominant inheritance pattern with variable expressivity and marked penetrance. The adenomatous polyposis coli (APC) gene is responsible for Gardner syndrome and is located on the long arm of chromosome 5 regions 21-22 (5q21-22). One of the basic components is the presence of osteomas in various bones, especially the frontal bones, mandible, and maxilla. Osteomas of the facial skeleton, when expanding, will obliterate the sinuses and induce facial asymmetry. Osteomas also can occur in the long bones of the skeleton but with less frequency than in the bones of the face.

In addition to osteomas, multiple odontomas can occur in the jawbones, especially the mandible **(Figure 6-22)**. Teeth can exhibit hypercementosis and can fail to erupt.

The most serious component of this syndrome is the presence of intestinal polyps, which become malignant at age 30 and after. Polyposis primarily affects the colon and rectum and generally develops before puberty. Some authors advocate intestinal resection when the polyps appear because their malignant transformation into adenocarcinoma is invariable, especially with increasing age.

Mandibulofacial dysostosis

The inheritance pattern of **mandibulofacial dysostosis** is autosomal dominant with incomplete penetrance and variable expressivity. The gene for this syndrome has been mapped to the long arm of chromosome 5 regions 32-33.1 (5q32-33.1). The facies shows downward sloping of the palpebral fissures, a hypoplastic nose, hypoplastic malar bones with hypoplasia or absence of the zygomatic process, abnormal and misplaced ears, and a receding chin. The mouth appears fishlike, with downward sloping of the lip commissures. The lower eyelids show a cleft (coloboma) of

Figure 6-20 Infant with Ellis-van Creveld syndrome (chondroectodermal dysplasia). The anterior maxillary vestibular sulcus is absent.

Figure 6-21 Multiple extracted supernumerary teeth from a patient with cleidocranial dysplasia.

the outer third, with a lack of lashes medial to it. The ears may exhibit tags, which on occasion can also be seen near the angle of the mouth.

Deafness is a constant feature resulting from a lack of otic ossicles. Mental development is within normal limits; difficulty in learning arises from deafness. Oral manifestations include a markedly hypoplastic mandible with flattened condyles and coronoid processes and an obtuse mandibular angle. Teeth are malposed, and malocclusion with open bite is quite evident. The palate is high or a cleft is present in about 30% of affected patients **(Figure 6-23)**. Gingival disease is common and is related to the dental abnormalities.

Nevoid basal cell carcinoma syndrome

The **nevoid basal cell carcinoma syndrome,** also known as **Gorlin syndrome,** has an autosomal dominant inheritance pattern with high penetrance and variable expressivity. The gene for this syndrome maps to the long arm of chromosome 9 region 22.3 (9q22.3). The facies is characterized by mild hypertelorism (increased distance between the eyes) and mild prognathism, with frontal and parietal enlargement and a broad nasal root.

The cutaneous manifestations, which are called *nevi,* are typically basal cell carcinomas. The term *nevus* (plural, *nevi*), as defined here, is a congenital lesion characterized by skin pigmentation. These basal cell carcinomas appear early in life and continue to develop over the nose, eyelids, cheeks, neck, arms, and trunk. They can be flesh colored or pale brown and develop singly or in clusters. Histologically they are basal cell carcinomas. The palms and soles show small pits that become filled with dirt and appear as dark spots on those surfaces.

The oral manifestations of this syndrome consist of multiple cysts of the jaws **(Figure 6-24)** that (histologically) are odontogenic keratocysts (see Chapter 5). These cysts vary in size; they can be very large and have a marked tendency to recur after surgical removal. Occasionally an ameloblastoma arises in these cysts as part of this syndrome. The cysts develop as early as 5 to 6 years of age in some affected patients and interfere with normal development of the jawbones and teeth.

A great variety of skeletal anomalies have been reported in association with the nevoid basal cell carcinoma syndrome, the most constant being bifurcation or splaying of one or more ribs. Other frequent abnormalities of bone include shortening of the metacarpals, spina bifida occulta (defective closure of the bone encasement of the spinal cord), and kyphoscoliosis (a combination of scoliosis, which is a lateral curving of the spine, and kyphosis, which is an abnormal vertical curvature of the spine or "hunchback").

Many different neoplasms have been reported in association with this syndrome. Medulloblastoma (brain tumor) has been seen in many cases. Children surviving the medulloblastoma eventually present other manifestations of the syndrome. Other less frequent findings include calcified ovarian fibromas and mesenteric cysts.

Figure 6-22 Panoramic radiograph of a patient with Gardner syndrome shows multiple osteomas and odontomas. (Courtesy Dr. Carl J. Witkop.)

Osteogenesis imperfecta

Osteogenesis imperfecta is known to have an autosomal dominant inheritance pattern with variable expressivity. However, only 30% of patients have a family history of this condition. The remaining 70% represent sporadic cases and cases suggesting autosomal recessive inheritance. The basic defect is produced by different mutations affecting the genes that encode for type I collagen, resulting in abnormally formed bones that fracture easily. The genes responsible for the inherited varieties of osteogenesis imperfecta are mapped as follows: collagen type I alpha 2 is in the long arm of chromosome 7 region 22.1 (7q22.1), collagen type I alpha 1 is in the long arm of chromosome 17 region 21.31-22.05 (17q21.31-22.05). Osteogenesis imperfecta occurs in about 1 in 20,000 births, and major syndromes have been classified in four types: I, II, III and IV.

The clinical manifestations are markedly variable from patient to patient. The sporadic cases tend to be more severe than those with an autosomal dominant inheritance pattern. The basic defect involves collagen and results in abnormally formed bones that fracture easily. Multiple bone fractures are the main clinical complication of this syndrome. In the congenital form, newborns can have several fractured bones at birth. Infants with this condition have experienced fractures just by being moved. In the most severe cases, all bones can be affected, presenting a plethora of abnormalities, including bowing of the legs, curvature of the spine (kyphosis and scoliosis), deformity of the skull, shortening of arms and legs, and other abnormalities. In the mildest cases, individuals show only blue sclerae (a blue appearance of the white of the eye).

The oral manifestation of this syndrome is a dentinogenesis imperfecta–like condition (a description of dentinogenesis imperfecta follows later in this chapter). Primary teeth are affected in 80% of patients, whereas permanent teeth are affected in only 35% of these individuals **(Figure 6-25)**. The crowns, roots, and pulp chambers are generally smaller than normal. Teeth appear opalescent or translucent at

Figure 6-23 Markedly high-arched palate and malpositioned teeth in a patient with mandibulofacial dysostosis.

Figure 6-24 Multiple mandibular radiolucencies in a patient with nevoid basal cell carcinoma syndrome. These lesions are odontogenic keratocysts.

time of eruption, but they darken with age. The enamel is lost because the abnormal dentin cannot provide adequate support.

Torus mandibularis

Mandibular tori (singular, torus) have an autosomal dominant inheritance pattern with variable expressivity and marked penetrance. This anomaly can be unilateral or bilateral. These tori occur on the lingual aspect of the mandible in the area of the premolar teeth **(Figure 6-26)**. Occurrence before age 15 years is extremely rare. The size of the torus is variable, and occasionally it can be multilobulated. Mandibular tori are symptomless and generally require no treatment. Surgical removal may be necessary if the patient needs a denture. Intraoral radiographs usually show a radiopacity in the area of the mandibular premolars if mandibular tori are present. (Mandibular tori are also discussed in Chapters 1 and 7.)

Torus palatinus

Autosomal dominance with variable expressivity and almost 100% penetrance characterizes **torus palatinus.** A bony overgrowth occurs at the midline of the hard palate **(Figure 6-27)**. A marked predilection exists for women (2:1), and a higher prevalence exists among Native Americans, including Inuits. Torus palatinus becomes evident around the time of puberty and is only rarely seen in children younger than 14 years of age. The size of this anomaly varies from nearly undetectable to large masses that occupy almost the entire hard palate. Some palatal tori are multilobular. Torus palatinus is symptomless. However, the surface mucosa is thin and easily traumatized. The torus may need to be removed if the patient needs a full denture. (Torus palatinus is also described in Chapters 1 and 7.)

Maxillary exostosis

Exostoses have an autosomal dominant inheritance pattern. **Maxillary exostoses** represent tori that generally develop on the buccal aspect of the maxillary alveolar ridge, usually in the molar and premolar area **(Figure 6-28)**. They are generally symptomless unless traumatized. They may be single, multiple, unilateral, and bilateral and occur less frequently than either palatal or mandibular tori. (Exostoses are also described in Chapters 1 and 7.)

Inherited Disorders Affecting the Oral Mucosa

Isolated cleft palate and cleft lip with or without cleft palate

The majority of cases of facial clefting are multifactorial in origin; they occur in about 1 in 800 births. A large number of inherited syndromes can include cleft lip and palate or isolated cleft palate as a component. When clefting is part of an inherited syndrome, its occurrence within affected families will be in accordance with the inheritance pattern of the

Figure 6-26 Bilateral lobulated mandibular tori.

Figure 6-27 Torus palatinus.

Figure 6-25 Patient with osteogenesis imperfecta. Teeth are yellowish with chipped enamel.

syndrome. The majority of these syndromes are very rare. **Cleft lip-palate** and **congenital lip pits** (Van der Woude syndrome) is the syndrome that is considered to occur most frequently; therefore it is the only one described here. It has an autosomal dominant inheritance pattern with 80% penetrance for any of its components. In the majority of cases the gene has been mapped to the long arm of chromosome 1 regions 32 to 41 (1q32-41). The labial pits **(Figure 6-29)** are bilateral and are located near the midline of the vermilion border of the lower lip. They may be 3 mm or more in diameter and generally finish in a blind end. Occasionally, they exude saliva because of their association with a labial minor salivary gland. These pits are rarely unilateral, and the clefting is bilateral in about 80% of patients. Some patients without clefting have agenesis (lack of development) of the maxillary lateral incisors or peg lateral incisors. Other oral findings that have been seen include fibrous adhesions between the maxilla and mandible, a cleft uvula, and ankyloglossia.

Hereditary hemorrhagic telangiectasia

The inheritance pattern of **hereditary hemorrhagic telangiectasia**, also known as **Osler-Rendu-Parkes Weber syndrome**, is autosomal dominant. Recent studies indicate that this syndrome may have two different responsible loci: one at the long arm of chromosome 9 (9q3) and the other in chromosome 12. It is characterized by multiple capillary dilations of the skin and mucous membranes **(Figure 6-30)**. The skin of the face shows numerous pinpoint and spiderlike telangiectases, especially on the lips, eyelids, and around the nose. The scalp and ears are also affected. Similar lesions are present in the nasal mucosa and are responsible for frequent and sometimes serious nosebleeds **(epistaxis)** that can last for several days. Any organ or mucous membrane can be the site of telangiectasia.

Telangiectases of the oral mucosa are especially prominent on the tip and anterior dorsum of the tongue. The palate, gingiva, and buccal mucosa are often affected but to a lesser degree. Hemorrhage from sites in the oral cavity, mainly the lips and tongue, is second in frequency to epistaxis. Gingival bleeding has been reported and is a possible complication of dental hygiene treatment. The risk of gingival hemorrhage should be a concern of the dental hygienist when treating a patient with this syndrome.

Multiple mucosal neuroma syndrome

The combination of **multiple mucosal neuromas, medullary carcinoma of the thyroid gland,** and **pheochromocytoma** is identified as **multiple endocrine neoplasia, type 2B (MEN 2B).** The inheritance pattern is autosomal dominant with decreased penetrance. This syndrome is the result of mutations in the receptor tyrosine kinase (RET) that maps to chromosome 10q11.2. Patients are tall with characteristic thick, large lips and, often, everted upper eyelids. The mucosal neuromas are prominent on the lips and the anterior dorsal surface of the tongue **(Figure 6-31).** They generally appear in the first few years of life. Additionally, neuromas can occur on the buccal mucosa and also on the

Figure 6-28 Maxillary exostoses are inherited as autosomal dominant.

Figure 6-29 Paramedial pits in the lower lip. Note the scar of the repaired cleft of the left upper lip

eyelids. The mucosal neuromas are seen as multiple, mobile, firm lumps covered by normal mucosa. Histologically they are aggregates of nerve tissue.

Medullary carcinoma of the thyroid has been diagnosed in more than 75% of patients with this syndrome; it generally develops in the second decade of life. Metastatic lesions develop frequently, and about 20% of patients die as a consequence of metastasis. The thyroid carcinoma produces calcitonin (a hormone normally produced by the C cells of the thyroid gland). The carcinoma can be detected by evaluating plasma levels of this hormone.

Pheochromocytoma is a benign neoplasm that generally develops in ganglia around the adrenal glands. The tumor is often bilateral and is responsible for night sweats, high blood pressure, and episodes of severe diarrhea. It generally develops in the second or third decade of life. The pheochromocytoma induces increased urinary levels of epinephrine and other substances. Other findings in this syndrome have included cutaneous pigmentation and a host of skeletal abnormalities.

Early diagnosis of this syndrome is imperative because of the high malignant potential of the thyroid carcinoma. Some authors recommend preventive thyroidectomy when this syndrome is diagnosed so that the development of carcinoma is avoided. The neuromas of the oral mucosa may be the earliest visible manifestation of this syndrome.

Neurofibromatosis of von Recklinghausen

Neurofibromatosis of von Recklinghausen, also called **von Recklinghausen disease,** has an autosomal dominant inheritance pattern and is probably a disorder of neural crest origin. The gene for this syndrome maps to the long arm of chromosome 17 region 11.2 (17q11.2). Several varieties exist; however, only the classic form is described here.

Multiple neurofibromas, which appear as papules and growths of various sizes, are seen on the facial skin, especially the eyelids. The tumors can arise anywhere, including the oral cavity, and can be present at birth or develop early in life, increasing in number and size at puberty. Malignant transformation of the neurofibromas occurs in an estimated 3% to 15% of patients with neurofibromatosis. Neurofibromas also develop in the central nervous system, eyes, ears, viscera, and intraosseous locations. Mental retardation is occasionally observed, and multiple skeletal anomalies are common.

Oral involvement is seen in about 10% of patients and is characterized by single or multiple tumors at any location in the oral mucosa, the most frequent being the lateral borders of the tongue. Gingival neurofibromas can also occur in these patients **(Figure 6-32).** Intramandibular neurofibromas have also been reported and present as radiolucencies in the mandible.

Figure 6-30 Multiple telangiectases of lips and tongue in a patient with hereditary hemorrhagic telangiectasia. Gingival bleeding can be profuse in cases like this. (From Sedano HO, Sauk JJ, Gorlin RJ: *Oral manifestations of inherited disorders,* Boston, 1977, Butterworth. Used with permission.)

Figure 6-31 Patient with MEN 2B syndrome with multiple mucosal neuromas on the tip of the tongue and upper lip. (From Sedano HO, Sauk JJ, Gorlin RJ: *Oral manifestations of inherited disorders,* Boston, 1977, Butterworth. Used with permission.)

Café au lait (the color of coffee with milk) pigmentation of skin is present from the first decade of life in 90% of patients with neurofibromatosis. This pigmentation is quite marked in the axilla and can also affect other areas of the skin. Café au lait skin pigmentation generally precedes the development of the neurofibromas.

Peutz-Jeghers syndrome

Autosomal dominant inheritance characterizes the **Peutz-Jeghers syndrome.** The gene for this syndrome maps to the short arm of chromosome 19 region 13.3 (19p13.3). It consists of multiple melanotic macular pigmentations of the skin and mucosa, which are associated with gastrointestinal polyposis. The pigmentations occur around the eyes, nose, and mouth **(Figure 6-33).** These macules are a few millimeters in diameter and vary in number and degree of pigmentation. They tend to diminish with age. Intraorally, larger areas of pigmentation are observed on the lips and buccal mucosa of about 98% of affected patients.

Pigmentation of the hands, nasal mucosa, and eyes can also occur. The intestinal polyps are hamartomas (an abnormal growth of normal tissue in its normal location). They develop mostly in the small intestine; only rarely do they undergo malignant transformation.

White sponge nevus

Autosomal dominant inheritance with complete penetrance characterizes **white sponge nevus (Cannon disease,** or **familial white folded mucosal dysplasia).** The cause of white sponge nevus is a mutation in the mucosal keratin pair K4 or K13. The disorder can be present at birth or develop around puberty. Clinically it is characterized by a white, corrugated, soft, folding oral mucosa. The buccal mucosa is always affected, and in most patients the lesions are bilateral. A thick layer of keratin, which at times desquamates and leaves a raw mucosal surface, produces the whitening. Other areas of the oral mucosa can also be affected, but the free gingiva is spared.

Inherited Disorders Affecting the Teeth

Amelogenesis imperfecta

A group of inherited conditions affecting the enamel of teeth and having no associated systemic defects characterizes **amelogenesis imperfecta.** Witkop and Sauk classified amelogenesis imperfecta into four types:

- Type I: Hypoplastic amelogenesis imperfecta
- Type II: Hypocalcified amelogenesis imperfecta
- Type III: Hypomaturation amelogenesis imperfecta
- Type IV: Hypoplastic-hypomaturation amelogenesis imperfecta

The **hypoplastic type** of amelogenesis imperfecta is characterized by tooth enamel that does not

Figure 6-32 Multiple neurofibromas of the maxillary gingiva and palate in a patient with neurofibromatosis of von Recklinghausen.

Figure 6-33 Multiple small- to medium-sized pigmented macules on the labial mucosa of a patient with Peutz-Jeghers syndrome.

develop to a normal thickness because of failure of the ameloblasts to lay down enamel matrix properly. On radiographs the abnormal enamel contrasts normally with dentin. Several varieties of this type of amelogenesis imperfecta are further classified according to their clinical presentation: pitted, local, smooth, rough, and enamel agenesis. Combined with the clinical appearance, the classification also includes the inheritance pattern. Thus an autosomal dominant and an autosomal recessive variety exist for the local hypoplastic type. Among this group of enamel defects, the most frequent one is the pitted autosomal dominant variety **(Figure 6-34)**, which is characterized by teeth that have random pits on the enamel. The size of these pits varies from pinpoint to pinhead, and the pits are observed mostly on the labial and buccal surfaces of the permanent teeth. The pits are frequently arranged in rows or columns, or both. Occasionally, more than one tooth has a normal clinical appearance. The gene for the local hypoplastic autosomal dominant type of amelogenesis imperfecta maps to the long arm of chromosome 4 (4q11-13).

An enamel of normal thickness that is poorly calcified characterizes the **hypocalcified type** of amelogenesis imperfecta **(Figure 6-35)**. Two varieties of hypocalcified amelogenesis imperfecta exist: (1) an autosomal dominant variety and (2) an autosomal recessive variety. The autosomal recessive pattern is more severe in its clinical manifestations. At eruption, teeth present a yellow to orange enamel that is very soft and rapidly lost, leaving exposed dentin. On radiographs the enamel has a moth-eaten appearance and is less radiopaque than dentin. Cervical enamel is better calcified and generally remains on the crown. This type of amelogenesis imperfecta is frequently associated with an anterior open bite.

An enamel of mottled appearance but normal thickness characterizes the **hypomaturation type** of amelogenesis imperfecta. This type of amelogenesis imperfecta is composed of large amounts of enamel matrix; therefore the enamel is softer than normal. With pressure the tip of an explorer will penetrate the enamel. The basic defect seems to be in the enamel rod sheath. The enamel chips easily from the crown. On radiographs it has almost the same radiodensity as dentin. Four varieties of the hypomaturation type of amelogenesis imperfecta exist; however, only the snowcapped type is discussed here.

A type of hypomaturation amelogenesis imperfecta, called **snow-capped amelogenesis imperfecta,**

apparently has an X-linked recessive inheritance pattern in some families and an autosomal dominant pattern in others. Clinically, both varieties are identical and are characterized by a hypomaturation of the surface enamel of the occlusal third of all the teeth of both dentitions. The maxillary teeth are more severely affected with this whitish discoloration **(Figure 6-36)**. The enamel in those areas is of regular hardness and smooth. It does not fracture or chip from the crown.

Its association with taurodontic teeth (described later in this chapter and also in Chapter 5) characterizes the **hypoplastic-hypomaturation type** of amelogenesis imperfecta. The thin enamel is yellow to brown and pitted. On radiographs the enamel has a radiodensity similar to dentin, and single-rooted teeth have large pulp chambers.

Dentinogenesis imperfecta

Dentinogenesis imperfecta is usually subdivided into three types. One type is dentinogenesis imperfecta associated with osteogenesis imperfecta (previously described in this chapter). The other two types are not associated with osteogenesis imperfecta. The teeth in all three types have a similar clinical appearance.

Dentinogenesis imperfecta type II is also known as hereditary opalescent dentin. The inheritance pattern is autosomal dominant and the gene maps to the long arm of chromosome 4 (4q13-21). Teeth have bulbous crowns with a color that varies from opalescent brown to brownish blue **(Figure 6-37)**. The primary

Figure 6-34 Pitted autosomal dominant amelogenesis imperfecta. Multiple pits on the labial surface of the teeth should be noted. Some of the pits have been filled with composite. (From Young WG, Sedano HO: *Atlas of oral pathology,* Minneapolis, 1981, University of Minnesota Press. Used with permission.)

teeth are usually affected more severely than the permanent teeth. Twenty percent of patients have enamel hypoplasia as well. The dentin is very soft, which produces chipping of enamel that results in tooth attrition. Occasionally this attrition can cause the teeth to be worn down to the alveolar process. Radiographically no pulp chambers or root canals are seen **(Figure 6-38)**. Roots are short and thin with periapical radiolucencies. Patients may lose teeth prematurely because of complications produced by the attrition and the short roots. The basic defect lies with the odontoblasts, which lay down an abnormal matrix and then degenerate. Cells derived from the dental pulp, which lay down abnormal dentin, later replace these odontoblasts.

Dentin dysplasia

Dentin dysplasia is subdivided into type I (radicular dentin dysplasia) and type II (coronal dentin dysplasia).

Figure 6-35 Loss of enamel is exhibited in the teeth of a patient with hypocalcified amelogenesis imperfecta.

Figure 6-36 Uniform whitening of incisal edges and occlusal cusps is exhibited in a case of snow-capped amelogenesis imperfecta.

RADICULAR DENTIN DYSPLASIA. Teeth with normal crowns and abnormal roots and an autosomal dominant inheritance pattern characterize this condition. The basic defect seems to lie in a disturbance in the Hertwig epithelial root sheath, which guides the formation of the root. Radiographs show total or partial lack of pulp chambers and root canals **(Figure 6-39)**. Primary and secondary dentitions are affected equally. The color of the teeth is normal. Because of the short roots, the teeth are generally exfoliated prematurely, especially in the event of even minor trauma. The pulp chambers of the permanent teeth generally are not obliterated fully and have a half-moon appearance on the radiograph. Occasionally, periapical cysts can be associated with this condition.

CORONAL DENTIN DYSPLASIA. Dentin dysplasia type II has an autosomal dominant inheritance pattern. The basic defect in this condition is a mutation in the gene termed dentin sialophosphoprotein (DSPP) that maps to the long arm of chromosome 4 (4q13-21). Recently it has been shown that dentinogenesis imperfecta type II and dentin dysplasia type II share the DSPP gene loci and the proteins encoded by that gene. Translucent teeth with an amber color characterize the primary dentition. Radiographs show a lack

Figure 6-37 Opalescent bluish hue in the anterior teeth typical of dentinogenesis imperfecta. The yellow color seen in the molars is from exposed abnormal dentin due to loss of enamel.

of pulp chambers and small root canals. Primary teeth are quite similar to those observed in dentinogenesis imperfecta. Permanent teeth present normal crown formation with normal color. Radiographs show thistle-shaped pulp chambers in single-rooted teeth and a bow-tie appearance of the pulp chambers of permanent molars **(Figure 6-40)**. Permanent teeth may or may not have pulp stones.

Hypohidrotic ectodermal dysplasia

This syndrome represents a genetic heterogeneity. Although in the majority of families it is inherited as an X-linked recessive trait, in some families it is inherited as an autosomal recessive trait. The clinical manifestations for both the X-linked and autosomal recessive forms are identical. The gene for the X-linked variety of this syndrome maps to the long arm of the X chromosome region 12-13.1 (Xq12-13.1). The autosomal recessive variety maps to the long arm of chromosome 2 (2q11-q13).

This entity represents the most severe form of ectodermal dysplasia. Its major components are hypodontia (partial anodontia), hypotrichosis (less than the normal amount of hair), and hypohidrosis (abnormally diminished secretion of sweat). Affected children are born without lanugo (body hair present at birth), and many have episodes of fevers of unknown

causes because of the almost complete lack of sweat glands. Some patients die of hyperthermia (greatly increased body temperature) after prolonged exposure to the sun or heavy exercise. The clinical characteristics may not be apparent until the second year of life.

The facies is quite typical, with marked frontal bossing, depressed nasal bridge (saddle nose), protuberant lips, and almost complete lack of scalp hair. The hair that is present is usually blond, short, fine, and stiff. The skin is soft, thin, and very dry. Sebaceous glands are also lacking. Linear wrinkles and increased pigmentation are seen around the eyes and mouth. The eyelashes and eyebrows are often missing entirely. After puberty, the beard is generally normal, but axillary and pubic hair is scanty.

The oral manifestations of hypohidrotic ectodermal dysplasia consist of hypodontia or, rarely, anodontia. When present, incisors and canines have small, conical crowns **(Figure 6-41)**. The alveolar bone is formed only when teeth are present, and therefore patients lacking alveolar processes have loss of vertical dimension with markedly protruding lips. There may also be partial lack and aplasia of minor salivary glands in the buccal, labial, and lower respiratory tract mucosa.

Female carriers of the X-linked form of hypohidrotic ectodermal dysplasia have minor clinical

Figure 6-38 Panoramic radiograph of a patient with dentinogenesis imperfecta shows marked short roots and almost complete lack of pulp chambers. (From Young WG, Sedano HO: *Atlas of oral pathology,* Minneapolis, 1981, University of Minnesota Press. Used with permission.)

manifestations, such as thin and slightly sparse hair, cone-shaped teeth, hypodontia, and variable degrees of reduced sweating. This is in accordance with the Lyon hypothesis of variability of expression.

Hypophosphatasia

The inheritance pattern of this disorder is autosomal recessive. The gene for this syndrome maps to the short arm of chromosome 1 regions 36.1-34 (1p36.1-34). The basic defect in this condition is a decrease in serum alkaline phosphatase levels with increased urinary and plasma levels of phosphoethanolamine. Alkaline phosphatase participates in the process of calcification of bone and cementum; therefore those two tissues will be altered in patients with hypophosphatasia. Agenesis or abnormal formation of cemen-

Figure 6-39 Radiographs of a patient with radicular dentin dysplasia shows blunted and short tooth roots. The few remaining pulp chambers have a half-moon appearance. (Courtesy Dr. Carl J. Witkop.)

Figure 6-40 Obliteration and partial lack of coronal pulp chambers and small root canals can be seen in teeth of a patient affected with coronal dentin dysplasia. (Courtesy Dr. Carl J. Witkop.)

tum in these patients leads to spontaneous premature shedding of primary teeth, especially mandibular incisors **(Figure 6-42)**. Teeth are exfoliated without evidence of periodontal or gingival disease. The primary molars and permanent teeth are rarely if ever affected, which is probably associated with the greater mechanical fixation resulting from the larger size of their roots. The total lack of cementum observed in exfoliated teeth implies a lack of periodontal fiber attachment, with consequent exfoliation of single-rooted teeth. The most important alteration in this syndrome is the improper formation of mature bone. Therefore individuals who survive the neonatal period experience rachitic-like changes, such as bowing of legs and multiple fractures.

Hypophosphatemic vitamin D–resistant rickets

This condition, which is quite common, has an X-linked dominant inheritance pattern and it is the result of a mutation in the PHEX gene. It consists of low serum levels of phosphorus, which are produced by low absorption of inorganic phosphate in the renal tubules, rickets or osteomalacia, resistance to treatment with usual doses of vitamin D, and a lack of other abnormalities. Affected individuals are generally of short stature and have bowlegs, especially if the condition is present from childhood. Adult-onset forms also exist, and the clinical manifestations in these patients are minor or even lacking, with the exception of low serum levels of inorganic phosphate.

The characteristic radiographic oral findings are large pulp chambers with very long pulp horns. Additionally the dentin exhibits pronounced cracks that extend to the dentinoenamel junction. These cracks induce fracture of the enamel with microexposure of the pulp and subsequent pulpal infection.

Figure 6-41 Patient with hypohidrotic ectodermal dysplasia has only three abnormally shaped teeth.

Figure 6-43 Pegged maxillary lateral incisor. The conical shape should be noted.

Figure 6-42 Histologic section of a tooth from a patient with hypophosphatasia shows only dentin. Cementum is entirely lacking.

Figure 6-44 Intraoral radiograph of taurodontic teeth shows large pulp chambers and low bifurcation of the roots in this pyramid-shaped molar.

Eventually, with the progress of the infectious inflammatory pulpal disease, periapical abscess formation occurs. Gingival abscesses are also frequent. Regional lymphadenitis accompanies these processes.

Pegged or absent maxillary lateral incisors

The inheritance pattern of this trait is generally autosomal dominant with variable expressivity. The lateral incisor can be small, peg shaped, or congenitally lacking, either unilaterally or bilaterally **(Figure 6-43)**. Both primary and secondary dentitions can be affected, but mostly the latter. This condition has a prevalence of 1% to 3% in the white population and about 7% in Asians. In addition, the premolar teeth are congenitally lacking in 10% to 20% of affected individuals.

Taurodontism

This is a genetic heterogeneous condition with dominant and recessive inheritance. It is characterized by very large, pyramid-shaped molars with large pulp chambers **(Figure 6-44)**. (Taurodontic teeth [bull teeth] are also described in Chapter 5.) Taurodontism is most frequent among Native Americans, including Inuits. The furcation of the roots is displaced apically, and these teeth are classified according to the degree of furcation displacement. It is frequently found in Klinefelter syndrome (XXY) and is associated with many other syndromes as well.

Selected References

Books

Cummings MR: *Human heredity: principles and issues,* St Paul, MN, 1988, West Publishing.

Fitzgerald MJT, Fitzgerald M: *Human embryology,* London, 1994, WB Saunders.

Gorlin RJ, Cohen MM, Hennekam RCM: *Syndromes of the head and neck,* ed 4, New York, 2001, Oxford University Press.

Sadler TW: *Langman's medical embryology,* ed 7, Baltimore, 1995, Williams & Wilkins.

Sapp JP, Eversole LR, Wisocki GP: *Contemporary oral and maxillofacial pathology,* St Louis, 1997, Mosby.

Thompson MW: *Thompson and Thompson genetics in medicine,* ed 5, Philadelphia, 1991, WB Saunders.

Witkop CJ Jr, Sauk JJ Jr: *Dental and oral manifestations of hereditary disease,* Washington, DC, 1971, American Academy of Oral Pathology (monograph).

Witkop CJ Jr, Sauk JJ Jr: Heritable defects of enamel. In Stewart RE, Prescott GH, editors: *Oral facial genetics,* St Louis, 1976, Mosby.

Young WG, Sedano HO: *An atlas of oral pathology,* Minneapolis, 1981, University of Minnesota Press.

Journal Articles

Barnet ML, Friedman D, Kastner T: The prevalence of mitral valve prolapse in patients with Down's syndrome: implications for dental management, *Oral Surg Oral Med Oral Pathol* 66:445, 1988.

Bozzo L, Scully C, Aldred MJ: Hereditary gingival fibromatosis, *Oral Surg Oral Med Oral Pathol* 78:452, 1994.

Chadwick B et al: Laband syndrome: report of two cases, review of the literature, and identification of additional manifestations, *Oral Surg Oral Med Oral Pathol* 78:57, 1994.

Crawford PJM, Aldred MJ: Clinical features of a family with X-linked amelogenesis imperfecta mapping to a new locus (AIH3) on the long arm of the X chromosome, *Oral Surg Oral Med Oral Pathol* 76:187, 1993.

Ghaffar KA et al: Papillon-Lefèvre syndrome, *Oral Surg Oral Med Oral Pathol Oral Radiol Endod* 88:320, 1999.

Koury ME, Stella JP, Epker BN: Vascular transformation in cherubism, *Oral Surg Oral Med Oral Pathol* 76:20, 1993.

O'Connell AC, Marini JC: Evaluation of oral problems in an osteogenesis imperfecta population, *Oral Surg Oral Med Oral Pathol Oral Radiol Endod* 87:189, 1999.

Szilágyi A et al: Oral manifestations of patients with Turner syndrome, *Oral Surg Oral Med Oral Pathol Oral Radiol Endod* 89:577, 2000.

Yuasa K et al: Computed tomography of the jaws in familial adenomatosis coli, *Oral Surg Oral Med Oral Pathol* 76:251, 1993.

Review Questions

1. The constriction present in all chromosomes, which joins the short and long arms, is called the:
   A. Equatorial plate
   B. Chromatid
   C. Centromere
   D. Chiasmata
   E. Barr body

2. The process by which a primitive germ cell becomes a gamete is called:
   A. Meiosis
   B. S phase
   C. Haploid
   D. Mitosis
   E. Nondisjunction

3. *Trisomy* means:
   A. Three times the amount of chromosome complement
   B. A pair of chromosomes with an identical extra chromosome
   C. The presence of two extra X chromosomes in a male
   D. One extra chromosome in each pair
   E. An extra set of chromosomes

4. The Lyon hypothesis is applied to:
   A. Autosomal dominant traits
   B. Autosomal recessive traits
   C. X-linked dominant traits
   D. X-linked recessive traits
   E. Males only

5. Barr bodies are seen at the:
   A. Periphery of the cytoplasm in all human cells
   B. Nuclear periphery of cells in women
   C. Nuclear periphery of all human cells
   D. Periphery of the cytoplasm in all cells from women
   E. Nuclear periphery of all cells in men

6. The karyotype of a patient with Turner syndrome shows:
   A. 44 autosomes and XO
   B. 43 autosomes and XYY
   C. 44 autosomes and XXY
   D. 44 autosomes and XYY
   E. 44 autosomes and XX

7. Hypothetically, an autosomal dominant trait would be clinically present in:
   A. 25% of the offspring of an affected parent
   B. 50% of the offspring of an affected parent
   C. 75% of the offspring of an affected parent
   D. Only in males, never in female offspring
   E. All offspring of an affected parent

8. Patients with an X-linked hereditary condition:
   A. Are always men
   B. Have cells with many Barr bodies
   C. Are always women
   D. Are generally affected more severely if they are men
   E. Have numerical chromosomal abnormalities

9. The major concern for a dental hygienist when treating a patient with cyclic neutropenia should be:
   A. Preventing dental caries
   B. Viral infections
   C. Chipping away of enamel

D. Exfoliating teeth because of short roots
E. Number of circulating neutrophils

10. A 9-year-old boy exhibits markedly swollen red and bleeding gingiva. In addition, he has tooth mobility and the intraoral radiographs show marked alveolar bone atrophy with vertical periodontal pockets. Which of the following will be found in this child if he were to have the Papillon-Lefèvre syndrome?
    A. Diminished sweating
    B. Lack of anterior vestibular sulcus
    C. Blue sclerae
    D. Palmar and plantar hyperkeratosis
    E. Cysts of the jaws

11. In all inherited varieties of gingival fibromatosis, the gingival enlargement is characterized by a marked:
    A. Collagenization of the connective tissue
    B. Hyperplasia of the covering epithelium
    C. Chronic inflammatory cellular infiltrate
    D. Alveolar bone hypertrophy
    E. Reaction to medication

12. A 14-year-old boy is seen in consultation because of bilateral mandibular swelling. Radiographs show a bilateral multilocular lesion in the ascending mandibular rami. The mother of this patient has similar findings. The most likely diagnosis is:
    A. Ellis-van Creveld syndrome
    B. Nevoid basal cell carcinoma syndrome
    C. Cleidocranial dysplasia
    D. Cherubism
    E. Gardner syndrome

13. A 19-year-old woman is diagnosed with cleidocranial dysplasia. She has absent clavicles and a mushroom-shaped skull. Which of the following conditions is she also most likely to have?
    A. Taurodontism
    B. Pegged lateral incisors
    C. Supernumerary teeth
    D. Large pulp chambers
    E. Hypercementosis

14. Which of the following is the most serious component of Gardner syndrome?
    A. Mandibular osteomas
    B. Multiple odontomas
    C. Intestinal polyposis
    D. Teeth hypercementosis
    E. Sinus obliteration

15. Two characteristic clinical components of mandibulofacial dysostosis are:
    A. Lack of clavicles and delayed teeth eruption
    B. Hypoplastic mandible and deafness
    C. Hypodontia and dysplastic nails
    D. Cleft lip and fistulas of lower lip
    E. Mandibular prognathism and enamel hypoplasia

16. Odontogenic keratocysts are a clinical component of:
    A. Nevoid basal cell carcinoma syndrome
    B. Neurofibromatosis of von Recklinghausen
    C. MEN 2B syndrome
    D. Cherubism
    E. Gardner syndrome

17. Torus mandibularis and torus palatinus are similar in that both:
    A. Are inherited as an autosomal dominant trait
    B. Are more prevalent in females
    C. Are inherited as an autosomal recessive trait
    D. Develop in childhood
    E. Usually require removal

18. The cause of all forms of labial and palatal clefting is considered to be:
    A. Autosomal dominant
    B. Autosomal recessive
    C. Environmental
    D. Drug induced
    E. Multifactorial

19. The major concern for a dental hygienist when treating a patient with Osler-Rendu-Parkes Weber syndrome should be:
    A. Severe infections
    B. Spontaneous ulcerations
    C. Gingival hemorrhage
    D. Epithelial desquamation
    E. The need for premedication

20. The most serious clinical manifestation of the MEN 2B syndrome is considered to be:
    A. Carcinoma of the colon
    B. Mucosal neuromas
    C. Pheochromocytoma
    D. Basal cell carcinomas
    E. Carcinoma of the thyroid gland

21. Which of the following is true for von Recklinghausen disease?
    A. It is inherited as an autosomal recessive trait.
    B. Patients have multiple neurofibromas.

    C. Patients have gingival fibromatosis.
    D. Patients experience a generalized whitening of the oral mucosa.
    E. No known risk exists for malignant transformation of the skin lesions.

22. Teeth in snowcapped amelogenesis imperfecta have:
    A. A thin, brown enamel
    B. Obliterated pulp chambers
    C. Short, blunted roots
    D. White hypocalcified enamel at the incisal and occlusal thirds
    E. Unusually shaped crowns

23. In dentinogenesis imperfecta type II, teeth have:
    A. Roots that are shorter than normal
    B. Obliterated pulp chambers and canals
    C. Markedly brittle enamel
    D. Larger than normal roots
    E. Dilacerated roots

24. The characteristic finding in permanent teeth affected with coronal dentin dysplasia is:
    A. Crowns with amber color
    B. Thistle-shaped pulp chambers on radiographs
    C. Markedly short roots
    D. Large, square pulp chambers
    E. Crowns that resemble dentinogenesis imperfecta

25. Patients with hypohidrotic ectodermal dysplasia characteristically have:
    A. Multiple tongue nodules
    B. Lack of anterior vestibular sulcus
    C. Excessive amounts of hair
    D. Blue sclerae
    E. Hypodontia

26. Patients with hypophosphatasia characteristically have:
    A. Absence of root cementum
    B. Obliterated pulp chambers
    C. Gangrenous gingivitis
    D. Marked gingival keratinization
    E. Elevated serum alkaline phosphatase levels

27. Taurodontic teeth:
    A. Are supernumerary
    B. Have long roots
    C. Have no pulp chambers
    D. Have thistle-shaped pulp chambers
    E. Are pyramidal in shape

Chapter 6 Synopsis

Condition/ Disease	Cause	Age/Race/Sex	Location
Trisomy 21	One extra chromosome #21	From birth	Systemic
Trisomy 13	One extra chromosome # 13	From birth	Systemic
Turner Syndrome	One X chromosome missing	From birth, women	Systemic
Klinefelter Syndrome	One extra X chromosome	From birth, men	Systemic
Cat Cry Syndrome	Deletion 5p	From birth, M=F	Systemic
Cyclic Neutropenia	AD	From birth, M=F	Oral mucosas and periodontium
Papillon-Lefèvre Syndrome	AR, gene 11q14-q21	From birth, M=F	Gingiva, periodontal ligament, palms, and soles
Focal Palmoplantar Gingival Hyperkeratosis	AD	From birth, M=F	Gingiva, palms, and soles
Laband Syndrome	AD	From birth, M=F	Gingiva
Gingival Fibromatosis, Hypertrichosis, Epilepsy, and Mental Retardation	AD	From birth, M=F	Gingiva, hair, central nervous system
Gingival Fibromatosis and Multiple Hyaline Fibromas	AD	From birth, M=F	Gingiva, nails, mucosas, and skin
Cherubism	AD, gene 4p16	From birth, M=F	Mandible bilaterally

AD, autosomal dominant.
AR, autosomal recessive.
M=F, Male/females 50/50%.

Clinical Features	Radiographic Features	Microscopic Features	Treatment	Diagnostic Process
Slanted eyes, gingivoperiodontitis, fissured tongue, hypodontia	None	None	Root planing, scaling	Karyotype shows trisomy 21
Bilateral CL/P, polydactyly microphthalmia	Extra fingers in hand	None	None	Karyotype shows trisomy 13
Short stature, webbing of neck, edema of hands	None	No Barr bodies in buccal smear	None	Karyotype shows absent X chromosome
Tall stature, gynecomastia	Hypoplastic mandible	One Barr body, in buccal smear	None	Karyotype shows two X chromosomes
Catlike cry, severe mental retardation	None	None	Dental care for mentally handicapped	Deletion of short arm of chromosome 5
Gingivitis, periodontitis ulcers, hemorrhage	Alveolar bone loss, pocket formation	Diminished neutrophils in peripheral blood	Root planing, scaling, antibiotics	Clinical and blood studies
Teeth mobility, pockets, palmoplantar hyperkeratosis	Alveolar bone loss, severe periodontal disease	Profuse inflammatory infiltrate of soft dental tissues	Root planing, scaling, tooth fixation, retinoid for skin lesions	Clinical, genetic evaluation
Keratosis of gingiva, palms, and soles	None	Hyperorthokeratosis of affected areas	Maintain oral hygiene	Clinical and family history
Marked gingival hyperplasia, abnormal nails, short fingers and toes	Hypoplasia of terminal phalanges of fingers and toes	Profuse fibrosis and increase collagen of affected gingiva	Maintain oral hygiene, surgical remodeling of gingiva (recurrence)	Clinical and family history
Gingival hyperplasia, abundant body hair, epilepsy	None	Profuse fibrosis and increase collagen of affected gingiva	Maintain oral hygiene, surgical remodeling of gingiva (recurrence)	Clinical and family history
Gingival hyperplasia, nails' hypertrophy, multiple tumors	None	Fibrosis of gingiva, hyaline fibromas	Maintain oral hygiene, removal of fibromas	Clinical and family history
Bilateral enlargement of face	Multiple bilateral radiolucencies of mandibular ramus	Multinucleated giant cells in a loose connective tissue	Lesions fill in after puberty	Clinical, radiographs, and family history

Continued

Chapter 6   Synopsis—cont'd

Condition/ Disease	Cause	Age/Race/Sex	Location
Chondroectodermal Dysplasia (Ellis-van Creveld Syndrome)	AR, gene 4p16	From birth, M=F	Gingival, teeth, alveolar ridge, hands
Cleidocranial Dysplasia	AD, gene 6p21	From birth, M=F	Teeth, clavicles, skull
Gardner Syndrome	AD, gene 5q21-q22	From birth, M=F	Maxilla and mandible
Mandibulofacial Dysostosis	AD, gene 5q32-q33.1	From birth, M=F	Mandible, teeth, ears
Nevoid Basal Cell Carcinoma Syndrome	AD, gene 9q22.3-q31	From birth, M=F	Mandible, maxilla, skin
Osteogenesis Imperfecta	AD and AR genes 7q22.1 and 17q 21.31, q 22.05	Variable	Bones and teeth
Hereditary Hemorrhagic Telangiectasia	AD, gene 9q3	Starts after teens	Mucous membranes and skin
Multiple Mucosal Neuromas	AD, gene 10 (RET)	From birth, M=F	Oral mucosas, especially tongue
Neurofibromatosis of von Recklinghausen	AD, gene 17q11.2	From birth, M=F	Skin, oral mucosas, especially tongue
Peutz-Jeghers Syndrome	AD, gene 19p13.3	From birth, M=F	Skin, oral mucosas, small intestine
White Sponge Nevus	AD, mutation mucosal keratin K4 or K13	At birth or develops at puberty	Buccal mucosas

AD, autosomal dominant.
AR, autosomal recessive.
M=F, Male/females 50/50%.

Clinical Features	Radiographic Features	Microscopic Features	Treatment	Diagnostic Process
Absent upper vestibule, serrated lower alveolar ridge, polydactyly	Thinning of enamel	None	Reconstruction of upper vestibule, amputation of extra fingers	Clinical and family history
Supernumerary teeth absent clavicles, open fontanelles	Multiple impacted teeth	Absent cellular cementum	Extractions, orthodontia	Clinical, radiographs, and family history
Multiple osteomas, colon polyps, adenocarcinoma	Odontomas and osteomas in the jaws	Review osteoma and colonic cancer	Surgery of: polyps and/or carcinoma, odontomas, osteomas	Clinical, radiographs, and family history
Hypoplastic mandible, malposed teeth, deafness	Obtuse mandibular angle, small condyle	None	Plastic surgery, orthodontia, maintain oral hygiene	Clinical, radiographs, and family history
Multiple: odontogenic keratocysts and basal cell carcinoma	Multiple radiolucencies of the jaws, bifid rib	Review odontogenic keratocyst (Chapter 5) and basal cell carcinoma (Chapter 7)	Surgical removal of cysts and basal cell carcinomas	Clinical, radiographs and family history Microscopic
Multiple bone fractures, dentinogenesis imperfecta	Fractures, no pulp chambers, small teeth	Abnormal globular dentin	Maintain oral hygiene	Clinical, radiographs, and family history
Telangiectases, gingival bleeding	None	Capillary dilations	Care must be taken during scaling because of marked bleeding tendency	Clinical and family history
Multiple nodes on tongue tip, lips, and cheek mucosas	None	Review neurofibroma and thyroid carcinoma	Preventive thyroidectomy and excision of oral neurofibromas	Clinical and family history, microscopic
Multiple nodes on tongue and other mucosas	Spine anomalies	Review neurofibroma and neurofibrosarcoma	Surgical removal of neurofibromas	Clinical and family history, microscopic
Pigmented macules in perioral skin and oral mucosas	Intestinal polyps	Melanin apposition in skin and oral mucosas	Removal of intestinal polyps if needed	Clinical and family history
Bilateral whitening of buccal mucosas	None	Thick layer of orthokeratin and clear cells	Maintain oral hygiene	Clinical and family history, microscopic

Continued

Chapter 6 Synopsis—cont'd

Condition/ Disease	Cause	Age/Race/Sex	Location
Amelogenesis Imperfecta Pitted Hypoplastic	AD	Visible when teeth erupt, M=F	All primary and permanent teeth
Amelogenesis Imperfecta Hypocalcified Type	AD and AR	When teeth erupt, M=F	All primary and permanent teeth
Amelogenesis Imperfecta Hypomaturation Type	AD, AR and X-linked recessive	When teeth erupt, AD and AR, M= F, X-linked, more men	All primary and permanent teeth
Amelogenesis Imperfecta Snow Capped (Hypomaturation)	AD and X-linked recessive	When teeth erupt, AD, M=F, X-linked, more men	All primary and permanent teeth
Dentinogenesis Imperfecta	AD gene 4q13-q21	When teeth erupt	All primary and permanent teeth
Radicular Dentin Dysplasia	AD	When teeth erupt	All primary and permanent teeth
Coronal Dentin Dysplasia	AD gene 4q13-q21	When teeth erupt	All primary and permanent teeth
Hypohidrotic Ectodermal Dysplasia	X-linked recessive and AR gene Xq12-q13.1 AR 2q11-q13	From birth, X-linked all males, AR, M=F	Skin, sweat, hair, both dentitions
Hypophosphatasia	AR, gene 1p36.1-p34	From birth, M=F	Bones, teeth
Hypophosphatemic Vitamin D– Resistant Rickets	X-linked dominant	From birth, more males	Bones, teeth

AD, autosomal dominant.
AR, autosomal recessive.
M=F, Male/females 50/50%.

Clinical Features	Radiographic Features	Microscopic Features	Treatment	Diagnostic Process
Random pinpoint pits on labial and lingual	Enamel thinner than normal	Abnormal enamel matrix thinner than normal	Aesthetic dentistry operative procedures	Clinical and family history
Cheesy soft enamel, rapidly lost, anterior open bite	Enamel has "moth-eaten" appearance	Enamel of normal thickness, poorly calcified	Jacket crowns, metal crowns, aesthetic dentistry	Clinical and family history
Enamel softer than normal and chips easily	Enamel has same radiolucency as dentin	Large amounts of enamel matrix	Jacket crowns, metal crowns, aesthetic dentistry	Clinical and family history
White discoloration surface enamel occlusal one third	None	Not available	Aesthetic dentistry if the patient wants it	Clinical and family history
Bulbous crowns, opalescent brown bluish color	Short pointed roots, absent pulp chambers	Abnormal globular dentin, trapped odontoblasts	Aesthetic dentistry crowns, operative procedures	Clinical and family history
Normal crowns in size and color	Short pointed roots, absent pulp chambers	Abnormal tubular dentin and osteodentin	Prosthesis if teeth are lost	Radiographs and family history
Primary teeth amber in color, permanent normal	Primary absent pulp chambers, permanent molars "bow tie" pulp, uniradicular teeth, "thistle-shaped" pulp	Abnormal dentin in primary teeth, permanent teeth with pulp stones	Regular dental and dental hygiene care	Clinical, radiographs, and family history
Few teeth are formed, little sweat, few hairs	Almost no teeth present	Reduced and abnormal sweat pores	Dental implants and/or dental prosthesis	Clinical, radiographs, and family history
Premature loss of primary anterior teeth	Large pulp chambers	Absence of root cementum	Space retainers or dental prosthesis	Clinical, radiographs, and family history
Multiple periapical radiolucencies (cyst, granuloma)	Large pulp chambers, large pulp horns	Abnormal globular dentin, large cracks in dentin	Endodontics and regular dental hygiene care	Clinical, radiographs, and family history

Neoplasia

Anne Cale Jones
Paul D. Freedman
Joan A. Phelan

Objectives

After studying this chapter, the student will be able to:

1. Define each of the words in the vocabulary list for this chapter.
2. Explain the difference between a benign tumor and a malignant tumor.
3. Define leukoplakia and erythroplakia.
4. Define the following neoplasms, describe the clinical features of each, and explain how they are treated: papilloma, squamous cell carcinoma, verrucous carcinoma, basal cell carcinoma, pleomorphic adenoma, monomorphic adenoma, adenoid cystic carcinoma, mucoepidermoid carcinoma, ameloblastoma, calcifying epithelial odontogenic tumor (CEOT), adenomatoid odontogenic tumor (AOT), odontogenic myxoma, central cementifying and ossifying fibromas, benign cementoblastoma, ameloblastic fibroma, ameloblastic fibro-odontoma, odontoma, peripheral ossifying fibroma, lipoma, neurofibroma and schwannoma, granular cell tumor, congenital epulis, rhabdomyosarcoma, hemangioma, lymphangioma, Kaposi sarcoma, melanocytic nevi, malignant melanoma, torus, exostosis, osteoma, osteosarcoma, chondrosarcoma, leukemia, lymphoma, multiple myeloma, and metastatic jaw tumors.

Vocabulary

Anaplastic (an′ĕplas′tik) Characterized by a loss of differentiation of cells and their orientation to one another; a characteristic of malignant tumors.

Benign (be-nīn′) Not malignant; favorable for recovery.

Carcinoma (kar″si-no′mah) Malignant tumor of epithelium.

Central (sen′tral) Occurring within bone.

Dysplasia (dis-pla′ze-ah) Disordered growth; alteration in size, shape, and organization of adult cells.

Encapsulated (en-kap′su-lt-ed) Surrounded by a capsule of fibrous connective tissue.

Hyperchromatic (hi″per-kro-mat′āik) Staining more intensely than normal.

Hyperplasia (hi″per-pla′zĕ-ah) Abnormal increase in the number of cells in an organ or tissue.

Immunoglobulin (im′yĕnō-gläb′yĕlin) Antibody.

In situ (in sĭtoo) Confined to the site of origin without invasion of neighboring tissues.

Invasion (in-va′zhun) Infiltration and active destruction of surrounding tissues.

Leukoplakia (loo-kō-plā′kē-ah) Clinical term used to identify a white, plaquelike lesion of the oral mucosa that cannot be wiped off and cannot be diagnosed as any other disease.

Malignant (mah-lig′nant) In reference to tumors—having the properties of anaplasia, invasion, and metastasis.

Malignant tumor (mah-lig′nant too′mor) Cancer; a tumor that is resistant to treatment and may cause death; a tumor that has the potential for uncontrolled growth and dissemination or recurrence, or both.

Metastasis (mĕ-tas′tah-sis) (*plural,* **metastases [mĕ-tas′tah-sēz]**) Transport of neoplastic cells to parts of the body remote from the primary tumor and the establishment of new tumors in those sites.

Metastatic tumor (met″ah-stat′ik too′mor) Tumor formed by cells that have been transported from the primary tumor to sites not connected to the original tumor.

Mitotic figure (mi-tot′ik fig′ur); mitosis (mi-to′sis) Dividing cells caught in the process of mitosis.

Neoplasia (ne″o-pla′ze-ah) New growth; the formation of tumors by the uncontrolled proliferation of cells.

Neoplastic (nē′ō-plas′tik) Pertaining to the formation of tumors by the uncontrolled proliferation of cells.

Neoplasm (ne′o-plazm) Tumor; a new growth of tissue in which growth is uncontrolled and progressive.

Nevus (ne′vus) (plural, nevi [ne′vi]) Circumscribed malformation of the skin or oral mucosa presumed to be of hereditary origin.

Odontogenic (o-don″to-jen′ik) Tooth forming.

Oncology (ong-kol′o-je) Study of tumors or neoplasms.

Pedunculated (pidungk′yĕlā′tid) Attached by a stalk.

Peripheral (pĕ-rif′er-al) Occurring outside of bone.

Pleomorphic (ple″o-mor′fik) Occurring in various forms.

Primary tumor (pri′mer-e too′mor) Original tumor; the source of metastasis.

Sarcoma (sar-ko′mah) Malignant tumor of connective tissue.

Sessile (ses′il) Attached by a base.

Tumor (too′mor) Neoplasm; also, a swelling or enlargement.

Undifferentiated (un-dif′ĕr-en′shē-āt′ed) Absence of normal differentiation; anaplasia; a characteristic of malignant tumors.

Description

Neoplasia means new growth. It is a process in which cells exhibit uncontrolled proliferation. A **neoplasm** is a mass of such cells. Although the word **tumor** means swelling, it is commonly used as a synonym for neoplasm. The study of tumors is called **oncology.** *Onco,* in Greek, means swelling or mass.

For neoplasia to occur, an irreversible change must take place in the cells and this change must be passed on to new cells, resulting in uncontrollable cell multiplication. For most neoplasms the initial stimulus that triggers the process of cell change is not known. Regulatory processes maintain the size of normal tissues. The regulatory processes that maintain the size of normal tissues do not control a neoplasm; therefore it exhibits unlimited and unregulated growth.

Like hyperplasia, which is described in Chapter 2, neoplasia is an abnormal process. With hyperplasia, normal cells proliferate in a normal arrangement in response to tissue damage, and the proliferation stops when the stimulus is removed. Although the size of the tissue may be greater than normal, the growth of the tissue is still under control. Reactive lesions, such as the irritation fibroma, denture-related hyperplasia (epulis fissuratum), and the pyogenic granuloma, described in Chapter 2, are examples of hyperplasia. Neoplasia, in contrast, is a completely abnormal process; the cells are abnormal, and the proliferation of those cells is uncontrolled and unlimited.

Causes of Neoplasia

Many agents—principally chemicals, viruses, and radiation—have been shown to cause neoplastic transformation of cells in the laboratory. Hundreds of chemicals have been shown to cause cancer in animals. In addition, certain chemicals, viruses, and radiation have been shown to cause some cancers in humans. Neoplastic transformation can also occur spontaneously secondary to a genetic mutation.

Viruses that cause tumors are called **oncogenic viruses.** Radiation from sunlight, x-rays, nuclear fission, or other sources is well established as a cancer-producing agent in humans.

Classification of Tumors

Tumors are divided into two categories: benign and malignant. A **benign tumor** or **neoplasm** remains localized. It may be **encapsulated**, which means that it is walled off by surrounding fibrous connective tissue. Sometimes a benign tumor can invade adjacent structures, but it does not have the ability to spread to distant sites. A **malignant tumor,** in contrast, both invades and destroys surrounding tissue and also has the ability to spread throughout the body. **Cancer** is synonymous with malignancy.

Benign tumors almost always resemble normal cells, whereas malignant tumors vary in their histologic appearance. Malignant tumors composed of neoplastic cells that resemble normal cells are called well-differentiated tumors. Malignant tumors may also be poorly differentiated. The cells of these tumors have only some of the characteristics of the tissue from which they were derived. Still other malignant tumors may be undifferentiated or anaplastic and do not resemble at all the tissue from which they were derived. Malignant tumors are often composed of cells that vary in size and shape **(pleomorphic) (Figure 7-1).** The nuclei of these cells are darker than those of normal cells **(hyperchromatic)** and exhibit an increased nuclear cytoplasmic ratio (see Figure 7-1, *A* and *B*). Normal and abnormal **mitotic figures** are seen in the nucleus of the neoplastic cells (see Figure 7-1, *A*). Abnormal mitotic figures are those that are not dividing normally; therefore the shape of the dividing nucleus does not follow the shape of a normal mitotic figure. **Table 7-1** compares benign and malignant tumors.

Names of Tumors

The prefix of the name of a tumor is determined by the tissue or cell of origin. The suffix *oma* is used to indicate a tumor. For example, a benign tumor of fat is called a **lipoma**, and a benign tumor of bone is called an **osteoma**. Malignant tumors are named in a similar fashion. Malignant tumors of epithelium are called **carcinomas**, and malignant tumors of connective tissue are called **sarcomas**. The prefix of the name of a malignant tumor is also determined by the

Figure 7-1 Photomicrographs of malignant tumors shows pleomorphic *(P)* and hyperchromatic *(H)* nuclei and mitotic figures *(MI)*. **A,** Squamous cell carcinoma. **B,** Osteosarcoma.

Table 7-1 Comparison of Benign and Malignant Tumors

Benign	Malignant
Usually well differentiated	Well differentiated to anaplastic
Usually slow growing	Slow to rapid growth
Mitotic figures are rare	Mitotic figures may be numerous
Usually encapsulated	Invasive and unencapsulated
No metastasis	Metastasis is likely

tissue or cell of origin. Therefore a malignant tumor of squamous epithelium is called a **squamous cell carcinoma** or an **epidermoid carcinoma**, and a malignant tumor of bone is called an **osteosarcoma**. Carcinomas are about 10 times more common than sarcomas. **Table 7-2** lists tumors according to their tissue or cell of origin.

Treatment of Tumors

Benign tumors are generally treated by surgical excision, which can be accomplished through wide local excision or enucleation. Malignant tumors are treated by surgery, chemotherapy, or radiation therapy; a combination is often used.

Because many different types of tissues are present in the oral cavity, many different types of tumors can arise in this location. These neoplasms can be either benign or malignant. In this chapter the neoplasms are classified according to their tissue of origin. Benign tumors are described first, followed by their malignant counterparts.

Epithelial Tumors

Three different types of epithelial tumors occur in the oral cavity: (1) tumors derived from squamous epithelium, (2) tumors derived from salivary gland epithelium, and (3) tumors derived from odontogenic epithelium. A few of the lesions included in this section are not true tumors. The reasons for their inclusion are explained in their descriptions.

Tumors of Squamous Epithelium

PAPILLOMA

The **papilloma** is a benign tumor of squamous epithelium that presents a small exophytic pedunculated or sessile growth. These tumors are composed of numerous papillary projections that may be either white or the color of normal mucosa **(Figure 7-2)**. They are often described as cauliflower-like in appearance. Most cases arise on the soft palate or tongue. A papilloma may occur at any age, and

Figure 7-2 A, Clinical appearance of a papilloma of the oral mucosa shows a cauliflower-like appearance and rough surface resulting from fingerlike projections. Microscopic appearance of a papilloma shows fingerlike projections. **B,** Microscopic appearance of a papilloma shows fingerlike projections surfaced by squamous epithelium and supported by thin cores of fibrous connective tissue.

Table 7-2 Names of Tumors

Tissue of Origin	Benign Tumor	Malignant Tumor
Epithelium		
Squamous cells	Papilloma	Squamous cell or epithelial carcinoma
Basal cells		Basal cell carcinoma
Glands or ducts	Adenoma	Adenocarcinoma
Neuroectoderm		
Melanocytes	Nevus	Melanoma
Connective Tissue		
Fibrous	Fibroma	Fibrosarcoma
Cartilage	Chondroma	Chondrosarcoma
Bone	Osteoma	Osteosarcoma
Fat	Lipoma	Liposarcoma
Endothelium		
Blood vessels	Hemangioma	Angiosarcoma
Lymphatic vessels	Lymphangioma	Lymphangiosarcoma
Muscle		
Smooth muscle	Leiomyoma	Leiomyosarcoma
Striated muscle	Rhabdomyoma	Rhabdomyosarcoma

A B

Figure 7-3 Clinical appearance of leukoplakia. **A,** Floor of the mouth. **B,** Maxillary alveolar mucosa and palate. The cause of these lesions could not be identified.

an equal sex predilection is noted. Microscopic examination demonstrates numerous fingerlike or papillary projections surfaced by normal stratified squamous epithelium. A central core of fibrous connective tissue supports each papillary projection. The color of the lesion depends on the amount of surface keratin; the more keratin, the whiter the surface.

Other oral lesions that may look like a papilloma clinically are verruca vulgaris (common wart) and condyloma acuminatum (venereal wart). These two lesions are caused by human papillomaviruses (HPV) and are described in Chapter 4. They are differentiated from the papilloma by microscopic examination. Special staining procedures can be used to identify viral particles in these lesions.

The papilloma is treated by surgical excision, which must include the base of the growth. With adequate excision, the papilloma usually does not recur.

PREMALIGNANT LESIONS

Leukoplakia

In any discussion of premalignant lesions of the oral mucosa, it is important to define the term **leukoplakia**. Leukoplakia is a clinical term and does not refer to a specific histologic appearance. It is defined as a white plaquelike lesion of the oral mucosa that cannot be rubbed off and cannot be diagnosed as a specific disease **(Figure 7-3).**

Leukoplakia is sometimes referred to as idiopathic leukoplakia to emphasize that the specific cause of the lesion is not known. The white lesion il-

Figure 7-4 Clinical appearance of a white lesion that was associated with tobacco chewing (tobacco pouch keratosis). This lesion developed on the lower labial mucosa at the site where the tobacco was held.

lustrated in **Figure 7-4** is more accurately called **tobacco pouch keratosis** rather than a leukoplakia because the direct cause of the lesion is known.

The microscopic appearance of leukoplakia varies; therefore a biopsy is essential to establish a definitive diagnosis. Most leukoplakias are the result of hyperkeratosis (thickening of the keratin layer) or a combination of epithelial hyperplasia (thickening of the prickle cell or spinous layer) and hyperkeratosis. When examined microscopically, a leukoplakia may also show epithelial dysplasia, a premalignant condition, or even squamous cell carcinoma, a malignant tumor of squamous epithelium. Depending on the study, approximately 5% to 25% of leukoplakias examined microscopically demonstrated epithelial dysplasia. Studies have also revealed that leukoplakia found on the floor of the mouth, ventrolateral tongue, and lip are more likely to represent epithelial dysplasia or squamous cell carcinoma than leuko-plakia occurring in other areas of the oral cavity.

When a white lesion is identified in the oral cavity, the first goal is to identify the cause. Any associated irritation should be removed. If the lesion does not resolve, a biopsy and histologic examination of the tissue must be performed. Any white lesion that is diagnosed as epithelial dysplasia or that cannot be diagnosed as a specific disease should be completely removed. When leukoplakia is found on the floor of the mouth, ventrolateral tongue, or lip, the lesion should be removed even if the histologic appearance is hyperkeratosis or epithelial hyperplasia because of the increased risk of squamous cell carcinoma in these areas.

The treatment of leukoplakia is dependent on the histologic diagnosis. The treatment of epithelial dysplasia and squamous cell carcinoma is discussed in the sections that follow.

Erythroplakia

Erythroplakia is a clinical term that is used to describe an oral mucosal lesion that appears as a smooth red patch or a granular red and velvety patch. A lesion that shows a mixture of red and white areas is generally called **speckled leukoplakia** rather than erythroplakia. Most cases of erythroplakia occur in the floor of the mouth, tongue, and soft palate. Erythroplakia is much less common than leukoplakia. In one study, 60 cases of leukoplakia were seen for every 1 case of erythroplakia. When examined microscopically, 90% of cases of erythroplakia demonstrate epithelial dysplasia or squamous cell carcinoma. Because of these microscopic findings, erythroplakia is considered a more serious clinical finding than leukoplakia (a biopsy must be performed to establish a definitive diagnosis).

Treatment of erythroplakia depends on the histologic diagnosis.

Epithelial Dysplasia

Epithelial dysplasia is a histologic diagnosis that indicates disordered growth. It is considered a premalignant condition. Lesions that microscopically exhibit epithelial dysplasia frequently precede squamous cell carcinoma. Unlike squamous cell carcinoma, the cellular changes in epithelial dysplasia may revert to normal if the stimulus, such as tobacco smoking, is removed. Epithelial dysplasia may pres-

Figure 7-5 Microscopic appearance of epithelial dysplasia. Loss of the normal stratification of the epithelium, hyperplasia of the basal cells, and enlarged and hyperchromatic nuclei are seen.

ent clinically as an erythematous lesion (erythroplakia), as a white lesion (leukoplakia), or as a mixed erythematous and white lesion (speckled leukoplakia). Lesions often arise in the floor of the mouth or tongue. The term *dysplasia* may also be used to describe lesions that occur in tissues other than epithelium.

Dysplasia in other tissues (such as bone) is not considered a premalignant process. Microscopic examination of epithelial dysplasia demonstrates abnormal maturation of epithelial cells with disorganization of the epithelial layers; hyperplasia of the basal cells; and epithelial cells with enlarged and hyperchromatic nuclei, increased nuclear cytoplasmic ratios, abnormal keratinization, and increased numbers of normal and abnormal mitotic figures **(Figure 7-5)**. Microscopically, epithelial dysplasia differs from squamous cell carcinoma in that no invasion of the abnormal epithelial cells occurs through the basement membrane into the underlying tissue. Severe dysplasia involving the full thickness of the epithelium is called **carcinoma in situ**.

All dysplastic lesions should be surgically excised. Close long-term follow-up examinations are indicated because of the potential for recurrence.

SQUAMOUS CELL CARCINOMA

Squamous cell carcinoma, or epidermoid carcinoma, is a malignant tumor of squamous epithelium. It is the most common primary malignancy of the oral cavity and, like other malignant tumors, can infiltrate adjacent tissues and metastasize to distant sites.

Squamous cell carcinoma usually metastasizes to lymph nodes of the neck and then to more distant sites such as the lungs and liver. Clinically, squamous cell carcinoma is usually an exophytic ulcerative mass **(Figure 7-6)**, but early tumors may be erythematous and plaquelike (erythroplakia), white and plaquelike (leukoplakia), or a mixture of erythematous and white areas (speckled leukoplakia). Squamous cell carcinoma can infiltrate and destroy bone (see Figure 7-6, *D*).

The essential microscopic feature of squamous cell carcinoma is the invasion of tumor cells through the epithelial basement membrane into the underlying connective tissue **(Figure 7-7, *A*)**. Invasive sheets and nests of neoplastic squamous cells characterize the tumor. Although squamous cell carcinoma is a malignant tumor, it exhibits features that allow the cells to be recognized as squamous epithelial cells. In well-differentiated tumors, these features are easily recognized; however, in a poorly differentiated squamous cell carcinoma, they may not be easily seen. Because keratin is a product of squamous epithelium, well-differentiated tumors show keratin formation. In addition to normal surface keratin, the keratin may be seen in individual cells within the tumor and as structures called **keratin pearls** **(Figure 7-7, *B*)**. The neoplastic cells are not normal cells. They contain large hyperchromatic nuclei and numerous mitotic

Figure 7-6 A, Clinical appearance of a squamous cell carcinoma of the posterolateral tongue shows an exophytic, ulcerated mass. **B,** Clinical appearance of a squamous cell carcinoma of the left side of the soft palate and fauces. **C,** Clinical appearance of a squamous cell carcinoma on the floor of the mouth. **D,** Left side of a panoramic radiograph shows destruction of the mandible by a squamous cell carcinoma. (**C** courtesy Dr. Edward V. Zegarelli.)

figures. Some of the mitotic figures appear normal, whereas others are bizarre (see Figure 7-7, *B*).

Squamous cell carcinomas may occur anywhere in the oral cavity, but most tumors occur on the floor of the mouth, ventrolateral tongue, soft palate, tonsillar pillar, and retromolar areas. The clinical appearance of squamous cell carcinoma occurring in several different locations is seen in Figure 7-6.

Squamous cell carcinomas may occur on the vermilion border of the lips and skin of the face **(Figure 7-8).** In this location they are associated with sun exposure (actinic cheilitis) and tend to be more common in individuals with fair skin. The prognosis for

squamous cell carcinoma of the lips and skin is much better than that for squamous cell carcinoma of the oral mucosa. Sun exposure causes recognizable changes of the vermilion border of the lips. The color changes from dark pink and uniform to mottled grayish pink. The interface of the vermilion border and the skin becomes blurred, and linear fissures are seen at right angles to the line of the interface. Histologically, damage from sun exposure is seen as changes that range from degeneration of the collagen under the epithelium to a condition called **solar cheilitis,** in which mild to severe epithelial dysplasia occurs. Fair-skinned individuals are prone to the development of squamous cell carcinoma of the lips

Figure 7-7 A, Microscopic appearance (low power) of a squamous cell carcinoma shows infiltration of the tumor into the connective tissue. **B,** High-power photomicrograph shows abnormal keratinization *(K).*

Figure 7-8 Clinical appearance of squamous cell carcinoma of the lower lip. The reader should also note actinic (solar) cheilitis *(arrow)* in **A**. (Courtesy Dr. Edward V. Zegarelli.)

Table 7-3 TNM Staging System for Oral Squamous Cell Carcinoma

T—Tumor

T_1—Tumor less than 2 cm in diameter
T_2—Tumor 2-4 cm in diameter
T_3—Tumor greater than 4 cm in diameter
T_4—Tumor invades adjacent structures

N—Node

N_0—No palpable nodes
N_1—Ipsilateral (same side as primary tumor) palpable nodes (same side as tumor)
N_2—Contralateral (opposite side from primary tumor) or bilateral nodes
N_3—Fixed palpable nodes

M—Metastasis

M_0—No distant metastasis
M_1—Clinical or radiographic evidence of metastasis

From Regezi JA, Sciubba JJ: Oral pathology: clinical pathologic correlations, ed 3, Philadelphia, 1999, WB Saunders. Used with permission.

Table 7-4 TNM Staging System

Stage I	T_1	N_0	M_0
Stage II	T_2	N_0	M_0
Stage III	T_3	N_0	M_0
	T_1	N_1	M_0
	T_2	N_1	M_0
	T_3	N_1	M_0
Stage IV	T_1	N_2	M_0
	T_2	N_2	M_0
	T_3	N_2	M_0
	T_1	N_3	M_0
	T_2	N_3	M_0
	T_3	N_3	M_0
	T_4	N_0	M_0
Any patients with M_1			

From Regezi JA, Sciubba JJ: Oral pathology: clinical pathologic correlations, ed 3, Philadelphia, 1999, WB Saunders. Used with permission.

and skin resulting from sun exposure and therefore should be advised either to avoid the sun or to use a sun block.

The majority of squamous cell carcinomas occur in patients over 40 years of age. In the past, men have outnumbered women; however, in the last 30 years, there has been an increased incidence of squamous cell carcinoma in women. This is most likely a result of the increased number of women who smoke and the fact that women outnumber men in older age groups.

Risk Factors

Several risk factors have been associated with the development of squamous cell carcinoma. The most significant is tobacco—including cigar, pipe, and cigarette smoking, snuff dipping, and tobacco chewing. Alcohol consumption appears to add to the risk of oral squamous cell carcinoma. It has been suggested that chronic irritation is related to the development of oral cancer. However, no evidence indicates that it is an initiating factor.

Treatment and Prognosis

Squamous cell carcinoma is generally treated by surgical excision. Radiation therapy or chemotherapy may be used in combination with surgery. Occasionally, radiation therapy is used alone. The prognosis of squamous cell carcinoma is related to the size and location of the tumor and the presence or absence of metastases. The smaller the tumor at the time of treatment, the better the prognosis. For oral squamous cell carcinoma, determining the size of the tumor and the presence or absence of cervical lymph node involvement and distant metastasis are important in predicting the patient's prognosis. These are assessed using a system called the **TNM staging system;** the higher the stage, the worse the prognosis **(Tables 7-3** and **7-4)**. Metastasis to cervical lymph nodes is associated with a much poorer prognosis as is the presence of distant metastasis. Therefore it is important to identify asymptomatic areas of leukoplakia and erythroplakia while they are small and remove all potentially premalignant lesions.

Patients who have undergone radiation therapy for malignant tumors of the head and neck often experience severe xerostomia (dry mouth) as a result of radiation damage to the salivary gland tissue.

Figure 7-9 **A,** Clinical appearance of a verrucous carcinoma, occurring on the commissure and anterior buccal mucosa. **B,** Maxillary alveolar ridge.

These patients require preventive dental care, consisting of nutritional counseling, topical fluoride application, and meticulous home care.

VERRUCOUS CARCINOMA

Verrucous carcinoma is a form of squamous cell carcinoma that is separated from other squamous cell carcinomas because it has a much better prognosis. Clinically it appears as a slow-growing exophytic tumor with a pebbly white and red surface **(Figure 7-9).** Most cases occur in men over 55 years of age and involve the vestibule and buccal mucosa. Microscopic examination demonstrates a tumor composed of numerous papillary epithelial proliferations. The spaces between these papillary projections are filled with keratin. The epithelium is well differentiated, does not contain atypical cells, and exhibits broad-based rete pegs that penetrate deeply into the connective tissue. The epithelial basement membrane is intact, and the tumor does not show invasion of tumor cells through the basement membrane, as is seen in squamous cell carcinoma.

Verrucous carcinoma is treated by surgical excision. Although it is a carcinoma, it usually does not metastasize; therefore the prognosis is better for verrucous carcinoma than for squamous cell carcinoma. If it is not treated, it can cause extensive local damage. Close long-term follow-up is necessary for patients with this condition.

Figure 7-10 Clinical appearance of a basal cell carcinoma *(arrow)* illustrating the characteristic "rolled" borders.

BASAL CELL CARCINOMA

Basal cell carcinoma is a malignant skin tumor associated with excessive sun exposure. This particular neoplasm does not occur in the oral cavity. Basal cell carcinoma frequently arises on the skin of the face and appears as a nonhealing ulcer with characteristic rolled borders **(Figure 7-10).** Most cases occur in Caucasian adults, and no sex predilection is seen.

A basal cell carcinoma is composed of basal cells derived from squamous epithelium. Microscopic examination demonstrates a proliferation of basal epithelial cells into the underlying connective tissue. In most cases, the tumor cells are well differentiated.

The basal cell carcinoma is a locally invasive tumor that can become large and disfiguring if it is not removed. Surgical excision is the treatment of choice, and radiation therapy may be used to treat large le-

sions. Only rarely does a basal cell carcinoma metastasize. Patients should be referred to a dermatologist, or a biopsy should be performed on any ulcer of the skin or lips that does not heal within 10 days.

Salivary Gland Tumors

Benign and malignant tumors can arise in either the major or the minor salivary glands. Tumors may oc-

Figure 7-11 A, Benign salivary gland tumor of the palate (pleomorphic adenoma). **B,** Malignant salivary gland tumor of the palate (adenoid cystic carcinoma). Biopsy site should be noted. **C,** Benign salivary gland tumor of the upper lip (pleomorphic adenoma). **D,** Malignant salivary gland tumor of the buccal mucosa (mucoepidermoid carcinoma). **E,** Malignant salivary gland tumor of the tongue (adenoid cystic carcinoma).

cur within the parotid, submandibular, or sublingual glands, or they may involve any of the minor salivary glands located throughout the oral cavity. Intraorally, minor salivary gland tumors are most commonly located at the junction of the hard and soft palates. They can also occur on the labial and buccal mucosa, the retromolar area, the floor of the mouth, and, rarely, the tongue **(Figure 7-11).** Tumors of minor salivary gland origin are much more common in the upper lip than in the lower lip.

Because the origin of these tumors is glandular epithelium, benign tumors of salivary gland origin are called **adenomas.** Although some malignant salivary gland tumors are called **adenocarcinomas,** most have more specific names such as **adenoid cystic carcinoma** and **mucoepidermoid carcinoma.** All salivary gland tumors are diagnosed based on their microscopic appearance. A biopsy and microscopic examination of the tissue are required to establish a specific diagnosis.

PLEOMORPHIC ADENOMA (BENIGN MIXED TUMOR)

The **pleomorphic adenoma** is a benign salivary gland tumor. It is the most common salivary gland neoplasm and accounts for about 90% of all benign salivary gland tumors. Microscopic examination reveals an encapsulated tumor composed of tissue that appears to be a mixture of both epithelium and connective tissue **(Figure 7-12).** For this reason, the tumor is often called the **benign mixed tumor.** The

connective tissuelike part can vary from loose and dense fibrous connective tissue to cartilage. The tissue that looks like connective tissue is derived from a salivary gland cell called a **myoepithelial cell.**

The most common extraoral location for the pleomorphic adenoma is the parotid gland. The most common intraoral site is the palate. However, these tumors can occur wherever salivary gland tissue is present. Clinically, the pleomorphic adenoma appears as a slowly enlarging, nonulcerated, painless, dome-shaped mass (see Figure 7-11, *A* and *C*). The surface can be ulcerated if traumatized. Its size can range from a few millimeters to several centimeters. Most pleomorphic adenomas occur in individuals over 40 years of age, and a female predilection has been noted. Pleomorphic adenomas have also been reported in children.

The pleomorphic adenoma is treated by surgical excision. The extent of the surgery depends on the location of the tumor. Clinicians treat parotid gland tumors by removing the part of the parotid gland containing the tumor (partial parotidectomy), whereas minor salivary gland tumors are treated by more conservative surgical excision. The pleomorphic adenoma grows by extension of projections of tumor into the surrounding tissue. Therefore some tumors are difficult to remove completely. Recurrence rates vary and are related to the adequacy of the initial surgical removal. Pleomorphic adenomas have been known to undergo malignant transformation, and this occurrence is known as a **carcinoma arising in a pleomorphic adenoma.**

A   B

Figure 7-12 Microscopic appearance of a pleomorphic adenoma. **A,** Low-power photomicrograph shows a capsule *(C)*. **B,** High-power photomicrograph shows a mixture of epithelium *(E)* and connective tissue *(CT)*.

MONOMORPHIC ADENOMA

The **monomorphic adenoma** is a benign encapsulated salivary gland tumor that occurs less frequently than the pleomorphic adenoma. It is composed of a uniform pattern of epithelial cells **(Figure 7-13)**. These tumors do not have the connective tissuelike component seen in pleomorphic adenomas. They occur most commonly in adult females, with a predilection for the upper lip and buccal mucosa. The **papillary cystadenoma lymphomatosum** is a unique type of monomorphic adenoma. It is also called a **Warthin tumor**. Microscopic examination demonstrates an encapsulated tumor composed of two types of tissue: epithelial and lymphoid **(Figure 7-14)**. The epithelial component is neoplastic. The epithelial component lines papillary projections that protrude from cystic structures. Sheets of lymphocytes surround the cystic structures. In some cases the lymphoid component demonstrates germinal center formation. The tumor is a painless, soft, compressible or fluctuant mass, usually in the parotid gland and very rarely in the oral cavity. It often develops bilaterally and occurs predominantly in adult men.

Monomorphic adenomas are treated by surgical excision. Recurrence is rare.

ADENOID CYSTIC CARCINOMA (CYLINDROMA)

The **adenoid cystic carcinoma** (see Figure 7-11, *E*) is a malignant tumor of salivary gland origin that can originate from either major or minor salivary gland tissue. It is unencapsulated and infiltrates surrounding tissue. This tumor is composed of small, deeply staining, uniform epithelial cells arranged in perforated round to oval islands. The microscopic appearance of adenoid cystic carcinoma has been likened to that of Swiss cheese **(Figure 7-15)**. These round and oval islands represent cylinders of tumor, and therefore this tumor has also been called a **cylindroma**. Although it is malignant, pleomorphic cells and mitotic figures are rarely seen. Malignancy is recognized based on the unique microscopic features. The adenoid cystic carcinoma is a slow-growing malignant tumor.

Metastasis occurs late in the course of the disease. The most common extraoral site for an adenoid cystic carcinoma is the parotid gland. The most

Figure 7-13 Microscopic appearance (low power) of a monomorphic adenoma shows a capsule and a uniform pattern of epithelial cells.

Figure 7-14 Microscopic appearance of a papillary cystadenoma lymphomatosum (Warthin tumor) shows spaces lined by epithelium and surrounded by lymphocytes.

Figure 7-15 Microscopic appearance of an adenoid cystic carcinoma shows perforated islands of uniform cells. Tumor *(T)* is seen infiltrating the adjacent adipose tissue.

common intraoral site is the palate. Most tumors appear as slowly growing masses that can exhibit surface ulceration (see Figure 7-11, *B* and *E*). Pain is often present because of the tendency of these tumors to surround nerves. Adenoid cystic carcinoma is more common in women than in men and is a tumor of adults, the majority occurring in the fifth and sixth decades of life.

The treatment of choice for adenoid cystic carcinoma is complete surgical excision. Radiation treatment has been attempted and has been shown to be of benefit in some cases. However, recurrence and persistent local invasion are common. About 30% of patients experience cervical lymph node involvement. Distant metastases, most often involving the lungs, can occur after many years. In these cases the prognosis is poor.

MUCOEPIDERMOID CARCINOMA

The **mucoepidermoid carcinoma** is a malignant salivary gland tumor. It is an unencapsulated, infiltrating tumor composed of a combination of mucous cells interspersed with squamouslike epithelial cells called **epidermoid cells (Figure 7-16).**

Mucoepidermoid carcinomas involving the major glands occur most often in the parotid gland, whereas minor gland tumors are most common on the palate. They appear clinically as slowly enlarging masses (see Figure 7-11, *D*). Occasionally a mucoepidermoid carcinoma may occur centrally within bone (see Figure 7-16, *B*), usually in the mandibular premolar and molar region. In this location, they appear as either a unilocular or a multilocular radiolucency (see Figure 7-16, *B*). A central mucoepidermoid carcinoma is derived from either salivary gland tissue trapped within bone or from the transformed epithelial lining of a dentigerous cyst (a developmental odontogenic cyst that forms around the crown of an unerupted or impacted tooth; see Chapter 5).

A mucoepidermoid carcinoma may occur over a wide age range. Although it usually occurs in adults after middle age, this tumor is the most common malignant salivary gland tumor in children. A female predilection is noted.

Treatment of the mucoepidermoid carcinoma consists of complete surgical excision, with close long-term follow-up for signs of recurrence and metastasis. The behavior of any one tumor is difficult to predict and is related to the histologic appearance of the tumor. Low-grade tumors have a 92% 5-year survival rate after initial treatment. For high-grade (more malignant) tumors, only 49% of patients survive 5 years after the initial treatment.

OTHER MALIGNANT SALIVARY GLAND TUMORS

In addition to the adenoid cystic carcinoma and the mucoepidermoid carcinoma, several other malignant salivary gland tumors exist, including polymorphous low-grade adenocarcinoma (lobular carcinoma), acinic cell adenocarcinoma, and other adenocarcinomas.

A

B

Figure 7-16 A, Microscopic appearance (low power) of a mucoepidermoid carcinoma shows cystic structures, mucous cells, and epidermoid cells. **B,** Radiograph of a central mucoepidermoid carcinoma shows a multilocular radiolucency.

Table 7-5 Classification of Central Odontogenic Tumors

Epithelial Odontogenic Tumors	Mesenchymal Odontogenic Tumors	Mixed Odontogenic Tumors
Ameloblastoma	Odontogenic myxoma	Ameloblastic fibroma
Calcifying epithelial odontogenic tumor (CEOT)	Cementifying fibroma	Ameloblastic fibro-odontoma
Adenomatoid odontogenic tumor (AOT or OAT)	Ossifying fibroma	Odontoma
	Peripheral ossifying fibroma	
	Benign cementoblastoma	

Odontogenic Tumors

Odontogenic tumors are derived from tooth-forming tissues. Tooth formation results from an interaction between odontogenic epithelium and odontogenic mesenchyme. Some odontogenic tumors are composed of epithelium only, some are composed of mesenchyme only, and others are composed of a mixture of both elements. Most odontogenic tumors are benign. Malignant odontogenic tumors occur but are rare. **Table 7-5** presents a classification scheme for odontogenic tumors based upon the derivation of the odontogenic tissue.

In addition to the odontogenic tumors described in this text, other uncommon odontogenic tumors exist, such as the squamous odontogenic tumor and the central odontogenic fibroma. (See the references at the end of this chapter for more detailed information on these tumors.)

EPITHELIAL ODONTOGENIC TUMORS

Ameloblastoma

The **ameloblastoma** is a benign, slow-growing but locally aggressive epithelial odontogenic tumor that may arise in either the maxilla or the mandible. It is an unencapsulated tumor that infiltrates into surrounding tissue and can cause extensive destruction. When it occurs in the maxilla, death can result from direct extension into vital structures. It is composed of ameloblast-like epithelial cells that surround areas resembling stellate reticulum. These cells are

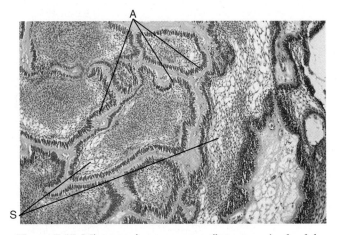

Figure 7-17 Microscopic appearance (low power) of a follicular ameloblastoma shows dental follicle-like islands composed of epithelial cells consisting of peripheral ameloblast-like cells *(A)* and stellate reticulum-like areas *(S)*.

arranged in either dental follicle-like islands or interconnecting strands **(Figure 7-17)**. An ameloblastoma may also exhibit other, less common, microscopic patterns.

The classic radiographic appearance of an ameloblastoma is a multilocular soap-bubblelike or honeycombed radiolucency **(Figure 7-18)**. In smaller tumors, the radiolucency may be unilocular. An ameloblastoma may arise anywhere in the jaws and can occur in association with a dentigerous cyst **(Figure 7-19)**. However, 80% of ameloblastomas

A

B

C

Figure 7-18 A, Radiograph of an ameloblastoma shows multilocular radiolucency in the molar area of the mandible. **B,** Radiograph of an ameloblastoma shows a multilocular radiolucency in the molar area of the mandible. **C,** Radiograph of an ameloblastoma shows a small but multilocular radiolucency in the mandibular cuspid and bicuspid region.

arise in the mandible, most often in the molar and ramus area. The molar area is also the most common location when they occur in the maxilla. The tumor may cause expansion of bone. The usual initial presentation is a slowly developing, asymptomatic swelling of the affected bone. The age range of individuals affected is broad, but most ameloblastomas occur in adults. No sex predilection is noted.

Ameloblastomas are treated by complete surgical removal. Recurrence is common. Occasionally these tumors occur in the gingiva and do not involve bone, in which case they are called **peripheral ameloblastomas.** These are also treated by surgical excision and differ from the central ameloblastomas in that they generally do not recur.

Figure 7-19 Radiograph of an ameloblastoma that formed in association with an impacted tooth and dentigerous cyst.

Calcifying Epithelial Odontogenic Tumor (CEOT)

The **CEOT**, also known as a **Pindborg tumor**, is a benign epithelial odontogenic tumor that occurs much less frequently than the ameloblastoma. It is a unique odontogenic tumor because the proliferating cells do not resemble odontogenic epithelium. The tumor is composed of islands and sheets of polyhedral (multisided) epithelial cells. Deposits similar to amyloid are seen in the tumor, and calcifications are seen within these deposits. The amyloid-like material is thought to represent a form of abnormal enamel protein (**Figure 7-20**, *A*). Radiographically the CEOT is a unilocular or multilocular radiolucency (**Figure 7-20**, *B*). Calcifications that form within the tumor appear as radiopacities within the radiolucency.

The majority of patients affected with this tumor are adults. However, the CEOT affects a broad age range, which extends from young adults to elderly individuals. No sex predilection is noted. Reports of this tumor occurring in the mandible are twice as common as reports of those occurring in the maxilla. Although it can occur anywhere in the maxilla or mandible, the bicuspid and molar area is the most common location. Many neoplasms are associated with impacted teeth.

Treatment of the CEOT depends on the size and location of the tumor and involves complete surgical excision. Recurrence has been reported, but the recurrence rate is lower than that for ameloblastoma.

Adenomatoid Odontogenic Tumor (AOT)

The **AOT**, also known as an **odontogenic adenomatoid tumor (OAT)**, is an encapsulated, benign epithelial odontogenic tumor that has a distinctive age, sex, and site distribution. It also differs from other epithelial odontogenic tumors in that it does not recur. The tumor is surrounded by a dense, fibrous connective tissue capsule and consists of ductlike structures, whorls, and large masses of cuboidal and spindle-shaped epithelial cells (**Figure 7-21**, *A*). The ductlike structures are one of the distinctive features of this tumor and are the reason for the name **adenomatoid**, or glandlike.

These structures are not ducts but actually ameloblast-like cells that resemble ducts because of their circular arrangement. Eosinophilic material is seen in the centers of these structures, and calcifications also form in this tumor.

Approximately 70% of AOTs occur in females younger than 20 years of age, and 70% involve the anterior part of the jaws. The maxilla is more commonly involved than the mandible. Many AOTs are associ-

Figure 7-20 Calcifying epithelial odontogenic tumor. **A,** Microscopic appearance (low power) of a calcifying epithelial odontogenic tumor shows sheets of epithelial cells *(E)*, amorphous material *(A)*, and calcifications *(C)*. **B,** Radiograph of a calcifying epithelial odontogenic tumor shows a multilocular radiolucency.

ated with impacted teeth. Although localized swelling may be present, most AOTs are asymptomatic and are discovered on routine radiographic examination.

Radiographically the AOT appears as a well-circumscribed radiolucency (**Figure 7-21**, *B*). Because of the frequent association with an impacted tooth, an AOT often simulates a dentigerous cyst. However, unlike the dentigerous cyst (see Chapter 4), the AOT extends beyond the cementoenamel junction and can involve 50% to 60% of the root. As calcifications form within the tumor, radiopaque areas of varying size are visible on radiographs.

The clinician should treat AOT conservatively by a process called enucleation, in which the tumor is removed in its entirety. The tumor is easily separated from the surrounding bone, and recurrence is rare.

Calcifying Odontogenic Cyst

The **calcifying odontogenic cyst** is usually a nonaggressive cystic lesion lined by odontogenic epithelium with an associated, characteristic, ghost cell keratinization (**Figure 7-22**, *A*). The epithelium resembles that seen in an ameloblastoma, consisting

Figure 7-21 Adenomatoid odontogenic tumor. **A,** Microscopic appearance of an adenomatoid odontogenic tumor shows the capsule *(C)*, epithelial cells, and ductlike structures *(D)*. **B,** Radiograph of an adenomatoid odontogenic tumor shows a unilocular radiolucency surrounding the crown of an unerupted maxillary cuspid.

Figure 7-22 Calcifying odontogenic cyst. **A,** Microscopic appearance of a calcifying odontogenic cyst shows a cystic structure lined by odontogenic epithelium *(E)* with associated ghost cells *(G)*. **B,** Radiograph of a calcifying odontogenic cyst shows a unilocular radiolucency of the mandible.

of ameloblast-like cells and stellate reticulum-like areas. Ghost cells are round structures with clear centers. The calcifying odontogenic cyst is usually a radiographically well-defined lesion that can present as either a unilocular or a multilocular radiolucency (**Figure 7-22**, *B*). Calcifications can occur and are seen as radiopaque areas. The calcifying odontogenic cyst affects a broad age range but is most commonly seen in individuals younger than 40 years of age. No sex predilection has been noted.

A solid variant of the calcifying odontogenic cyst has been reported and has been suggested to represent a neoplasm rather than a cyst.

The calcifying odontogenic cyst is generally treated by surgical enucleation; although a few recurrences have been reported, it usually does not recur. The solid variant may exhibit more aggressive behavior and may be treated with a more extensive surgical procedure.

MESENCHYMAL ODONTOGENIC TUMORS

Odontogenic Myxoma

The **odontogenic myxoma** is a benign nonencapsulated infiltrating tumor composed of a pale-staining mucopolysaccharide ground substance that contains dispersed cells with long cytoplasmic processes (**Figure 7-23**, *A*). This tissue closely resembles tissue seen in the dental papilla, the mesenchymal component of tooth-forming tissue.

The odontogenic myxoma most often occurs in young people between 10 and 29 years of age. No sex predilection is noted.

The odontogenic myxoma exhibits a multilocular, honeycombed radiolucency with poorly defined margins (**Figure 7-23**, *B*). The tumor may become quite large and cause tooth displacement. Although most cases occur in the mandible, the odontogenic myxoma may occur anywhere in the maxilla or mandible.

The odontogenic myxoma is treated by complete surgical excision. The extent of the surgery depends on the size of the tumor. The recurrence rate is 25%. When they recur, most myxomas recur within the first 2 years after treatment.

Central Cementifying and Ossifying Fibromas

The central **cementifying fibroma** is a benign well-circumscribed tumor composed of fibrous connective tissue and rounded or globular calcifications resembling cementum (**Figure 7-24**, *A*). Because microscopic examination demonstrates fibrous connective

Figure 7-23 **A,** Photomicrograph of an odontogenic myxoma shows background substance containing widely dispersed cells with long cytoplasmic processes. **B,** Radiograph of an odontogenic myxoma shows a multilocular, honeycombed radiolucency.

tissue and calcifications, it is classified as a fibro-osseous lesion. The central cementifying fibroma and central ossifying fibroma are variants of the same tumor. In the central **ossifying fibroma**, the calcifications more closely resemble bone trabeculae. Some tumors have bone trabeculae and globular calcifications resembling cementum. These are called central **cemento-ossifying fibromas**. This variation in microscopic appearance results from the potential of periodontal ligament cells to produce either cementum or bone. The tumor usually occurs in adults in the third and fourth decades of life. Females are affected more often than males. Affected patients may be asymptomatic or demonstrate bone expansion or facial asymmetry. Radiographically it is well defined and varies from radiolucent to radiopaque, depending on the amount of calcified tissue present (**Figure 7-24**, *B* and C). The majority of cases occur in the mandible.

Other fibro-osseous lesions, such as periapical cemento-osseous dysplasia (discussed in Chapter 8) and fibrous dysplasia (discussed in Chapter 9), may be histologically identical to the central cementifying and central ossifying fibroma. The radiographic appearance of these individual lesions is important in distinguishing them from each other.

The central cementifying and central ossifying fibromas are treated by surgical excision. Because these lesions are well delineated, they separate easily from the surrounding bone. Recurrence is rare.

Figure 7-24 A, Photomicrograph of a central cementifying fibroma shows rounded, globular calcifications *(GC)* and cellular fibrous connective tissue *(FCT)*. **B,** Radiograph of a central cementifying fibroma shows a well-circumscribed radiolucent lesion. **C,** Radiograph of a central cementifying fibroma shows a radiolucent and radiopaque lesion.

Benign Cementoblastoma

The **benign cementoblastoma** is a cementum-producing lesion that is found fused to the root or roots of a vital tooth. The radiographic appearance is distinctive and consists of a well-defined radiopaque mass with a surrounding radiolucent halo **(Figure 7-25)**. The neoplasm is seen in continuity with the root or roots of a mandibular molar or premolar tooth. Obliteration of the apex of the affected tooth is common. Occasional cases may cause localized bone expansion. The tumor typically occurs in young adults. Unlike other odontogenic tumors, pain is a frequent symptom. Microscopic examination reveals a proliferation of cellular cementum fused to the root or roots of the affected tooth.

Treatment of the benign cementoblastoma consists of enucleation of the tumor and removal of the involved tooth. It does not recur.

MIXED ODONTOGENIC TUMORS

Ameloblastic Fibroma

The **ameloblastic fibroma** is a benign, nonencapsulated odontogenic tumor composed of both strands and small islands of odontogenic epithelium and tissue that resembles the dental papilla **(Figure 7-26)**. The ameloblastic fibroma occurs in young children and adults. However, most cases occur in individuals younger than 20 years of age. A male sex predilection is noted. The most common location is the mandibular bicuspid and molar region. Most patients are asymptomatic, but bone expansion or swelling may be noted.

Radiographically the ameloblastic fibroma appears as either a well-defined or a poorly defined

A

B

Figure 7-26 A, Microscopic appearance of an ameloblastic fibroma shows a combination of odontogenic epithelium *(E)* and mesenchymal tissue *(M)*. **B,** Radiograph of an ameloblastic fibroma shows a poorly defined unilocular radiolucency.

Figure 7-25 Radiograph of a benign cementoblastoma shows a well-circumscribed radiopaque mass surrounded by a radiolucent halo and attached to the roots of a mandibular first molar.

unilocular or multilocular radiolucency (see Figure 7-26, *B*).

The ameloblastic fibroma is treated by surgical excision. The recurrence rate is low.

Ameloblastic Fibro-odontoma

The **ameloblastic fibro-odontoma** is a benign odontogenic tumor that has features of an ameloblastic fibroma and an odontoma. Most cases occur in young adults with an average age of 10 years. No sex predilection is noted. The ameloblastic fibro-odontoma typically arises in the posterior jaws and is often asymptomatic. However, some patients may experience swelling of the affected area.

Radiographic examination reveals a well-delineated radiolucent lesion that may be unilocular or multilocular. Calcifications of various size and shape are noted within the radiolucency. These calcifications represent tooth formation.

Microscopic examination demonstrates features similar to those described in the ameloblastic fibroma combined with structures that resemble teeth. Therefore various amounts of enamel, dentin, cementum, and pulp tissue are noted.

The ameloblastic fibro-odontoma is a well-circumscribed lesion that usually separates easily from the surrounding bone and therefore can be treated by conservation surgical excision. Recurrence is unusual.

Odontoma

The **odontoma** is an odontogenic tumor composed of mature enamel, dentin, cementum, and pulp tissue. The odontoma is the most common of the odontogenic tumors. The two types of odontomas are compound and complex. A **compound odontoma** consists of a collection of numerous small teeth. A **complex odontoma** consists of a mass of enamel, dentin, cementum, and pulp that does not resemble a normal tooth.

Most odontomas are detected in adolescents and young adults. No sex predilection is noted. The compound odontoma is usually located in the anterior maxilla, and the complex odontoma most commonly occurs in the posterior mandible. The most common clinical manifestation of an odontoma is the failure of a permanent tooth to erupt. Most odontomas are small, but large lesions can cause swelling and displacement of erupted teeth. Odontomas can be associated with impacted or unerupted teeth and with odontogenic cysts and tumors.

Radiographically, compound odontomas appear as a cluster of numerous miniature teeth surrounded by a radiolucent halo **(Figure 7-27)**. A complex

Figure 7-27 Radiograph of a compound odontoma shows a collection of numerous, small, toothlike radiopacities surrounded by a radiolucent halo.

odontoma appears as a radiopaque mass surrounded by a thin radiolucent halo **(Figure 7-28).**

Treatment of an odontoma consists of surgical excision. Odontomas generally do not recur.

Figure 7-28 Radiograph of a complex odontoma shows a radiopaque mass surrounded by a radiolucent halo.

PERIPHERAL ODONTOGENIC TUMORS

Peripheral Ossifying Fibroma

The **peripheral ossifying fibroma** is usually a well-demarcated sessile or pedunculated lesion that appears to originate from the gingival interdental papilla and is most likely derived from cells of the periodontal ligament (**Figure 7-29,** *A*). It is more common in females than in males and often occurs in young individuals. It has been reported in children and adults.

It is composed of cellular fibrous connective tissue interspersed with scattered bone and cementum-like calcifications (**Figure 7-29,** *B*). The peripheral ossifying fibroma is microscopically similar to the central cementifying fibroma and central ossifying fibroma.

Treatment of the peripheral ossifying fibroma consists of surgical excision with thorough scaling of the adjacent teeth to remove any irritants that can induce regrowth of the lesion. The recurrence rate for the peripheral ossifying fibroma is about 16%.

Figure 7-29 A, Clinical appearance of a peripheral ossifying fibroma shows an exophytic lesion involving the palatal gingiva of the maxillary anterior teeth. **B,** Photomicrograph of a peripheral ossifying fibroma shows bonelike calcifications *(B)* in cellular fibrous connective tissue *(CT)*. A small amount of surface epithelium *(E)* is also visible.

Other Peripheral Odontogenic Tumors

Several other odontogenic tumors have been reported to occur in the gingiva without underlying bone involvement. Although rare, these lesions are of importance to the dental hygienist because of their gingival location. The peripheral ameloblastoma and the peripheral CEOT have been reported to occur in this location.

Treatment for the tumors described previously is surgical excision. After appropriate treatment, recurrence is rare.

Tumors of Soft Tissue

Tumors of soft tissue include benign and malignant tumors of adipose tissue (fat), nerve, muscle, blood, and lymphatic vessels.

LIPOMA

The **lipoma** is a benign tumor of mature fat cells. Clinically it appears as a yellowish mass that is surfaced by a thin layer of epithelium (**Figure 7-30**, *A*). Because of this thin epithelium, a delicate pattern of blood vessels is usually seen on its surface. The majority of lipomas occur in individuals over 40 years of age, and no sex predilection is noted. The most common intraoral locations are the buccal mucosa and the vestibule. Microscopic examination reveals a well-delineated tumor composed of lobules of mature fat cells that are uniform in size and shape (**Figure 7-30**, *B*).

The lipoma is treated by surgical excision and generally does not recur.

TUMORS OF NERVE TISSUE

Neurofibroma and Schwannoma

The **neurofibroma** (**Figure 7-31**, *A*) and the **schwannoma** are benign tumors derived from nerve tissue. The schwannoma is also called a **neurilemmoma**. Both of these tumors are derived from Schwann cells, which are a component of the connective tissue surrounding a nerve. Although the neurofibroma and schwannoma are distinct tumors microscopically, they are quite similar in their clinical presentation and behavior and are therefore discussed together. The tongue is the most common intraoral location. Neurofibromas and schwannomas may occur at any age, and no sex predilection is noted. Microscopic examination of a neurofibroma reveals a fairly well-delineated, diffuse proliferation of spindle-shaped Schwann cells (**Figure 7-31**, *B*), whereas a schwannoma exhibits spindle-shaped Schwann cells arranged in palisaded whorls around a central pink zone. A connective tissue capsule surrounds the schwannoma.

The treatment for a neurofibroma or schwannoma is surgical excision. They generally do not recur. Malignant tumors of nerve tissue occur but are extremely rare.

Multiple neurofibromas occur in a genetically inherited disorder known as **neurofibromatosis of von Recklinghausen** or **von Recklinghausen disease**. Patients with this syndrome have numerous

Figure 7-30 A, Clinical appearance of a lipoma. **B,** Photomicrograph of a lipoma shows mature fat cells. (**A** courtesy Dr. Edward V. Zegarelli.)

Figure 7-31 A, Clinical appearance of a neurofibroma shows a nonulcerated mass on the lateral border of the tongue. **B,** Photomicrograph of a neurofibroma.

neurofibromas on the skin and other sites in addition to other abnormalities. This syndrome is genetically inherited and is described in detail in Chapter 6.

Granular Cell Tumor

The **granular cell tumor** is a benign tumor composed of large cells with a granular cytoplasm. It most likely arises from neural or primitive mesenchymal cells. The granular cell tumor most often occurs on the tongue followed by the buccal mucosa. The tumor appears as a painless, nonulcerated nodule (**Figure 7-32**, *A*). The majority of cases occur in adults, and a female sex predilection is noted. Microscopic examination reveals large oval-shaped cells with a granular cytoplasm. The granular cells are found in the connective tissue and between striated muscle fibers

Figure 7-32 A, Clinical appearance of a granular cell tumor of the tongue shows a nonulcerated mass. **B,** Photomicrograph of a granular cell tumor showing granular cell(s) *(G)* between striated muscle fiber(s) *(M).* **C,** Photomicroscope of a granular cell tumor showing overlying pseudoepitheliomatous hyperplasia. (**A** courtesy Dr. Sidney Eisig.)

(**Figure 7-32,** *B*). The overlying surface epithelium exhibits pseudoepitheliomatous hyperplasia, which is a benign proliferation of epithelium into the connective tissue (**Figure 7-32,** *C*).

This tumor is treated by surgical excision and does not recur.

Congenital Epulis

The **congenital epulis,** or **congenital epulis of the newborn,** is a benign neoplasm composed of cells that closely resemble those seen in the granular cell tumor. The neoplasm most likely arises from a primitive mesenchymal cell. This tumor is present at birth and appears as a sessile or pedunculated mass on the gingiva. It usually occurs on the anterior maxillary gingiva and almost always occurs in girls.

The congenital epulis is treated by surgical excision and does not recur. Occasional examples have regressed without treatment.

TUMORS OF MUSCLE

Tumors of muscle are extremely uncommon in the oral cavity. The **rhabdomyoma,** a benign tumor of striated muscle, has been reported to occur on the tongue. The **leiomyoma,** a benign tumor of smooth muscle, may occur in association with blood vessels. These tumors are called **vascular leiomyomas** and occasionally occur in the oral cavity. The **rhabdomyosarcoma,** a malignant tumor of striated muscle, is the most common malignant soft tissue tumor of the head and neck in children. It typically occurs in individuals under 10 years of age and has a male sex predilection. It is a rapidly growing, destructive tumor.

The rhabdomyosarcoma is an aggressive, malignant tumor that is best treated by a combination of multidrug chemotherapy, radiation therapy, and surgery. Despite treatment, the prognosis is poor.

VASCULAR TUMORS

Hemangioma

The **hemangioma** is a benign proliferation of capillaries (**Figure 7-33,** *A* and *B*). It is a common vascular lesion considered by many to represent a developmental lesion rather than a tumor because hemangiomas do not generally exhibit an unlimited growth potential. Some contain numerous small

A

B

C

Figure 7-33 Clinical appearance of a hemangioma of the lower lip **(A)** and of the buccal mucosa **(B). C,** Microscopic appearance of a cavernous hemangioma showing large dilated blood vessels *(B)* filled with red blood cells *(RBC).*

capillaries and are called **capillary hemangiomas.** Others contain larger blood vessels and are called **cavernous hemangiomas (Figure 7-33,** *C*).

Most are present at birth or arise shortly thereafter. More than half of the hemangiomas that occur in the body occur in the head and neck area. The tongue is the most common intraoral location. Involvement of the tongue often leads to marked enlargement (macroglossia). Hemangiomas are more common in girls than in boys. They also occur in adults as a response to trauma and represent an abnormal proliferation of blood vessels during the healing process. They appear as variably sized, deep-red or blue lesions that frequently blanch when pressure is applied.

Many hemangiomas undergo spontaneous remission. Others can enlarge rapidly because of hemorrhage, thrombosis, or inflammation. Treatment is variable and includes surgery or the injection of a sclerosing solution into the lesion, which causes it to resolve.

Lymphangioma

The **lymphangioma** is a benign tumor of lymphatic vessels. It is less common than the hemangioma. Most lymphangiomas are present at birth, and half arise in the head and neck area. No sex predilection is noted. The most common intraoral location is the tongue, where the lymphangioma is an ill-defined mass with a pebbly surface. Involvement of the tongue may lead to macroglossia. A cystic lymphangioma in the neck is called a *cystic hygroma*. It is usually present at birth or develops shortly thereafter.

Lymphangiomas are generally treated by surgical excision and tend to recur.

Malignant Vascular Tumors

Malignant vascular tumors, such as angiosarcoma, may occur in the oral cavity but are rare. **Kaposi sarcoma** is a malignant vascular tumor and may arise in multiple sites, including the skin and oral mucosa. Classic Kaposi sarcoma occurs as multiple purplish tumors of the lower extremities in older men. The condition in these patients progresses slowly, usually resolves with low doses of radiation, and rarely causes death. With the advent of the human immunodeficiency virus (HIV) epidemic in the 1980s, Kaposi sarcoma has appeared in a much more aggressive form. In HIV-positive patients, these lesions are often seen in the oral cavity where they present as purple macules, plaques, or exophytic tumors. The hard palate and gingiva are the most common intraoral sites. Kaposi sarcoma associated with HIV infection is described in Chapter 4. Kaposi sarcoma may also occur in patients with other forms of immunodeficiency, specifically patients who have received immunosuppressive drug therapy.

Kaposi sarcoma is caused by a human herpesvirus (HHV) that is called both human herpesvirus type 8 (HHV-8) and Kaposi sarcoma–associated herpesvirus (KSAH). Men are more often affected than women. Microscopic examination reveals a neoplasm composed of spindle-shaped cells mixed with slitlike spaces containing red blood cells.

Kaposi sarcoma is treated by surgical excision, radiation therapy, chemotherapy, or a combination of these therapies. In HIV-positive patients, recurrence is common and the disease may be rapidly progressive.

Tumors of Melanin-Producing Cells

MELANOCYTIC NEVI

The word **nevus** (plural, nevi) has two meanings. Here the word is used to mean a developmental tumor of melanocytes (melanin-producing cells), which are called **nevus cells.** Nevus also refers to a pigmented congenital lesion (a lesion present at birth). A hemangioma present at birth is an example of this type of nevus.

Melanocytic nevi can arise on the skin or the oral mucosa. Intraoral tumors consist of tan to brown macules or papules that occur most often on the hard palate. The buccal mucosa is the second most common intraoral location **(Figure 7-34).** They occur twice as often in women as in men and are usually first identified in individuals between 20 and 50 years of age.

Most pigmented lesions that occur in the oral cavity are benign. Pigmented lesions that exhibit ulceration, an increase in size, or a change in color may be malignant.

A biopsy, followed by microscopic examination, is indicated for pigmented lesion of unknown cause, unknown duration, or recent onset. Surgical excision is the treatment of choice for intraoral melanocytic nevi. Recurrence is rare.

MALIGNANT MELANOMA

Malignant melanoma is a malignant tumor of melanocytes **(Figure 7-35).** Although the name malignant melanoma suggests that a benign counterpart exists, all melanomas are malignant. Most malignant melanomas arise on the skin as a result of prolonged exposure to sunlight. Primary malignant melanoma of the oral cavity is rare. However, malignant melanomas that arise on the skin may metastasize to the oral cavity.

Malignant melanoma is usually a rapidly enlarging blue-to-black mass. Malignant melanoma is a very aggressive tumor that exhibits an unpredictable behavior and early metastasis. The most common intraoral locations are the palate and maxillary gingiva. These neoplasms usually occur in adults older than 40 years of age.

Malignant melanomas are treated by surgical excision. Chemotherapy may be used in conjunction with surgery. The prognosis for oral malignant melanoma is poor.

Tumors of Bone and Cartilage

TORUS

A **torus** (plural, tori) is a benign lesion composed of normal compact bone. Tori are located in the midline of the palate **(torus palatinus** or **palatal torus)** or on the lingual aspect of the mandible in the area of the premolars **(torus mandibularis** or **mandibular torus) (Figure 7-36,** *A* and *B*). Tori are not true tumors. Because they have a hereditary basis, they are also discussed in Chapter 6. They are described in this chapter because of their resemblance to osteomas. Tori occur in adults and are more common in females than in males. They present as asymptomatic, bony hard, lobulated masses covered by epithelium with very little underlying fibrous connective tissue. Surface ulceration may occur if a torus is traumatized. Palatal or mandibular tori may result in radiopaque areas superimposed on tooth roots. The diagnosis is confirmed by the presence of a torus on clinical examination.

No treatment is necessary for these lesions unless they interfere with the fabrication of a prosthetic appliance.

Figure 7-34 Clinical appearance of a melanocytic nevus shows a well-defined pigmented lesion on the labial mucosa.

Figure 7-35 Clinical appearance of a malignant melanoma shows a darkly pigmented lesion in the area of the fauces. (Courtesy Dr. Edward V. Zegarelli.)

Figure 7-36 A, Clinical appearance of bilateral lobulated mandibular tori. **B,** Clinical appearance of a lobulated torus palatinus.

EXOSTOSIS

An **exostosis** (plural, exostoses) is a small nodular excrescence of normal compact bone **(Figure 7-37).** Exostoses present as asymptomatic, bony hard nodules on the buccal aspect of the maxillary or mandibular alveolar ridges. Most cases occur in adults and no sex predilection is noted.

No treatment is indicated unless they interfere with the fabrication of a prosthetic appliance.

OSTEOMA

An osteoma is an asymptomatic benign tumor composed of benign compact bone. It is a slow-growing tumor that appears radiographically as either a sharply defined radiopaque mass within bone or a delineated mass attached to the outer surface of the bone **(Figure 7-38).** A large central osteoma may cause expansion of the involved bone. No sex predilection is noted. Osteomas are a component of Gardner syndrome that is genetically transmitted and described in Chapter 6.

Osteomas are treated by surgical excision and generally do not recur.

Figure 7-37 Clinical appearance of exostoses on the labial and buccal aspect of the maxilla. Less prominent exostoses are noted on the labial and buccal aspect of the mandible.

OSTEOSARCOMA

Osteosarcoma (osteogenic sarcoma) is a malignant tumor of bone-forming tissue. It is the most common primary malignant tumor of bone in patients less than 40 years of age. Tumors that involve the long bones occur at an average age of 27 years, whereas the average age of occurrence for tumors that involve the jawbones is about 37 years. These tumors occur in the mandible twice as frequently as in the maxilla and are more common in males than in females. Patients may experience a diffuse swelling or mass that is often painful **(Figure 7-39,** *A*). Some patients present initially with a toothache or exhibit tooth mobility. Paresthesia of the lip is common in tumors involving the mandible.

The radiographic appearance of an osteosarcoma varies from radiolucent to radiopaque (**Figure 7-39,** *B*). It is usually a destructive, poorly defined lesion and may or may not involve the adjacent soft tissue. Asymmetric widening of the periodontal ligament space and a sunburst pattern may be seen radiographically in some cases. Microscopic examination of this tumor shows pleomorphic and hyperchromatic cells and abnormal bone formation. Abnormal cartilage formation may also be present (**Figure 7-39,** *C*).

Figure 7-38 Radiograph of an osteoma shows a radiopacity of the posterior mandible. (Courtesy Dr. Sidney Eisig.)

Figure 7-39 A, Clinical appearance of an osteogenic sarcoma in another patient shows swelling. **B,** Radiograph of an osteogenic sarcoma in the left molar area shows a poorly defined radiopaque lesion. **C,** Microscopic appearance of an osteogenic sarcoma shows pleomorphic *(P)* and hyperchromatic cells and bone formation *(B).*

Currently, osteosarcomas are treated with preoperative multiagent chemotherapy followed by surgery. Jaw tumors frequently recur after treatment. Only about 20% of patients with osteosarcoma of the jaws survive 5 years.

TUMORS OF CARTILAGE

Cartilaginous tumors of the jawbones are extremely rare and are more likely to be malignant than benign. A **chondroma** is a benign tumor of cartilage. A **chondrosarcoma** is a malignant tumor of cartilage **(Figure 7-40)** that may occur in either the maxilla or the mandible and is more common in males than in females. Most patients have enlargement of the affected bone.

Chondrosarcomas are treated by wide surgical excision. Radiation therapy and chemotherapy are not effective. The prognosis is poor. Only about 30% of patients with chondrosarcoma involving the jaws survive 5 years after the diagnosis.

Tumors of Blood-Forming Tissues

LEUKEMIA

Leukemia comprises a broad group of disorders characterized by an overproduction of atypical white blood cells. The atypical white blood cells proliferate in the bone marrow and then spill into the circulating blood and tissues. Several types of leukemia are seen that are classified according to the kind of cells that are proliferating: myelocytes, lymphocytes, or monocytes.

Leukemias are divided into two forms: acute and chronic. Acute leukemia is most common in children and young adults and is characterized by a proliferation of immature white blood cells (blasts). Chronic leukemia exhibits an excess proliferation of mature white blood cells and most frequently occurs in middle-aged adults. Leukemia occurs more often in males than in females.

Although oral involvement may occur in any type of leukemia, the monocytic variant most often exhibits oral lesions. A common oral manifestation of monocytic leukemia is diffuse gingival enlargement with persistent bleeding **(Figure 7-41)**. (Leukemia is further described in Chapter 9.)

The treatment of leukemia consists of chemotherapy, radiation therapy, and corticosteroids. The prognosis depends on the type and the extent of disease.

LYMPHOMA (NON-HODGKIN'S LYMPHOMA)

Lymphoma is a malignant tumor of lymphoid tissue. Numerous types of lymphoma exist, each of which is differentiated based on microscopic findings. The characteristic clinical presentation is gradual enlargement of involved lymph nodes. Rarely a lymphoma may present as a primary lesion in the oral soft tissues or bone. However, most lymphomas involve either lymph nodes or aggregates of lymphoid tissue that are located in the digestive tract from the oral cavity to the anus. In the oral cavity, lymphoid tissue is located at the base of the tongue, soft palate, and pharynx (Waldeyer ring). The most common location for intraoral lymphoma is the ton-

Figure 7-40 Clinical appearance of a chondrosarcoma shows an exophytic mass in the anterior mandible.

Figure 7-41 Clinical appearance of a patient with leukemic infiltration of the gingiva resulting in diffuse enlargement. (Courtesy Dr. Edward V. Zegarelli.)

sillar area. Lymphomas usually occur in adults and are more common in males than in females.

Lymphoma is treated by radiotherapy, surgery, chemotherapy, or a combination of these therapies. The prognosis depends on the type of lymphoma and the extent of involvement.

MULTIPLE MYELOMA

Multiple myeloma is a systemic, malignant proliferation of plasma cells that causes destructive lesions in bone. The neoplastic plasma cells produce large amounts of immunoglobulin. Most patients are older than 40 years of age, and the disease occurs most commonly in the seventh decade of life. Males are affected more often than females. Patients usually experience bone pain and swelling. Pathologic fracture of an involved bone is common and typically occurs in bones weakened as a result of their destruction by the proliferation of neoplastic plasma cells (**Figure 7-42**, *A*).

Radiographically, the involved bones show multiple radiolucent lesions. The disease can involve the

Figure 7-42 Multiple myeloma. **A,** Microscopic appearance of multiple myeloma shows a proliferating of plasma cells. **B,** Radiograph shows multiple radiolucent lesions of the mandible in a patient with multiple myeloma.

skull, spine, ribs, pelvis, long bones, and jaws. The mandible is affected more often than the maxilla (see **Figure 7-42,** *B*). Most patients have an elevation of a single type of immunoglobulin, which is detected by a process called immunoelectrophoresis. This elevation is called a **monoclonal spike.** Patients may have fragments of immunoglobulins in the urine. These fragments are called **Bence Jones proteins.**

The tumors are composed of sheets of well- to poorly-differentiated plasma cells.

A localized tumor of plasma cells in soft tissue is called an **extramedullary plasmacytoma.** Although these are rare tumors, they are more common in the head and neck region than anywhere else in the body. Many patients with extramedullary plasmacytoma will eventually develop multiple myeloma. Therefore patients with a single tumor of plasma cells must be evaluated to determine if the lesion is solitary or part of multiple myeloma.

Patients with multiple myeloma are treated with chemotherapy and radiation. The prognosis is poor. The most common cause of death is infection followed by renal failure. Only 18% of patients survive 5 years after the diagnosis.

Figure 7-43 Radiograph shows diffuse radiolucent and radiopaque changes resulting from metastatic carcinoma of the prostate gland.

Metastatic Tumors of the Jaws

Metastatic tumors of the jaws from primary sites elsewhere in the body are rare. The majority of these tumors arise from the thyroid, breast, lungs, prostate gland, and kidneys. The most frequent intraoral site for metastatic tumors is the mandible. Patients display various signs and symptoms, including pain, paresthesia or anesthesia of the lip, swelling, expansion of the affected bone, and loosening of the teeth in the involved area. Metastatic lesions usually appear several years after the primary lesion is discovered. Occasionally the oral metastatic tumor is the first manifestation of a primary tumor elsewhere. Most patients are adults, and males are affected more often than females.

The radiographic appearance of metastatic tumors is variable **(Figure 7-43).** Lesions are usually poorly defined and radiolucent. The roots of the involved teeth may show a spiked appearance. Metastatic tumors from the breast, prostate gland, and lungs may form bone and therefore may show areas of radiopacity.

Histologically the metastatic tumor resembles the primary malignancy. The majority of metastatic tumors in the jaws is epithelial in origin, and most are adenocarcinomas.

Chemotherapy and radiation therapy are used to alleviate the discomfort of metastatic tumors in the jaws. The prognosis for patients with tumors that have metastasized to the jaws is poor.

Selected References

Books

Neville BW et al: *Oral and maxillofacial pathology,* ed 2, Philadelphia, 2001, WB Saunders.

Regezi JA, Sciubba JJ: *Oral pathology: clinical-pathologic correlations,* ed 4, Philadelphia, 2003, WB Saunders.

Robbins SL, Kumar V: *Basic pathology,* ed 6, Philadelphia, 1997, WB Saunders.

Journal Articles
Tumors of Squamous Epithelium

Abbey LM, Page DG, Sawyer DR: The clinical and histopathologic features of a series of 464 oral squamous cell papillomas, *Oral Surg Oral Med Oral Pathol* 49:419, 1980.

Damm DD et al: Leukoplakia of the maxillary vestibule—an association with Viadent? *Oral Surg Oral Med Oral Pathol Oral Radiol Endod* 87:61, 1999.

Kaugars GE et al: Actinic cheilitis: a review of 152 cases, *Oral Surg Oral Med Oral Pathol Oral Radiol Endod* 88:181, 1999.

Krutchkoff DF et al: Oral cancer: a survey of 566 cases from the University of Connecticut Oral Pathology Biopsy Service 1975-1986, *Oral Surg Oral Med Oral Pathol* 70:192, 1990.

Medina JE, Dichtel W, Luna MA: Verrucous-squamous carcinomas of the oral cavity. A clinicopathologic study of 104 cases, *Arch Otolaryngol* 110:437, 1984.

Padayachee A, Van Wyk CW: Human papillomavirus (HPV) in oral squamous cell papillomas, *J Oral Pathol* 16:353, 1987.

Shibuya H et al: Multiple primary cancer risk in patients with squamous cell carcinoma of the oral cavity, *Cancer* 60:3083, 1987.

Leukoplakia and Erythroplakia

Shafer WG, Waldron CA: Erythroplakia of the oral cavity, *Cancer* 36:1021, 1975.

Silverman S Jr, Gorsky M, Lozada F: Oral leukoplakia and malignant transformation. A follow-up study of 257 patients, *Cancer* 53:563, 1984.

Waldron CA, Shafer WG: Leukoplakia revisited. A clinicopathologic study of 3256 oral leukoplakias, *Cancer* 36:1386, 1975.

Salivary Gland Tumors

Eveson JW, Cawson RA: Tumours of the minor (oropharyngeal) salivary glands: a demographic study of 336 cases, *J Oral Pathol* 14:500, 1985.

Neville B et al: Labial salivary gland tumors, *Cancer* 61:2113, 1988.

Waldron CA, El-Mofty SK, Gnepp DR: Tumors of the intraoral minor salivary glands: a demographic and histologic study of 426 cases, *Oral Surg Oral Med Oral Pathol* 66:323, 1988.

Odontogenic Tumors

Ai-Ru L, Zhen L, Jian S: Calcifying epithelial odontogenic tumors: a clinicopathologic study of 9 cases, *J Oral Pathol* 11:399, 1982.

Buchner A, Ficarra G, Hansen LS: Peripheral odontogenic fibroma, *Oral Surg Oral Med Oral Pathol* 64:432, 1987.

Courtney RM, Kerr DA: The odontogenic adenomatoid tumor: a comprehensive study of 20 new cases, *Oral Surg Oral Med Oral Pathol* 39:424, 1975.

Daley TD, Wysocki GP: Peripheral odontogenic fibroma, *Oral Surg Oral Med Oral Pathol* 78:329, 1994.

Kaugars GE, Miller ME, Abbey LM: Odontomas, *Oral Surg Oral Med Oral Pathol* 67:172, 1989.

Shamaskin RG, Svirsky JA, Kaugars GE: Intraosseous and extraosseous calcifying odontogenic cyst (Gorlin cyst), *J Oral Maxillofac Surg* 47:562, 1989.

Ulmansky M et al: Benign cementoblastoma, *Oral Surg Oral Med Oral Pathol* 77:48, 1994.

Waldron CA, El-Mofty SK: A histopathologic study of 116 ameloblastomas with special reference to the desmoplastic variant, *Oral Surg Oral Med Oral Pathol* 63:441, 1987.

Vascular Tumors

Hernandez GA et al: Aneurysmal bone cyst versus hemangioma of the mandible, *Oral Surg Oral Med Oral Pathol* 76:790, 1993.

Tumors of Melanin-Producing Cells

Kaugars GE et al: Oral melanotic macules, *Oral Surg Oral Med Oral Pathol* 76:59, 1993.

Tumors of Bone

Forteza G, Colmenero A, Lopez-Barea F: Osteogenic sarcoma of the maxilla and mandible, *Oral Surg Oral Med Oral Pathol* 62:179, 1986.

Tumors of Blood-Forming Tissues

Lambertenghi-Deliliers G et al: Incidence of jaw lesions in 193 patients with multiple myeloma, *Oral Surg Oral Med Oral Pathol* 65:533, 1988.

Raubenheimer EJ, Dauth J, van Wilpe E: Multiple myeloma: a study of 10 cases, *J Oral Pathol* 16:383, 1987.

Metastatic Tumors

Hasimoto N et al: Pathological characteristics of metastatic carcinoma in the human mandible, *J Oral Pathol* 16:362, 1987.

Review Questions

1. Which of the following are associated with the neoplastic transformation of cells?
   A. Chemicals
   B. Sunlight
   C. Viruses
   D. All of the above
   E. Only A and B

2. Neoplasia involves:
   A. Abnormal proliferation of cells in response to tissue damage
   B. Controlled proliferation of cells
   C. Normal arrangement of proliferating cells
   D. Irreversible change that results in an uncontrolled multiplication of cells
   E. Cell proliferation associated with tissue repair

3. Which of the following statements concerning leukoplakia is *true*?
   A. Most cases represent examples of epithelial dysplasia.
   B. Sites that are at high risk for epithelial dysplasia include the palate and gingiva.
   C. A biopsy should be performed to establish a diagnosis.
   D. Leukoplakia is less common than erythroplakia.
   E. Leukoplakia is a term that describes a histologic appearance of epithelium.

4. Which of the following is a characteristic of benign tumors?
   A. Numerous mitotic figures
   B. Pleomorphic cells
   C. Slow growth
   D. Metastasis likely
   E. Invasive growth

5. A small exophytic lesion of the tongue that is the color of normal mucosa and is composed of papillary projections arranged in a cauliflower-like appearance is most likely a:
   A. Papilloma
   B. Fibroma
   C. Neurofibroma
   D. Granular cell tumor
   E. Hemangioma

6. Which of the following is a histologic characteristic of squamous cell carcinoma?
   A. Invasion of tumor cells into the connective tissue
   B. Pleomorphic epithelial cells
   C. Keratin pearls
   D. Cells with hyperchromatic nuclei
   E. All of the above

7. Which of the following are the most common locations for intraoral squamous cell carcinoma?
   A. Upper labial mucosa, buccal mucosa, and hard palate
   B. Lower labial mucosa, maxillary gingiva, and buccal mucosa
   C. Floor of the mouth, ventrolateral tongue, and soft palate
   D. Anterior tongue, mandibular gingiva, and retromolar area
   E. Commissure of the lips and anterior hard palate

8. A patient with squamous cell carcinoma of the lateral tongue exhibits metastatic disease in the lungs. What clinical stage correlates with these findings?
   A. Stage I
   B. Stage II
   C. Stage III
   D. Stage IV
   E. None of the above

9. Which of the following represents the earliest clinical example of squamous cell carcinoma?
   A. Exophytic mass
   B. Erythematous plaque
   C. Nonhealing ulceration
   D. Destructive radiolucency
   E. Recurrent ulceration

10. The most appropriate treatment for epithelial dysplasia is:
    A. Observation
    B. Chemotherapy
    C. Radiation therapy
    D. Repeat biopsy in 6 months
    E. Surgical excision

11. Verrucous carcinoma is differentiated from squamous cell carcinoma because it:
    A. Does not occur in the oral cavity
    B. Responds to chemotherapy
    C. Has a better prognosis
    D. Often metastasizes
    E. Grows more rapidly

12. The most common intraoral location for salivary gland tumors is the:
    A. Lower lip
    B. Buccal mucosa
    C. Junction of the hard and soft palate
    D. Anterior tongue
    E. Fauces

13. Which of the following is an example of a malignant salivary gland tumor?
    A. Pleomorphic adenoma
    B. Warthin tumor
    C. Monomorphic adenoma
    D. Adenoid cystic carcinoma
    E. Papillary cystadenoma lymphomatosum

14. Which of the following statements concerning an ameloblastoma is *true*?
    A. It often occurs in young children.
    B. It is a radiopaque lesion.
    C. It often occurs in the mandibular molar and ramus area.
    D. It should be treated with radiation therapy.
    E. It usually appears as unilocular radiolucencies.

15. The odontogenic tumor that characteristically appears as a well-circumscribed radiolucency located in the anterior maxilla of an adolescent girl is an:
    A. Ameloblastic fibroma
    B. Ameloblastoma
    C. Odontogenic myxoma
    D. Adenomatoid odontogenic tumor
    E. Adenoid cystic carcinoma

16. Which odontogenic tumor most closely resembles the mesenchyme of the dental follicle?
    A. Benign cementoblastoma
    B. Odontogenic myxoma
    C. Complex odontoma
    D. Adenomatoid odontogenic tumor
    E. Ossifying fibroma

17. A benign cementoblastoma may be radiographically recognized because:
    A. It is a well-circumscribed radiopaque lesion with a radiolucent halo attached to the root of a tooth.
    B. It has a radiolucent multilocular appearance.
    C. It is a radiolucent lesion surrounding the crown of an impacted tooth.
    D. It is an ill-defined radiolucent lesion containing scattered opacifications.
    E. It is usually associated with the root of an unerupted tooth.

18. Which of the following lesions characteristically occurs on the alveolar mucosa?
    A. Congenital epulis
    B. Granular cell tumor
    C. Lymphangioma
    D. Lipoma
    E. Neurofibroma

19. Human herpesvirus 8 (HHV-8) is associated with:
    A. Lymphangioma
    B. Rhabdomyosarcoma
    C. Kaposi sarcoma
    D. Schwannoma
    E. Papilloma

20. A compound odontoma differs from a complex odontoma in that a compound odontoma:
    A. Is composed of toothlike structures
    B. Has unlimited growth potential
    C. Is composed primarily of pulp tissue
    D. Is located in the posterior mandible
    E. Is composed of a mass of enamel, dentin, and pulp that does not resemble a normal tooth

21. Peripheral odontogenic tumors are located on the:
    A. Tongue
    B. Lower lip
    C. Buccal mucosa
    D. Gingiva
    E. Hard palate

22. A benign tumor of adipose tissue is called a:
    A. Lipoma
    B. Schwannoma
    C. Hemangioma
    D. Lymphangioma
    E. Fibroma

23. The most common malignant soft tissue tumor of the head and neck in children is:
    A. Squamous cell carcinoma
    B. Lymphoma
    C. Rhabdomyosarcoma
    D. Osteosarcoma
    E. Malignant melanoma

24. Malignant melanoma of the oral cavity is rare; however, the most common intraoral location is the:
    A. Palate and maxillary gingiva
    B. Tongue
    C. Buccal mucosa
    D. Retromolar area
    E. Floor of the mouth

25. Which of the following neoplasms often occurs in the buccal mucosa or vestibule?
    A. Lipoma
    B. Congenital epulis
    C. Lymphangioma
    D. Melanocytic nevus
    E. Pleomorphic adenoma

26. A malignant tumor of bone-forming tissue is called:
    A. Chondrosarcoma
    B. Melanoma
    C. Osteosarcoma
    D. Rhabdomyosarcoma
    E. Osteoma

27. An overproduction of atypical white blood cells in the circulating blood is called:
    A. Lymphoma
    B. Leukemia
    C. Malignant melanoma
    D. Multiple myeloma
    E. Neutropenia

28. Which of the following is a malignant tumor of lymphocytes?
    A. Multiple myeloma
    B. Malignant melanoma
    C. Lymphoma
    D. Kaposi sarcoma
    E. Lymphangioma

29. The cell involved in multiple myeloma is the:
    A. Lymphocyte
    B. Histiocyte
    C. Eosinophil
    D. Plasma cell
    E. Neutrophil

30. The most frequent intraoral site for metastatic tumors is the:
    A. Buccal mucosa
    B. Mandible
    C. Soft palate
    D. Floor of the mouth
    E. Posterior maxilla

31. Which of the following tumors is associated with von Recklinghausen disease?
    A. Pleomorphic adenoma
    B. Lipoma
    C. Neurofibroma
    D. Fibroma
    E. Malignant melanoma

32. Which of the following is the most common odontogenic tumor?
    A. Odontoma
    B. Ameloblastoma
    C. Ameloblastic fibroma
    D. Odontogenic myxoma
    E. Cementifying fibroma

33. Which of the following salivary gland tumors often occurs in adult males?
    A. Adenoid cystic carcinoma
    B. Monomorphic adenoma
    C. Papillary cystadenoma lymphomatosum
    D. Mucoepidermoid carcinoma
    E. Pleomorphic adenoma

34. A benign tumor composed of a proliferation of capillaries is called a:
    A. Schwannoma
    B. Hemangioma
    C. Lipoma
    D. Lymphangioma
    E. Lymphoma

35. A white plaquelike lesion that cannot be rubbed off or diagnosed as a specific disease is called:
    A. Speckled leukoplakia
    B. Erythroplakia
    C. Leukoplakia
    D. Epithelial dysplasia
    E. Hyperkeratosis

36. All of the following are benign lesions that histologically contain bone or bonelike material except a(n):
    A. Torus
    B. Osteoma
    C. Exostosis
    D. Central ossifying fibroma
    E. Odontoma

37. Which of the following malignant tumors may present as diffuse gingival enlargement with persistent bleeding?
    A. Multiple myeloma
    B. Leukemia
    C. Chondrosarcoma
    D. Osteosarcoma
    E. Squamous cell carcinoma

38. Which of the following malignancies is characterized by a monoclonal spike on immunoelectrophoresis?
    A. Malignant melanoma
    B. Squamous cell carcinoma
    C. Lymphoma
    D. Leukemia
    E. Multiple myeloma

39. Which of the following malignant tumors has been reported to show a characteristic sunburst pattern on radiographic examination?
    A. Malignant melanoma
    B. Osteosarcoma
    C. Squamous cell carcinoma
    D. Rhabdomyosarcoma
    E. Adenoid cystic carcinoma

40. All of the following neoplasms arise from squamous epithelium except a(n):
    A. Basal cell carcinoma
    B. Verrucous carcinoma
    C. Adenoid cystic carcinoma
    D. Papilloma
    E. Epidermoid carcinoma

Chapter 7 Synopsis

Condition/ Disease	Cause	Age/Race/Sex	Location
Papilloma	Neoplastic	M = F	Soft palate, tongue
Epithelial Dysplasia	Premalignant Smoking considered a risk factor	Adults	Floor of mouth, tongue
Squamous Cell Carcinoma	Neoplastic	Age > 40 M > F	Floor of mouth, tongue, lips—most common sites
Verrucous Carcinoma	Neoplastic	Age > 55 M > F	Vestibule, buccal mucosa—most common sites
Basal Cell Carcinoma	Neoplastic Associated with sun exposure	Age > 40 M = F Caucasian	Skin of face
Pleomorphic Adenoma	Neoplastic	Age > 40 F > M	Parotid gland Palate most comon intraoral site

Clinical Features	Radiographic Features	Microscopic Features	Treatment	Diagnostic Process
Exophytic, fingerlike projections	N/A	Papillary projections surfaced by stratified squamous epithelium covering connective tissue cores	Surgical excision	Microscopic
White, erythematous or mixed white and erythematous mucosal lesion	N/A	Abnormal maturation of epithelial cells Hyperplasia of basal cells, disorganization of epithelial layers, increased nuclear/cytoplasmic ratios, cells with enlarged and hyperchromatic nuclei Abnormal keratinization Increased numbers of normal and abnormal mitotic figures No invasion of abnormal cells into underlying tissue	Surgical excision	Microscopic
Exophytic mass, ulcerated leukoplakia erythroplakia	N/A	Invasion of tumor cells through basement membrane into underlying connective tissue Pleomorphic epithelial cells, normal and abnormal mitotic figures	Surgical excision Radiation therapy Chemotherapy	Microscopic
Slow-growing exophytic mass papillary projections	N/A	Papillary epithelial projections Well-differentiated epithelium with normal-appearing epithelial cells Broad-based rete pegs with intact basement membrane	Surgical excision	Microscopic
Nonhealing ulcer rolled borders	N/A	Proliferation of basal epithelial cells Broad rete pegs penetrate deeply into the connective tissue	Surgical excision Radiation therapy	Microscopic
Nonulcerated dome-shaped mass	N/A	Encapsulated tumor Mixture of epithelium and tissue that resembles varying forms of connective tissue	Surgical excision	Microscopic

Continued

Chapter 7 Synopsis—cont'd

Condition/ Disease	Cause	Age/Race/Sex	Location
Monomorphic Adenoma	Neoplastic	Adults F > M	Most common oral sites—upper lip and buccal mucosa
Adenoid Cystic Carcinoma	Neoplastic	Adults F > M	Parotid gland Most common oral site—palate
Mucoepidermoid Carcinoma	Neoplastic	F > M	Parotid gland Most common oral site—palate Some are central in mandible
Ameloblastoma	Neoplastic	Adults M = F	Intraosseous Peripheral tumors also occur Mandible > maxilla Posterior > anterior
Calcifying Epithelial Odontogenic Tumor	Neoplastic	Adults M = F	Posterior mandible
Adenomatoid Odontogenic Tumor	Neoplastic	Age < 20 F > M	70% involve anterior maxilla and mandible Maxilla > mandible
Calcifying Odontogenic Cyst	Cyst with neoplastic variant	Age < 40 M = F	Maxilla and mandible

Clinical Features	Radiographic Features	Microscopic Features	Treatment	Diagnostic Process
Smooth-surfaced mass	N/A	Encapsulated epithelial tumor with a uniform pattern of epithelial cells	Surgical excision	Microscopic
Mass, often painful Surface may be ulcerated	N/A	Unencapsulated, infiltrating tumor composed of small, deeply staining, uniform epithelial cells arranged in perforated round to oval islands	Surgical excision Radiation therapy	Microscopic
Asymptomatic swelling or mass	When intraosseous, unilocular or multilocular radiolucency	Unencapsulated, infiltrating tumor composed of a combination of mucous cells and squamouslike epithelial cells	Surgical excision	Microscopic
Slow growing, expansion of bone	Unilocular or multilocular radiolucency	Unencapsulated, infiltrating tumor composed of ameloblast-like epithelial cells surrounding areas resembling stellate reticulum	Surgical excision	Microscopic
Asymptomatic, slow-growing expansion of bone	Unilocular or multilocular radiolucency with scattered calcifications	Unencapsulated, infiltrating tumor composed of islands and sheets of polyhedral epithelial cells Calcifications and eosinophilic deposits in the tumor	Surgical excision	Microscopic
Asymptomatic swelling	Well-defined radiolucency associated with an impacted tooth Radiopacities within the radiolucency	Encapsulated tumor composed of ductlike epithelial structures, masses of cuboidal and spindle-shaped epithelial cells with eosinophilic material and calcifications	Surgical enucleation	Microscopic
Asymptomatic Swelling Root resorption	Unilocular or multilocular radiolucency Radiopacities within the radiolucency	Cyst lined by odontogenic epithelium with associated ghost cell keratinization Ameloblast-like cells and stellate reticulum-like areas	Enucleation	Microscopic

Continued

Chapter 7 Synopsis—cont'd

Condition/ Disease	Cause	Age/Race/Sex	Location
Odontogenic Myxoma	Neoplastic	Age 10-29 M = F	Mandible > maxilla
Central Cementifying and Ossifying Fibromas	Neoplastic	Adults F > M	Mandible (90%)
Benign Cementoblastoma	Neoplastic	Age < 25 M = F	Most occur associated with a mandible molar
Ameloblastic Fibroma	Neoplastic	Age < 20 M > F	Posterior mandible
Ameloblastic Fibro-odontoma	Neoplastic	Age < 10	Posterior Maxilla and mandible
Odontoma	Neoplastic	Age: children and young adults M = F	Most common locations—anterior maxilla, posterior mandible
Peripheral Ossifying Fibroma	Reactive	Age: children and young adults F > M	Gingiva

*Not covered in text.

Clinical Features	Radiographic Features	Microscopic Features	Treatment	Diagnostic Process
Asymptomatic expansion of bone	Multilocular, honeycombed radiolucency	Unencapsulated, infiltrating tumor composed of pale-staining substance containing widely dispersed cells with small nuclei	Surgical excision	Microscopic
Asymptomatic expansion, facial asymmetry	Wide-defined unilocular lesion, varying degrees of opacities	Well-circumscribed tumor composed of fibrous connective tissue and rounded globular calcifications, bone trabeculae, or both	Surgical excison	Radiographic Microscopic
Localized expansion, pain, vital teeth	Well-defined radiopaque mass in continuity with the root or roots of the affected tooth	*	Enucleation of the tumor Removal of the associated tooth	Radiographic Microscopic
Asymptomatic Swelling	Well-defined unilocular or multilocular radiolucency	Nonencapsulated tumor composed of both strands and small islands of odontogenic epithelium and tissue that resembles the dental papilla	Surgical excision	Microscopic
Asymptomatic Swelling	Well-defined radiolucency with associated calcifications Calcifications may resemble teeth	Strands and small islands of odontogenic epithelium and tissue that resembles the dental papilla combined with tooth structures	Surgical excision	Microscopic
Lack of eruption Swelling	Compound: cluster of miniature teeth Complex: radiopaque mass	Mature enamel, dentin, cementum, and pulp Compound: form multiple small teeth Complex: form irregular mass	Surgical excision	Radiographic Microscopic
Nodular, sessile, or pedunculated mass	N/A	Exophytic lesion composed of connective tissue interpersed with scattered bone or cementum-like calcifications	Surgical excision Scale teeth	Microscopic Clinical

Continued

Chapter 7 Synopsis—cont'd

Condition/ Disease	Cause	Age/Race/Sex	Location
Lipoma	Neoplastic	Age: most > 40 M = F	Most common intraoral locations— buccal mucosa, vestibule
Neurofibroma/ Schwannoma	Neoplastic	Age: any M = F	Most common intraoral location—tongue
Granular Cell Tumor	Neoplastic	Age: 30–50 F > M	Most common locations—tongue, buccal mucosa
Congenital Epulis	Neoplastic	Present at birth (congenital) F > M	Anterior maxillary gingiva
Rhabdomyosarcoma	Neoplastic	Age: frequently < 10 M > F	Head and neck
Hemangioma	Congenital/developmental Adults/response to trauma	Congenital F > M Also adults	Most common oral site—tongue
Lymphangioma	Neoplastic/developmental	Congenital M = F	Most common oral site—tongue
Kaposi Sarcoma	Neoplastic Human herpes virus 8 (HHV-8)	M > F	Most common oral sites—hard palate and gingiva
Melanocytic Nevi	Developmental	Age: 20-50 F > M	Most common oral sites—hard palate and buccal mucosa

*Not covered in text.

Clinical Features	Radiographic Features	Microscopic Features	Treatment	Diagnostic Process
Yellowish mass with delicate pattern of blood vessels on the surface	N/A	Well-delineated tumor composed of lobules of mature, uniform, fat cells	Surgical excision	Microscopic
Asymptomatic nodule	N/A	Neurofibroma: well-delineated, diffuse proliferation of spindle-shaped cells Schwannoma: encapsulated proliferation of Schwann cells arranged in palisaded whorls around central pink zones	Surgical excision	Microscopic
Asymptomatic nodule	N/A	Unencapsulated tumor composed of large cells with a granular cytoplasm Overlying epithelium exhibits pseudoepithe-liomatous hyperplasia	Surgical excision	Microscopic
Sessile or pedunculated mass	N/A	Unencapsulated tumor composed of large cells with granular cytoplasm (similar to cells in granular cell tumor)	Surgical excision	Microscopic
Rapidly growing destructive tumor	N/A	*	Surgical excision Multiagent chemotherapy Radiation therapy	Microscopic
Deep-red to blue mass Blanches with pressure	N/A	Vascular lesion composed of numerous small capillaries or larger blood vessels	Injection of sclerosing solution Spontaneous remission	Clinical Microscopic
Ill-defined mass with a pebbly surface	N/A	Lesion composed of lymphatic vessels	Surgical excision	Clinical Microscopic
Purple macules, plaques, or exophytic tumors	N/A	Unencapsulated tumor composed of spindle-shaped cells mixed with slit-like spaces containing red blood cells	Surgical excision Radiation therapy Chemotherapy	Microscopic Clinical
Tan/brown macules or papules	N/A	Benign tumor composed of nevus cells	Surgical excision	Clinical Microscopic

Continued

Chapter 7 Synopsis—cont'd

Condition/ Disease	Cause	Age/Race/Sex	Location
Malignant Melanoma	Neoplastic	Age > 40	Most common oral sites—hard palate and maxillary gingiva
Torus	Genetic	Adults F > M	Midline of hard palate Lingual aspect of mandible
Exostosis	Possibly reactive	Adults M = F	Buccal aspect of maxillary and mandibular ridges
Osteoma	Neoplastic	M = F	Intraosseous
Osteosarcoma	Neoplastic	Most common primary malignant tumor of bone in patients < 40 years old M > F	Mandible 2 × maxilla
Chondrosarcoma	Neoplastic	M > F	Maxilla and mandible
Leukemia	Neoplastic	M > F	Gingiva
Lymphoma	Neoplastic	Adults M > F	Most common oral site—tonsillar area
Multiple Myeloma	Neoplastic	Adults M > F	Mandible > maxilla
Metastatic Tumors	Neoplastic	Adults M > F	Mandible > maxilla

*Not covered in text.

Clinical Features	Radiographic Features	Microscopic Features	Treatment	Diagnostic Process
Rapidly enlarging blue to black mass	N/A	Malignant tumor	Surgical excision Chemotherapy	Microscopic
Asymptomatic, bony hard, lobulated mass	Radiopaque mass superimposed on tooth roots	Benign, compact bone	None unless necessary for fabrication of prosthetic appliance	Clinical
Asymptomatic, bony hard nodules	Occasionally seen as radiopacity	Benign, compact bone	None unless necessary for fabrication of prosthetic applicance	Clinical
Asymptomatic	Sharply defined radiopaque mass	Benign, compact bone	Surgical excision	Microscopic
Painful, diffuse swelling or mass Expansion of involved bone	Destructive, poorly defined radiolucency to radiopacity Asymmetric widening of the periodontal ligament space Sunburst pattern	Malignant tumor of bone *	Surgical excision Multiagent chemo-therapy	Microscopic
Enlargement of involved bone	*	Malignant tumor of cartilage*	Wide surgical excision	Microscopic
Diffuse gingival enlargement with persistent bleeding	N/A	Atypical white blood cells in circulating blood and tissues	Chemotherapy Radiation therapy Corticosteroids	Laboratory Microscopic
Enlargement of involved tissue	N/A	Malignant tumor of lymphoid tissue	Radiation therapy Chemotherapy	Laboratory Microscopic
Bone pain, swelling	Multiple radiolucent lesions	Malignant proliferation of plasma cells	Chemotherapy	Laboratory Microscopic
Pain Paresthesia Swelling Expansion of bone	Variable Usually poorly defined and radiolucent Tooth roots may show spiked appearance Some may show areas of radiopacity	Resemble primary malignancy	Chemotherapy Radiation	Microscopic

Nonneoplastic Diseases of Bone

Anne Cale Jones
Joan A. Phelan
Olga A.C. Ibsen

Objectives

After studying this chapter, the student will be able to:

1. Define benign fibro-osseous lesions.
2. Define dysplasia as it relates to bone diseases and differentiate the term from epithelial dysplasia.
3. Describe the clinical, radiographic, and microscopic features of periapical cemento-osseous dysplasia, focal cemento-osseous dysplasia, and florid cemento-osseous dysplasia.
4. Compare and contrast periapical cemento-osseous dysplasia, focal cemento-osseous dysplasia, and florid cemento-osseous dysplasia.
5. List the benign fibro-osseous lesions that occur in the jawbones.
6. Compare and contrast monostotic fibrous dysplasia with polyostotic fibrous dysplasia.

7. Compare and contrast the radiographic appearance, histologic appearance, and treatment of fibrous dysplasia of the jaws with those of ossifying fibroma of the jaws.
8. Compare and contrast the three types of polyostotic fibrous dysplasia.
9. Describe the histologic appearance of Paget disease of bone and describe its clinical and radiographic appearance when the maxilla or mandible is involved.
10. State the cause of osteomalacia and rickets.

Vocabulary

Benign fibro-osseous lesion (be-nīn′ fi″bro-os′ e-ĕs le′zhĕn) Benign lesion of bone characterized histologically by cellular fibrous connective tissue admixed with irregularly shaped bone trabeculae or cementoid material.

Dysplasia (dis-pla′ze-ah) Disordered growth.

Nonneoplastic diseases of bone that affect the maxilla and mandible fall into multiple categories. Inherited diseases that affect bone are discussed in Chapter 6, and benign and malignant neoplasms of bone are discussed in Chapter 7. Central and peripheral giant cell granulomas are included in Chapter 2, and aneurysmal bone cyst is included in Chapter 5. The purpose of this chapter is to delineate several other nonneoplastic diseases of bone that are important for a dental hygienist to understand but are not covered elsewhere in this text. These include three forms of cemento-osseous dysplasia: (1) periapical, (2) focal, and (3) florid. In addition, the dental hygienist should also be familiar with the various types of fibrous dysplasia and the clinical and radiographic features of Paget disease and osteomalacia.

The term **dysplasia,** as used in this chapter in the context of the cemento-osseous dysplasias and fibrous dysplasia, refers to the disordered production of cementum and bone. This term in this context should not be confused with dysplasia as used in the context of epithelial dysplasia. In the latter, epithelial dysplasia connotes a premalignant condition affecting squamous epithelium.

Benign Fibro-osseous Lesions

Fibro-osseous lesions that affect the maxilla and mandible include cementifying and ossifying fibromas (see Chapter 7), periapical cemento-osseous dysplasia, focal cemento-osseous dysplasia, florid cemento-osseous dysplasia, and fibrous dysplasia (**Table 8-1**).

PERIAPICAL CEMENTO-OSSEOUS DYSPLASIA

Periapical cemento-osseous dysplasia is a relatively common disease of unknown cause that affects periapical bone (**Figure 8-1**, *A* and *B*). The term cementoma is often used for this disease. However, because this disease does not represent a neoplasm, this term is inappropriate and should be avoided.

Clinical and Radiographic Features

The lesion is asymptomatic and is discovered on routine radiographic examination. It occurs most commonly in the anterior mandible of patients older than 30 years of age. It is more common in women than in men. Many studies have shown a predilection for this disease to arise in black women. Early lesions are well circumscribed and radiolucent and may mimic periapical disease. Teeth in the affected area are vital unless they are coincidentally carious or have been traumatized. With time the lesions become increasingly calcified; therefore older lesions are radiolucent with central opacifications.

Diagnosis and Treatment

The diagnosis of periapical cemento-osseous dysplasia is usually established based on observation of its characteristic clinical and radiographic features. A biopsy may be necessary in those cases where the characteristic radiographic features are not evident. Histologic examination reveals a fibro-osseous lesion. Like other fibro-osseous lesions, periapical cemento-osseous dysplasia is composed of a combination of fibrous tissue and calcifications. The calcifications in this lesion may resemble bone, cementum, or both. Early lesions consist mainly of fibrous tissue, whereas older lesions contain fibrous connective tissue interspersed with numerous calcifications (see **Figure 8-1**, *C*). If a patient demonstrates radiographic changes characteristic of an early lesion, close follow-up examinations may be necessary to ensure that a correct diagnosis was established. Once the condition is recognized, no treatment is necessary. The lesion remains asymptomatic and localized.

Table 8-1 Benign Fibro-osseous Lesions of the Jaws

Fibrous dysplasia
   Monostotic type
   Polyostotic types (Jaffe and Albright)
   Craniofacial type

Central ossifying fibroma

Cemento-ossifying fibroma

Cementifying fibroma

Peripheral ossifying fibroma

Periapical cemento-osseous dysplasia (cementoma)

Florid cemento-osseous dysplasia

FOCAL CEMENTO-OSSEOUS DYSPLASIA

Focal cemento-osseous dysplasia is an asymptomatic fibro-osseous lesion that shares similar histologic features with periapical cemento-osseous dysplasia and florid cemento-osseous dysplasia. However, it differs from these latter two lesions in that it has unique clinical and radiographic features.

Clinical and Radiographic Features

Focal cemento-osseous dysplasia usually occurs in women between 30 and 50 years of age, and unlike periapical cemento-osseous dysplasia, it is reported to be more common in white than in black individuals. It typically arises in the posterior mandible and appears as an isolated, well-delineated radiolucent to radiopaque lesion that is less than 1.5 cm in size.

Diagnosis and Treatment

Biopsy and histologic examination are usually necessary to establish a diagnosis of focal cemento-osseous dysplasia. A characteristic surgical feature of focal cemento-osseous dysplasia is that it is composed of numerous gritty pieces of soft and hard tissue. This tissue represents fibrous connective tissue interspersed with bone trabeculae and cementum-

Figure 8-1 A and **B,** Radiographs of periapical cemento-osseous dysplasia. **C,** Microscopic appearance of periapical cemento-osseous dysplasia shows a combination of cellular fibrous connective tissue *(F)* and calcified tissue *(C).*

like material. Once a definitive diagnosis has been established, no further treatment is necessary. The prognosis for focal cemento-osseous dysplasia is excellent. Occasional examples of this lesion have progressed to florid cemento-osseous dysplasia.

FLORID CEMENTO-OSSEOUS DYSPLASIA

Florid cemento-osseous dysplasia, another fibro-osseous lesion, is also a condition of disordered cementum and bone development that characteristically involves multiple quadrants in the maxilla and mandible.

Clinical and Radiographic Features

Florid cemento-osseous dysplasia occurs most often in middle-aged black women who are older than 40 years of age. The cause of this disease is unknown. Radiographically it differs from periapical cemento-osseous dysplasia in that it typically affects more than one quadrant of the maxilla and mandible, often in the posterior areas. Masses of irregular opacification are noted that are composed of dense, sclerotic bone, cementum, or both **(Figure 8-2).** In addition, the early radiolucent phase that is characteristic of periapical cemento-osseous dysplasia is generally not identified in florid cemento-osseous dysplasia.

Figure 8-2 Florid cemento-osseous dysplasia. Pantomographic radiograph shows irregular radiopaque masses in both the left and right mandible.

Diagnosis and Treatment

Florid cemento-osseous dysplasia is often diagnosed based on its characteristic clinical presentation and radiographic appearance. Because of these findings, treatment is often unnecessary. However, in an edentulous patient, the sclerotic masses may perforate the mucosa resulting in a communication between the oral environment and the underlying bone. This complication may lead to the development of an osteomyelitis, necessitating surgical intervention and antibiotic therapy.

FIBROUS DYSPLASIA

Fibrous dysplasia is a disease that is characterized by the replacement of bone with abnormal fibrous connective tissue interspersed with varying amounts of calcification. Although the cause is unknown, several theories have been proposed. One of the most widely accepted theories is that the unusual fibrous proliferation is the result of abnormal mesenchymal cell function. Several types of fibrous dysplasia exist; each type shares similar microscopic features, but the clinical presentation and associated systemic signs and symptoms differ. Histologically, fibrous dysplasia is a benign fibro-osseous lesion. It is composed of vascularized, cellular fibrous connective tissue interspersed with irregular trabeculae of bone emerging from the connective tissue.

Types of Fibrous Dysplasia

Monostotic fibrous dysplasia

Monostotic fibrous dysplasia, the most common type of fibrous dysplasia, is characterized by involvement of a single bone. The mandible and maxilla are commonly affected, and the maxilla is more frequently involved than the mandible. Other bones may be affected, including the ribs, femur, and tibia. Monostotic fibrous dysplasia is most commonly diagnosed in children and young adults; no sex predilection is seen. Clinical examination reveals a painless swelling or bulging of the buccal plate of the maxilla or mandible. The expanding nature of the lesion may lead to malocclusion, tipping, or displacement of adjacent teeth.

Polyostotic fibrous dysplasia

Polyostotic fibrous dysplasia is characterized by involvement of more than one bone. It typically occurs in children, and a definite female gender predilection is seen. The skull, clavicles, and long bones are often affected, and most cases are asymptomatic. When the long bones are involved, they may exhibit bowing and an associated dull aching pain. Patients with polyostotic fibrous dysplasia often demonstrate skin lesions. These lesions appear as light-brown macules called **café au lait spots.** Several forms of polyostotic fibrous dysplasia exist. **Craniofacial fibrous dysplasia** is the term used for polyostotic fibrous dysplasia that

Figure 8-3 Fibrous dysplasia. **A,** Radiograph of fibrous dysplasia demonstrating indistinct borders that blend into the adjacent normal bone. **B,** Microscopic appearance (high power) of fibrous dysplasia shows cellular fibrous connective tissue *(F)* and irregular trabeculae of bone *(B)*. (**A** courtesy Drs. Paul Freedman and Stanley Kerpel.)

involves the maxilla with extension into the sinuses and adjacent zygoma, sphenoid, and occipital bones. Another form of polyostotic fibrous dysplasia is called the **Jaffe type** (or **Jaffe-Lichtenstein type**). It involves multiple bones along with associated café au lait macules on the skin. The most severe type of polyostotic fibrous dysplasia is called **Albright syndrome** (or McCune-Albright syndrome). This condition is characterized by endocrine abnormalities, including precocious puberty in females, and stunting or deformity of skeletal growth in both sexes as a result of early epiphyseal plate closure. Precocious puberty is exhibited by menses, pubic hair, and breast development in children as young as 2 years of age. Other complications of Albright syndrome include diabetes mellitus and hyperthyroidism. Café au lait skin macules may occur in this and the Jaffe type of polyostotic fibrous dysplasia.

Clinical and Radiographic Features

Clinical examination reveals a painless enlargement of the affected bone or bones. Jaw involvement typically appears as a painless, progressive, unilateral enlargement of the maxilla or mandible. When fibrous dysplasia involves the maxilla, the disease usually extends into the maxillary sinuses. Involvement of the jaws may occur in any type of fibrous dysplasia. The classic radiographic appearance of fibrous dysplasia is a diffuse radiopacity that is described as "looking like ground glass" (**Figure 8-3,** *A*). The abnormal

bone blends into the adjacent normal bone. A unilocular or multilocular radiolucency, a patchy radiolucency with central opacifications, and a dense radiopacity have also been observed in fibrous dysplasia. The radiolucent or radiopaque appearance of fibrous dysplasia depends upon the degree of calcification present in the lesion.

Diagnosis and Treatment

The diagnosis of fibrous dysplasia is established by correlating the microscopic findings along with the characteristic clinical features and radiographic appearance. Histologic examination reveals a benign fibro-osseous lesion (**Figure 8-3,** *B*). The microscopic appearance is characterized by cellular fibrous connective tissue interspersed with irregularly shaped bone trabeculae. Fibrous dysplasia of the maxilla or mandible is distinguished from a cementifying or ossifying fibroma of the jaws based on review of the radiographic findings. In fibrous dysplasia, the radiographic changes blend into the surrounding normal bone. In a cementifying or ossifying fibroma, a tumor that can demonstrate microscopic features similar to fibrous dysplasia, the radiographic findings consist of a well-delineated lesion that is easily delineated from the surrounding normal bone. Likewise, other fibro-osseous lesions, such as periapical cemento-osseous dysplasia and florid cemento-osseous dysplasia, can be distinguished from fibrous dysplasia based on an examination of their distinct clinical and radiographic

A

B

C

Figure 8-4 Paget disease. **A,** Enlargement of the maxilla with spaces between the teeth. **B,** Radiograph demonstrating irregular opacification that is also referred to as a cotton-wool appearance. In areas, the lamina dura is obliterated. **C,** Microscopic appearance of Paget disease shows bone trabeculae surfaced by numerous osteoclasts and osteoblasts. The prominent reversal lines *(arrows)* seen here characterize the mosaic bone pattern of bone.

features. Fibrous dysplasia is treated surgically by recontouring the affected bone for cosmetic reasons. No treatment exists for severe and progressive polyostotic fibrous dysplasia. Radiation treatment of fibrous dysplasia is contraindicated because it has been associated with malignant transformation.

Paget Disease of Bone

Paget disease of bone, also called **osteitis deformans** and **leontiasis ossea,** is a chronic metabolic bone disease. It is characterized by resorption, osteoblastic repair, and remineralization of the involved bone. The cause is unknown. Several theories have been proposed and a viral cause is suspected. The disease occurs most commonly in men over the age of 50. It typically involves the pelvis and spinal column. When found in the jawbones, the maxilla is more commonly affected than the mandible.

CLINICAL AND RADIOGRAPHIC FEATURES

The clinical manifestations of Paget disease depend on the bone involved. Enlargement of the affected bone is common, and the patient often complains of pain. When the maxilla or mandible is involved, spacing between the teeth increases as the bone enlarges (**Figure 8-4,** *A*). Edentulous patients may complain that their dentures no longer fit. When other bones of the skull are involved, clinical manifestations include severe headache, dizziness, and deafness. The classic radiographic appearance is a patchy radiolucency and radiopacity that has been referred to as a cotton-wool appearance (**Figure 8-4,** *B*). However, this only occurs in the later stages of Paget disease. In earlier stages, the radiographic appearance is not as unique. Hypercementosis, loss of the lamina dura, and obliteration of the periodontal ligament may also occur.

DIAGNOSIS AND TREATMENT

Laboratory evaluation is important in establishing the diagnosis of Paget disease. The serum alkaline phosphatase level is significantly elevated in active disease. Two different measurements are used to evaluate the serum alkaline phosphatase level. In Bodansky units, the normal serum alkaline phosphatase value is 1.5 to 5.0. In Paget disease, the serum alkaline phosphatase value can be as high as 250 Bodansky units. Another measurement used for evaluating the serum alkaline phosphatase level is the King-Armstrong unit (KAU). Normal values are 5 to 10 KAU. In patients with Paget disease, KAU values may be as high as 200. Histologic examination reveals bone trabeculae surfaced by numerous osteoclasts and osteoblasts (**Figure 8-4,** *C*). The involved bone demonstrates prominent reversal lines that result from the resorption and deposition of bone; this pattern has been described as **mosaic bone.** The connective tissue between the bone trabeculae is so well vascularized that the overlying skin may feel warm when touched. Treatment of Paget disease is experimental. The disease is slowly progressive. Complications include fracture of the involved bone and development of malignant tumors, particularly osteosarcoma. Heart disease is a rare complication of Paget disease.

Osteomalacia

Osteomalacia is a disease of bone that develops over a long period of time as the result of a deficiency of calcium. When this disease occurs in young children, it is usually caused by a nutritional deficiency of vitamin D; the disease is termed *rickets.* An inherited form of vitamin D deficiency called *hypophosphatemic vitamin D–resistant rickets* is included in Chapter 6. In adults the disease may be related to various problems such as a malabsorption syndrome, drugs, liver and kidney disease, and the chronic use of antacids. Osteomalacia may also be induced by certain tumors.

CLINICAL AND RADIOGRAPHIC FEATURES

Delayed tooth eruption and periodontal disease have been associated with osteomalacia. Changes in bone trabeculation that occur in patients with osteomalacia may be subtle and difficult to detect. Pathologic fractures may also occur.

TREATMENT

Treatment is based on identification of the cause of the vitamin D deficiency and includes nutritional supplementation with vitamin D and dietary calcium.

Selected References

Books

Neville BW et al: *Oral and maxillofacial pathology,* ed 2, Philadelphia, 2001, WB Saunders.

Regezi JA, Sciubba JJ: *Oral pathology: clinical-pathologic correlations,* ed 4, Philadelphia, 2003, WB Saunders.

Journal Articles

Bessho K et al: Monostotic fibrous dysplasia with involvement of the mandibular canal, *Oral Surg Oral Med Oral Pathol* 68:396, 1989.

Hadjipavlou AG, Gaitanis IN, Kontakis GM: Paget's disease of the bone and its management, *J Bone Joint Surg* 84:160, 2002.

Regezi JA: Odontogenic cysts, odontogenic tumors, fibro-osseous, and giant cell lesions of the jaws, *Mod Pathol* 15:331, 2002.

Siris ES: Paget's disease of bone, *J Bone Miner Res* 13:1061, 1998.

Summerlin Don-John, Tomich CE: Focal cemento-osseous dysplasia: a clinicopathologic study of 221 cases, *Oral Surg Oral Med Oral Pathol* 78:611, 1994.

Review Questions

1. A 48-year-old black woman has multiple asymptomatic, radiopaque masses in the mandible and maxilla. No expansion of bone takes place. The most likely diagnosis is:
   A. Multiple odontomas
   B. Cementifying fibromas
   C. Periapical cemento-osseous dysplasia
   D. Florid cemento-osseous dysplasia
   E. Focal cemento-osseous dysplasia

2. All of the following are examples of benign fibro-osseous lesions *except:*
   A. Fibrous dysplasia
   B. Periapical cemento-osseous dysplasia
   C. Ossifying fibroma
   D. Odontoma
   E. Cementifying fibroma

3. Which of the following is characterized by precocious puberty in females?
   A. Monostotic fibrous dysplasia
   B. Albright syndrome
   C. Jaffe-Lichtenstein type polyostotic fibrous dysplasia
   D. Periapical cemento-osseous dysplasia
   E. Paget disease of bone

4. Periapical cemento-osseous dysplasia is characteristically located in the:
   A. Posterior quadrants of the maxilla and mandible
   B. Posterior maxilla
   C. Anterior maxilla
   D. Anterior mandible
   E. Mandibular bicuspid region

5. Periapical cemento-osseous dysplasia is also called:
   A. An odontoma
   B. A cementoblastoma
   C. A cementifying fibroma
   D. A fibrous dysplasia
   E. A cementoma

6. In which of the following diseases are café au lait spots seen on the skin?
   A. Polyostotic fibrous dysplasia
   B. Paget disease
   C. Monostotic fibrous dysplasia
   D. Osteomalacia
   E. Focal cemento-osseous dysplasia

7. Which type of fibrous dysplasia involves the maxilla and adjacent bones?
   A. Facial fibrous dysplasia
   B. Jaffe type of fibrous dysplasia
   C. Craniofacial fibrous dysplasia
   D. Monostotic fibrous dysplasia
   E. Albright syndrome

8. Bone resorption, osteoblastic repair, loss of the lamina dura, hypercementosis, and cotton-wool radiopacities are characteristics of:
   A. Albright syndrome
   B. Letterer-Siwe disease
   C. Paget disease
   D. Polyostotic fibrous dysplasia
   E. Florid cemento-osseous dysplasia

9. The most characteristic radiographic appearance of fibrous dysplasia is described as a:
   A. Cotton-wool appearance
   B. Ground glass appearance
   C. Well-circumscribed radiopacity
   D. Well-circumscribed radiolucency
   E. Mosaic bone

10. Which of the following are not present in the histologic appearance of the bone in Paget disease?
    A. Osteoblasts
    B. Bone with prominent irregular dark lines
    C. Osteoclasts
    D. Well-vascularized fibrous connective tissue
    E. Pleomorphic nuclei and atypical mitotic figures

11. Which of the following is diagnosed based on a characteristic radiographic appearance?
    A. Paget disease
    B. Osteomalacia
    C. Florid cemento-osseous dysplasia
    D. Focal cemento-osseous dysplasia
    E. Fibrous dysplasia

12. In patients with fibrous dysplasia, which of the following is the only recommended treatment modality?
    A. Surgery
    B. Radiation therapy
    C. Chemotherapy
    D. Bone marrow transplantation
    E. Antibiotics

13. Which of the following is helpful in the diagnosis of Paget disease?
    A. Complete blood count (CBC)
    B. Serum alkaline phosphatase
    C. Serum vitamin D
    D. Serum calcium
    E. Urinalysis

14. Osteomalacia is usually caused by a deficiency of:
    A. Vitamin C
    B. Vitamin B_{12}
    C. Vitamin D
    D. Alkaline phosphatase
    E. None of the above

15. Osteomalacia in children is called:
    A. Rickets
    B. Paget disease
    C. Fibrous dysplasia
    D. Osteogenesis imperfecta
    E. Albright syndrome

Chapter 8 Synopsis

Condition/ Disease	Cause	Age/Race/Sex	Location
Periapical Cemental Dysplasia	Reactive	Age > 30 F > M Race: > black	Anterior mandible
Focal Cemento-osseous Dysplasia	Reactive	Age 30-50 F > M Race: > white	Posterior mandible
Florid Cemento-osseous Dysplasia	Reactive	Age > 40 F > M Race: > black	Multiple areas Maxilla and mandible
Fibrous Dysplasia	Cause unknown Most widely accepted theory— 　abnormal mesencymal 　cell function	Children and young 　adults M = F	Monostotic (one bone) Maxilla > Mandible Other frequently affected bones Ribs, femur, tibia Polyostotic 　Jaffe type 　Albright syndrome
Paget Disease of Bone	Chronic metabolic bone disease Cause unknown	M > F Age > 50 yrs	Typically pelvis and spinal column When affecting the jaws: 　Maxilla > Mandible
Osteomalacia	Long-term deficiency of calcium Children: nutritional deficiency 　of vitamin D Adults: malabsorption syndromes 　drugs, liver disease, kidney 　disease, chronic use of antacids	Children: rickets Adults: osteomalacia	Generalized bone disease

*Not covered in text.

Clinical Features	Radiographic Features	Microscopic Features	Treatment	Diagnostic Process
Asymptomatic Vital teeth	Well-defined radiolucency to radiopacity at area of tooth apex	Fibrous connective tissue and calcifications	None	Radiographic
Asymptomatic	Well-defined radiolucency to radiopacity	Fibrous connective tissue with rounded globular calcifications and bone trabeculae	None	Radiographic Microscopic if diagnosis not certain
Asymptomatic	Multiple areas Radiolucency to radiopacity	Fibrous connective tissue with dense sclerotic masses of bone, cementum or both	None unless complicated by osteomyelitis	Radiographic
Oral/Facial: painless swelling or bulging of the jawbone Malocclusion, tipping or displacement of teeth More than one bone involved Café au lait macules on skin Extensive, progressive involvement of many bones Café au lait macules on skin Endocrine abnormalities	Diffuse "ground-glass"–appearing radiolucency Abnormal bone blends into normal bone Unilocular and multilocular radiolucencies have been described	Benign fibro-osseous lesions	Surgical recontouring of affected bone for cosmetic reasons	Radiographic Microscopic
Enlargement of the involved bone, patient may complain of pain in affected bone With involvement of the maxilla or mandible, spacing between teeth—when edentulous, dentures no longer fit	Patchy radiolucency/radiopacity ("cotton–wool" appearance) Hypercementosis and loss of lamina aura also described	Mosaic bone—reversal lines in bone with osteoblasts and osteoclasts lining the trabeculae Well-vascularized fibrous tissue	Experimental	Laboratory Radiographic
Children: delayed tooth eruption Pathologic fractures Periodontal disease	Subtle changes in bone trabeculation	*	Children: vitamin D and dietary calcium Adults: dependent on cause	*

Chapter 9

Oral Manifestations of Systemic Diseases

Olga A.C. Ibsen
Joan A. Phelan
Anthony T. Vernillo

Objectives

After studying this chapter, the student will be able to:

1. Define each of the words in the vocabulary list for this chapter.
2. Describe the difference between gigantism and acromegaly and list the physical characteristics of each.
3. State the oral manifestations of hyperthyroidism.
4. Describe the difference between primary and secondary hyperparathyroidism.
5. List the oral manifestations that occur in the uncontrolled diabetic state.
6. List the major clinical characteristics of type 1 and type 2 diabetes.
7. Define Addison disease and describe the changes that occur on the skin and oral mucosa in a patient with Addison disease.
8. Compare and contrast the cause, laboratory findings, and oral manifestations of each of the following: iron-deficiency anemia, pernicious anemia, folic acid deficiency, and vitamin B deficiency.
9. Compare and contrast the definitions and oral manifestations of thalassemia major and sickle cell anemia.
10. Define celiac sprue.
11. Describe the difference between primary and secondary aplastic anemia.
12. Describe the oral manifestations of polycythemia.
13. Explain why platelets may be deficient in polycythemia vera.
14. Describe the most characteristic oral manifestations of agranulocytosis.
15. Describe and contrast acute and chronic leukemia.
16. State the purpose of each of the following laboratory tests: platelet count, bleeding time, prothrombin time (PT), partial thromboplastin time (PTT), and international normalized ratio (INR).
17. List two causes of thrombocytopenic purpura.
18. Describe the oral manifestations of thrombocytopenia and nonthrombocytopenic purpura.
19. Define hemophilia and describe its oral manifestations and treatment.
20. Describe the difference between primary and secondary immunodeficiency.
21. Describe the oral problems that would be expected to occur in a patient with radiation-induced xerostomia.
22. List two drugs that are associated with gingival enlargement.

Vocabulary

Agranulocytosis (ah-gran″u-lo-si-to′sis) Marked decrease in the number of granulocytes, particularly neutrophils.

Anemia (ah-ne′me-ah) Reduction of the number of red blood cells, quantity of hemoglobin, or volume of packed red blood cells to less than normal.

Aplasia (ā-pla′zhe-ah) (adjective, aplastic) Lack of development.

Arthralgia (ar-thral′-ji-ah) Severe pain in a joint.

Autoimmunity (aw″to-ĭ-mu′nĭ-te) Immune-mediated destruction of the body's own cells and tissues; immunity against self.

Catabolism (kah-tab′ah-lizm) Component of metabolism that involves the breakdown of tissues.

Coagulation (ko-ag″u-la′shun) Formation of a clot.

Ecchymosis (ek″ĭ-mo′sis) Small, flat, hemorrhagic patch, larger than a petechia, on the skin or mucous membrane.

Fibrin (fi′brin) Insoluble protein that is essential to the clotting of blood.

Hematocrit (he-mat′ah-krit) Volume percentage of red blood cells in whole blood.

Hemolysis (he-mol′ĭ-sis) Release of hemoglobin from red blood cells by destruction of the cells.

Hemostasis (he″mo-sta′sis) Stoppage or cessation of bleeding.

Hepatomegaly (hep″ah-to-meg′ah-le) Enlargement of the liver.

Hormone (hor′mōn) Chemical substance produced in the body that has a specific regulatory effect on certain cells or a certain organ or organs.

Hypercalcemia (hi″per-kal-se′me-ah) Excess of calcium in the blood.

Hyperglycemia (hi″per-gli-se′me-ah) Excess of glucose in the blood.

Hypochromic (hi″po-kro′mik) Stained less intensely than normal.

Hypophosphatemia (hi″po-fos″fah-te′me-ah) Deficiency of phosphates in the blood.

Insulin (in′su-lin) Hormone produced in the pancreas by the beta cells in the islets of Langerhans; insulin regulates glucose metabolism and is the major fuel-regulating hormone.

Ketoacidosis (ke″to-ah″si-do′sis) Accumulation of acid in the body resulting from the accumulation of ketone bodies.

Microcyte (mi′kro-sīt) Red blood cell that is smaller than normal.

Myalgia (mi-al′-jē-ah) Muscle pain.

Neutropenia (nu″tro-pe′ne-ah) Decreased number of neutrophils in the blood.

Osteoporosis (os″te-o-po-ro′sis) Abnormal rarefaction of bone.

Parathormone (par″ah-thor′mōn) Parathyroid hormone.

Petechia (pe-te′ke-ah) Minute red spot on the skin or mucous membrane caused by escape of a small amount of blood.

Platelet (plāt′let) Disc-shaped structure, also called a thrombocyte, found in the blood; it plays an important role in blood coagulation.

Polycythemia (pol″e-si-the′me-ah) Increase in the total red blood cell mass in the blood.

Polydipsia (pol″i-dip′se-a) Chronic excessive thirst and intake of fluid.

Purpura (pur′pu-rah) Blood disorders characterized by purplish or brownish-red discolorations caused by bleeding into the skin or tissues.

Receptor (re-sep′ter) Cell surface protein to which a specific hormone can bind; such binding leads to biochemical events.

Splenomegaly (sple″no-meg′ah-le) Enlargement of the spleen.

Thrombocyte (throm′bo-sīt) Platelet.

Thrombocytopenia (throm″bo-si″to-pe′ne-ah) Decrease in the number of platelets in circulating blood.

Many diseases that affect the body as a whole are associated with alterations of the oral mucosa, maxilla, and mandible. Systemic diseases can cause mucosal changes such as ulceration or mucosal bleeding. Generalized immunodeficiency can lead to the development of opportunistic diseases such as infection and neoplasia. Bone disease can affect the maxilla and mandible, and systemic disease can cause dental and periodontal changes. Drugs prescribed for a systemic disease can affect the oral tissues.

Local factors are frequently involved in manifestations of systemic disease in the oral mucosa. In some systemic diseases the mucosa is more easily injured; therefore mild irritation and chronic inflammation can cause lesions that would not occur without the presence of the systemic disease.

This chapter discusses systemic diseases that have oral manifestations. Some overlapping occurs among the diseases included in this chapter and those included in other chapters, and some of the diseases discussed in this chapter could have been included in other chapters. Included here are endocrine disorders, disorders of red and white blood cells, disorders of platelets and other bleeding and clotting disorders, and immunodeficiency disorders. Oral changes can be similar for several different systemic diseases, and similar oral lesions can occur without the presence of systemic disease. Because of this, many oral lesions described in this chapter are also described elsewhere in this text.

Endocrine Disorders

The endocrine system consists of a group of integrated glands and cells that secrete hormones. The secretion of hormones by these glands is controlled by feedback mechanisms in which the amount of hormone circulating in blood triggers factors that control production. Diseases of this system can result from conditions in which too much or too little hormone is produced. Diseases of this system can also result from either dysfunction of the glands themselves or a problem in the mechanism that controls hormone production. Some of the endocrine gland diseases in which oral changes occur are included here.

HYPERPITUITARISM

Hyperpituitarism is excess hormone production by the anterior pituitary gland. It is caused most often by a benign tumor **(pituitary adenoma)** that produces growth hormone. If the increase in growth hormone production occurs during development, before the closure of the long bones, **gigantism** results. **Acromegaly** results when the hypersecretion occurs in adult life.

Gigantism includes excessive growth of the overall skeleton. Affected individuals can be more than 8 feet tall and weigh several hundred pounds, and as adults they experience headaches, chronic fatigue, and muscle and joint pain.

Clinical Features and Oral Manifestations

Acromegaly affects both men and women and most commonly occurs in the fourth decade of life. The onset is slow and insidious. Patients experience poor vision, sensitivity to light, enlargement of the hands and feet, and an increase in rib size. The facial changes include enlargement of the maxilla and mandible, frontal bossing (an enlargement of the bones of the forehead), and enlargement of the nasal bones. An enlargement of the maxillary sinus also occurs, which causes a characteristically deep voice. The enlargement of the maxilla and mandible causes separation of teeth and malocclusion. Mucosal changes such as thickened lips and macroglossia (enlarged tongue) have also been described in patients with acromegaly **(Figure 9-1).**

Diagnosis and Treatment

The diagnosis of hyperpituitarism involves measurement of growth hormone, and treatment often involves pituitary gland surgery.

Figure 9-1 Enlarged tongue (macroglossia) in a patient with acromegaly.

HYPERTHYROIDISM

Hyperthyroidism, also called **thyrotoxicosis,** is characterized by excessive production of thyroid hormone. It is much more common in women than in men. Hyperthyroidism has several different causes. The most common cause is Graves disease. The exact cause of Graves disease is not clear, but it appears to be due to an autoimmune disorder in which a substance that abnormally stimulates the thyroid gland is produced. Other causes of hyperthyroidism include hyperplasia of the gland, benign and malignant tumors of the thyroid, pituitary gland disease, and metastatic tumors.

Clinical Features

The clinical features of hyperthyroidism include rosy complexion, erythema of the palms, excessive sweating, fine hair, and softened nails. Exophthalmus (protrusion of the eyeballs) may be seen in hyperthyroidism. Anxiety, weakness, restlessness, and cardiac problems may be associated with the disorder.

Oral Manifestations

Hyperthyroidism in children may lead to premature exfoliation of deciduous teeth and premature eruption of permanent teeth. In adults, osteoporosis may occur, which may affect alveolar bone. Dental caries and periodontal disease appear to develop and progress more rapidly in these patients than in other patients. Burning discomfort of the tongue has also been reported in patients with hyperthyroidism.

Treatment

Treatment of hyperthyroidism may include surgery, medications to suppress thyroid activity, or the administration of radioactive iodine.

HYPOTHYROIDISM

Hypothyroidism is characterized by decreased output of thyroid hormone. When hypothyroidism is present during infancy and childhood, it is known as **cretinism.** In older children and adults, the condition is known as **myxedema.** Causes include developmental disturbances, autoimmune disease, iodine deficiency, drugs, and pituitary disease. In infants, facial and oral changes include thickened lips, enlarged tongue, and delayed eruption of teeth. Adults with hypothyroidism may have an enlarged tongue.

HYPERPARATHYROIDISM

Hyperparathyroidism results from excessive secretion of parathyroid hormone (parathormone [PTH]), which is secreted by the parathyroid glands. The four parathyroid glands are located near the thyroid gland. Parathyroid hormone plays an important role in calcium and phosphorus metabolism. Elevated blood levels of calcium **(hypercalcemia)**, low levels of blood phosphorus **(hypophosphatemia)**, and abnormal bone metabolism characterize hyperparathyroidism.

Hyperparathyroidism may be the result of hyperplasia of the parathyroid glands, a benign tumor of one or more of the parathyroid glands (parathyroid adenoma), or (less commonly) a malignant parathyroid tumor. The disease is found in middle-aged adults and is far more common in women than in men.

Calcium is obtained mainly from dairy products and plays an important role in the contraction of all types of muscle. Parathyroid hormone maintains normal blood levels of calcium through its effects on the kidney, gastrointestinal tract, and bone. It increases the uptake of dietary calcium from the gastrointestinal tract and is able to move calcium from bone to circulating blood when necessary. The hormone appears to be able to remove calcium from bone through the action of osteoclasts.

Hyperparathyroidism that results from an abnormality of the parathyroid glands is called **primary hyperparathyroidism. Secondary hyperparathyroidism** occurs when calcium is abnormally excreted by the kidneys and the parathyroid glands increase their production of parathyroid hormone to maintain adequate blood levels of calcium. The most common cause of secondary hyperparathyroidism is kidney failure.

Clinical Features

The clinical manifestations of hyperparathyroidism are varied. Patients with mild cases can be asymptomatic. Joint pain or stiffness may be present. The disease can affect the kidneys, skeletal system, and gastrointestinal system. In severe disease, lethargy and coma can occur.

Oral Manifestations

The oral manifestations of hyperparathyroidism include changes in the bone of the mandible and maxilla. The chief oral manifestation is the appearance of well-defined unilocular or multilocular radiolucencies **(Figure 9-2,** *A*). Microscopically these lesions appear indistinguishable from central giant cell granulomas (described in Chapter 2) **(Figure 9-2,** *B*). There have also been reports of a few cases of peripheral giant cell granulomas associated with hyperparathyroidism. Other radiographic changes that occur in hyperparathyroidism include a generalized mottled appearance of the bone and partial loss of the lamina dura. Loosening of teeth can also occur.

A   **B**

Figure 9-2 **A,** Radiograph of a mandibular lesion in a patient with hyperparathyroidism. **B,** Microscopic appearance of a jaw lesion occurring in a patient with hyperparathyroidism. The histologic appearance is identical to that of a central giant cell granuloma. (**A,** Courtesy Drs. Paul Freedman and Stanley Kerpel.)

Diagnosis and Treatment

The diagnosis of hyperparathyroidism involves the measurement of parathyroid hormone blood levels and can also include serum calcium and phosphorus measurements. Treatment is directed at correcting the cause of the increased production of the hormone. Causes of increased production of hormone can include tumors, renal disease, and vitamin D deficiency. Bone lesions resolve when the hyperparathyroidism is successfully treated.

DIABETES MELLITUS

Diabetes mellitus is a chronic disorder of carbohydrate (glucose) metabolism and is characterized by abnormally high blood glucose levels **(hyperglycemia)**, which result from a lack of the hormone insulin, defective insulin that does not work effectively to lower blood glucose levels, or increased insulin resistance because of obesity. Diabetes is appropriately considered a syndrome because it has several components, including both acute and chronic complications. This disorder of carbohydrate metabolism also leads to disorders of protein and fat metabolism. Normally, glucose signals the beta cells of the pancreas to make insulin. This hormone is then directly secreted into the blood stream to facilitate the uptake of glucose into fat and skeletal muscle cells. In the presence of insulin, fat and skeletal muscle cells can use glucose as an energy source. When insulin is lacking, these cells are starved of energy. Without insulin to meet the body's demand for carbohydrate, tissues are broken down (catabolism), and weight loss occurs, as well as severe hyperglycemia that can lead to diabetic coma. Furthermore, the production of ketone acid from the breakdown of fatty tissue is a life-threatening condition and is a common metabolic disturbance in type 1 (insulin-dependent) diabetes. These ketone acids (acetone) can lower the pH of the blood **(ketoacidosis)**, an acute condition that can lead to coma and death. White blood cell function is affected in patients with diabetes mellitus. Phagocytic activity of macrophages is reduced, and chemotaxis of neutrophils is delayed, increasing a patient's susceptibility to infection. In addition, collagen production is abnormal, thus affecting the healing process.

The precise cause of diabetes mellitus is unknown. Genetic and environmental factors have been implicated in its onset. Sixteen million Americans have been diagnosed with diabetes mellitus. It is estimated that an additional seven million Americans have undiagnosed diabetes and therefore are at risk for life-threatening complications of untreated diabetes.

Types of Diabetes

Insulin-dependent diabetes mellitus

Two major types of diabetes have been recognized and classified. The first type **(type 1 diabetes)** is called **insulin-dependent diabetes mellitus (IDDM)**. Autoimmunity appears to play a key role in the development of type 1 diabetes, leading to the destruction of the insulin-producing beta cells of the pancreas and, ultimately, profound insulin deficiency. Only 3% to 5% of all diabetic patients have this type of diabetes. IDDM can occur at any age, but its time of onset is usually at a peak age of 20 years. The onset is abrupt and can have the three Ps (or the complications of these signs): (1) **polydipsia** (excessive thirst and intake of fluid), (2) **polyuria** (excessive urination), and (3) **polyphagia** (excessive appetite). Patients usually have a thin body build.

Complications can occur in 90% of individuals with type 1 diabetes within 20 years of diagnosis. Difficulty in controlling blood glucose levels is a major problem for patients with IDDM. In recent years it has become increasingly evident that long-term, rigorous control of blood glucose levels is important in minimizing the extent of chronic complications (especially those of the eye, kidney, and nerves) in patients with IDDM. Rigorous control of glucose is more likely achieved with multiple injections of insulin throughout the day to simulate physiologic conditions rather than with a single daily injection. Multiple insulin injections, proper diet, exercise, and frequent determinations of blood glucose levels at home constitute the current approach to the management of the patient with IDDM. However, multiple insulin injections can more readily lead to low blood sugar **(hypoglycemia)**; severe hypoglycemia **(insulin shock)** constitutes a medical emergency. The disease is controlled by replacement of the hormone insulin; however, insulin injections are not a cure for diabetes. All patients with IDDM remain insulin-dependent for their entire lives. Studies are now in progress to assess the efficacy of nasal preparations of insulin. If these preparations are successful, some patients may be spared from injections of insulin. An increasing number of type 1 diabetics are now entering insulin pump therapy. The patient must still monitor blood sugar levels by testing several times a day. The insulin pump is external and approximately the size of a pager; it delivers insulin through a plastic tubing placed under the skin. The patient programs the pump to deliver small amounts of insulin on the hour over a 24-hour period according to the patient's metabolic needs. The pump can maintain even more rigorous, predictable control of blood sugar levels than multiple insulin injections. The diabetic patient using insulin pump therapy carries a back-up supply of syringes in case the pump fails to deliver insulin; such failure can lead to the rapid development of ketoacidosis, resulting in signs and symptoms of nausea, abdominal cramps, disorientation, and fatigue.

Noninsulin-dependent diabetes mellitus

The second type **(type 2 diabetes)** is **noninsulin-dependent diabetes mellitus (NIDDM)**. Increased insulin resistance, rather than profound insulin deficiency, is characteristic of type 2 diabetes. Approximately 95% of all diabetic patients have type 2 diabetes. The onset of this type of diabetes is gradual and usually occurs in patients who are 35 to 40 years of age or older. Obesity is a common finding in many of these individuals. Obesity probably decreases the number of receptors for insulin binding in sensitive tissues, such as fat and muscle, thereby leading to the development of the diabetic state. Complications are less common in this type of diabetes than in type 1 diabetes. Some patients achieve control of blood glucose levels with diet and weight reduction alone, whereas others require oral hypoglycemic agents. These medications also lower blood glucose levels but, unlike insulin, are not given by injection. However, some patients with type 2 diabetes require insulin injections to obtain control of blood glucose levels.

Clinical Features

The vascular system is the most severely affected in diabetes. Accelerated atherosclerosis (thickening of the blood vessel wall from fibrofatty plaques), a common complication of diabetes, can occur and lead to impaired circulation of blood, resulting in impaired transport of oxygen and nutrients to tissues. This increases the risk of ulceration and gangrene of the feet, high blood pressure, kidney failure, and stroke. Blood vessel changes in the eye (diabetic retinopathy) can lead to hemorrhage, which can result in blindness. The nervous system can also be affected in diabetes. This is partly the result of vascular damage and results in a variety of neurologic complaints. Decreased resistance to infection is seen, particularly in uncontrolled diabetes. Skin infections, especially furuncles (boils), urinary tract infections, and tuberculosis are common.

Oral Complications

The oral complications of diabetes are most severe when blood glucose levels are not controlled. In some patients, control is difficult, even with careful monitoring of these levels and insulin injections. These patients are said to have **brittle diabetes** and may benefit from recent advances with insulin pump therapy.

Increased colonization of the oral mucosa by *Candida albicans* and an increased prevalence of oral candidiasis have been reported in patients with diabetes mellitus, as has mucormycosis, a rare fungal infection that affects the palate and maxillary sinuses. These infections are generally seen in poorly or uncontrolled diabetes mellitus. (Both oral candidiasis and mucormycosis are described in Chapter 4.) The presence of such fungal infections is indicative of a compromised immune system that occurs in diabetes mellitus.

Bilateral, asymptomatic parotid gland enlargement occurs in some patients and results from both a deposition of fat and hypertrophy of the salivary gland tissue.

Xerostomia (dry mouth) is usually associated with uncontrolled diabetes mellitus. Dehydration of the oral tissues can result, increasing the risk of the development of oral candidiasis and dental caries. Altered subgingival flora have been described in diabetes and may be the result of immunologic or salivary changes.

Patients with diabetes mellitus have an accentuated response to plaque. The gingiva can be hyperplastic and erythematous, and acute and fulminating gingival abscesses can occur. Excessive periodontal bone loss, tooth mobility, and early tooth loss can also be associated with diabetes mellitus **(Figure 9-3)**. Slow wound healing and increased susceptibility to infection occur as a result of the immunologic changes and defective collagen production.

Figure 9-3 Periapical radiograph of a patient with diabetes mellitus shows severe alveolar bone loss.

The diabetic patient who is receiving good medical management and whose glucose levels are controlled can receive any indicated dental treatment. Early identification of oral infections is important. Infection aggravates diabetes because it often results in the loss of blood glucose control—thus creating a vicious cycle because susceptibility to infection is increased. Therefore elimination of infection is extremely important in diabetic patients. Antibiotic medication, calculus and plaque removal, effective oral hygiene care, and adequate nutrition are especially important in the management of the diabetic patient.

ADDISON DISEASE

Addison disease, also known as **primary adrenal cortical insufficiency**, is characterized by an insufficient production of adrenal steroids. A malignant tumor or tuberculosis may be responsible for destruction of the adrenal gland. However, in most cases, the cause of the destruction of the adrenal cortex is unknown. In these patients the condition may be an autoimmune disease.

As a result of the decreased production of adrenal steroids, the pituitary gland increases its production of adrenocorticotropic hormone (ACTH), which would normally increase the production of adrenal steroids. This hormone is similar to melanin-stimulating hormone and causes stimulation of melanocytes. Brown pigmentation (bronzing) of the skin occurs, and melanotic macules can develop on the oral mucosa. Treatment of Addison disease involves steroid administration (replacement therapy).

Blood Disorders

The **complete blood count (CBC)** is important in the diagnosis of blood disorders. The CBC is a series of tests that examines the red blood cells, white blood cells, and platelets. It provides information about the number of each type of cell, the ratio of types of cells, and the appearance of the cells. The information included in a CBC and normal values are included in **Table 9-1**.

DISORDERS OF RED BLOOD CELLS AND HEMOGLOBIN

Anemia

Anemia is defined as a reduction in the oxygen-carrying capacity of the blood that in most cases is related to a decrease in the number of circulating red blood cells. There are many different types and causes of anemia.

Nutritional anemias occur when a substance necessary for the normal development of red blood cells is in scant supply in the bone marrow. The most common deficiencies are of iron, folic acid, or vitamin B_{12}. These deficiencies can occur when the intake of the nutrient is insufficient or when disorders of absorption prevent its uptake. Anemia can also occur when suppression of the bone marrow stem cells takes place, resulting in an inability of the bone marrow to produce red blood cells.

Oral manifestations are similar for all types of anemia and include skin and mucosal pallor, angular cheilitis, erythema and atrophy of the oral mucosa, and loss of filiform and fungiform papillae on the dorsum of the tongue. Circumvallate papillae and foliate papillae are not affected.

Iron-Deficiency Anemia

Iron-deficiency anemia occurs when an insufficient amount of iron is supplied to the bone marrow for

Table 9-1 Complete Blood Count Normal Adult Values

Red Blood Cells (RBCs)

Count: The total number of RBCs mm^3 of whole blood

Males 4.6–6.2 × 10^6

Females 4.2–5.4 × 10^6

Hemoglobin: The amount of hemoglobin contained in 100 ml of whole blood

Males 13.5–18 g

Females 12.0–16 g

Hematocrit: The volume of packed RBCs in 100 ml of whole blood

Males 40%–54%

Females 38%–47%

Indices: Mean corpuscular (cell) volume (MCV): Describes the average size of an individual RBC

80–96 mm^3

Mean corpuscular (cell) hemoglobin (MCH): Indicates the amount of hemoglobin present in an RBC by weight

27–31 pg (picogram)

Mean corpuscular (cell) hemoglobin concentration (MCHC): Indicates the proportion of each cell occupied by hemoglobin

32%–36%

White Blood Cells (WBCs)

Count: 4000-11,000 mm^3

Differential count: The number of each type of WBC expressed as a percentage of the total number of WBCs

Mature neutrophils (granulocytes)	50%–60%
Immature neutrophils (bands)	2%–4%
Lymphocytes	30%–40%
Monocytes	1%–9%
Basophils	0%–1%
Eosinophils	2%–3%

---

red blood cell development. This type of anemia can occur as a result of a deficiency of iron intake, blood loss from heavy menstrual bleeding or chronic gastrointestinal bleeding, poor iron absorption, or an increased requirement for iron, as in pregnancy or infancy.

The Plummer-Vinson syndrome can develop as a result of long-standing iron-deficiency anemia. This syndrome includes dysphagia (difficulty swallowing), atrophy of the upper alimentary tract, and a predisposition to the development of oral cancer.

Clinical features and oral manifestations

Iron-deficiency anemia is most often asymptomatic. Nonspecific symptoms such as weakness and fatigue can occur. Oral mucosal signs in severe cases include angular cheilitis, pallor of the oral tissues, and an erythematous, smooth, painful tongue **(Figure 9-4).** The changes in the oral mucosa occur as a result of a lack of nutrients to the epithelium. The filiform papillae on the dorsum of the tongue disappear first because they have the highest metabolic requirements. Disappearance of the fungiform papillae can also occur in chronic and severe cases.

Diagnosis and treatment

The diagnosis of iron-deficiency anemia is made by laboratory tests, which show a low hemoglobin content of red blood cells and a reduced hematocrit value. Iron is needed for hemoglobin synthesis;

therefore in iron-deficiency anemia, the red blood cells appear smaller than normal (microcytic) and lighter in color than normal (hypochromic). Increasing the intake of iron is the treatment for iron-deficiency anemia; dietary supplements are usually used. The oral lesions resolve when the deficiency is corrected.

Figure 9-4 Iron-deficiency anemia. The tongue is devoid of filiform papillae. Angular cheilitis was also present in this patient.

Pernicious Anemia

Pernicious anemia is caused by a deficiency of intrinsic factor, a substance secreted by the parietal cells of the stomach. Intrinsic factor is necessary for the absorption of vitamin B_{12}. Normally, vitamin B_{12} is transported across the intestinal mucosa by intrinsic factor. An autoimmune mechanism is the most likely cause of pernicious anemia. Antibodies to components of gastric mucosa have been identified in patients with pernicious anemia. Other causes of pernicious anemia include surgical removal of the stomach (gastrectomy), gastric cancer, or gastritis. Vitamin B_{12} is needed for DNA synthesis; when it is lacking, the development of rapidly dividing cells, such as bone marrow cells and epithelial cells, is affected.

Clinical features and oral manifestations

The clinical signs of pernicious anemia are weakness, pallor, and fatigue on exertion. Other constitutional signs can include nausea, dizziness, diarrhea, abdominal pain, loss of appetite, and weight loss. Neurologic changes such as severe paresthesia may also occur in patients with pernicious anemia.

Oral manifestations of pernicious anemia include angular cheilitis; mucosal pallor; painful, atrophic and erythematous mucosa; mucosal ulceration; loss of papillae on the dorsum of the tongue; and burning and painful tongue (**Figure 9-5**, *A* and *B*).

A

B

Figure 9-5 Pernicious anemia. **A,** Angular cheilitis and depapillation of the tongue in a patient with pernicious anemia. **B,** The mucosa becomes atrophic in pernicious anemia and easily ulcerated. The reader should note the ulcer on the left lateral aspect of the tongue.

Diagnosis and treatment

The diagnosis of pernicious anemia is made by laboratory testing. The diagnostic features include low serum vitamin B_{12} levels and gastric achlorhydria (lack of hydrochloric acid). Pernicious anemia is a megaloblastic anemia. Megaloblastic anemia is characterized by red blood cells that are immature, abnormally large, and have nuclei **(megaloblasts)**. Immature neutrophils and platelets are also seen both in the bone marrow and in the circulating blood. The Schilling test, which detects an inability to absorb an oral dose of vitamin B_{12} (cyanocobalamin), is another method used in the diagnosis of pernicious anemia. The treatment consists of injections of vitamin B_{12}. The oral mucosa improves in time, but the papillae on the dorsum of the tongue may not completely regenerate.

Folic Acid and Vitamin B_{12} Deficiency Anemia

Dietary deficiencies of folic acid and vitamin B_{12} can result in anemia and can occur in association with malnutrition and increased metabolic requirements. Malnutrition can occur in association with alcoholism, and pregnant women can experience a deficiency because of increased metabolic demands. Folic acid is essential for DNA synthesis, as is vitamin B_{12}.

Oral manifestations

The oral manifestations are indistinguishable from those of pernicious anemia.

Diagnosis and treatment

The diagnosis of these anemias is based on laboratory test results that include serum assays of folic acid and vitamin B_{12}. These are also megaloblastic anemias. Thus as in pernicious anemia, the red blood cells are immature, abnormally large, and nucleated **(megaloblasts)**. Treatment involves dietary supplements.

Thalassemia

Thalassemia, also called **Mediterranean** or **Cooley anemia**, is the name of a group of inherited disorders of hemoglobin synthesis. It has an autosomal dominant inheritance pattern; therefore no predilection for either sex is seen. The heterozygous form (see Chapter 6), in which only one gene at a locus is involved, is called **thalassemia minor**

and can be asymptomatic or only mildly symptomatic. The homozygous form, in which the genes on both chromosomes are involved, is called **thalassemia major** and is associated with severe hemolytic anemia, which results from damage to the red blood cell membranes and destruction of the red blood cells.

Clinical features and oral manifestations

The severe form of the disease begins early in life. The child has a yellowish skin pallor, fever, malaise, and weakness. An enlarged liver and spleen are common. The characteristic facies includes prominent cheekbones, depression of the bridge of the nose, an unusual prominence of the premaxilla, and protrusion or flaring of the maxillary anterior teeth. Intraoral radiographs show a peculiar trabecular pattern of the maxilla and mandible. There is a prominence of some trabeculae and a blurring and disappearance of others, resulting in a "salt and pepper" effect. Thinning of the lamina dura and circular radiolucencies in the alveolar bone have also been described.

Treatment

Treatment of thalassemia major is experimental. Blood transfusions and splenectomy have provided periods of remission. The prognosis is poor. However, these supportive therapies have extended life from early childhood to about 20 years of age.

Sickle Cell Anemia

Sickle cell anemia is an inherited disorder of the blood that is found predominantly in black individuals and those of Mediterranean origin. Persons who are heterozygous for the disease are generally asymptomatic. This is called **sickle cell trait**. Those that are homozygous are much more severely affected. The disease occurs before age 30 years and is more common in women than in men. Sickle cell anemia occurs as a result of an abnormal type of hemoglobin in red blood cells. Because of this abnormal hemoglobin, the cells develop a sickle shape in the presence of decreased oxygen; hence, the name *sickle cell anemia*. Exercise, exertion, administration of a general anesthetic, pregnancy, or even sleep can trigger a sickling of the red blood cells. Because of the change in their shape, the red blood cells are no longer able to pass through small blood vessels and are destroyed more rapidly than normal.

Figure 9-6 Sickle cell anemia. Radiograph shows abnormal trabeculation. (Courtesy Dr. Edward V. Zegarelli.)

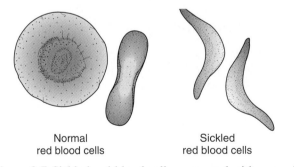

Normal
red blood cells

Sickled
red blood cells

Figure 9-7 Sickled red blood cells compared with normal red blood cells.

Clinical features and oral manifestations

The patient with sickle cell anemia experiences weakness, shortness of breath, fatigue, joint pain, and nausea. Oral manifestations are seen on dental radiographs **(Figure 9-6)**. A loss of trabeculation takes place, with the appearance of large, irregular marrow spaces. This change is most prominent in the alveolar bone.

Changes in the skull have been described as a hair-on-end pattern because the trabeculae radiate outward.

Diagnosis and treatment

The sickle-shaped cells are seen on a blood smear **(Figure 9-7)**. The number of red blood cells is usually low, as is the hemoglobin content. Management of sickle cell anemia is largely symptomatic and supportive and involves the administration of oxygen and intravenous and oral fluids. Sickle cell anemia can result in profound changes of the heart, such as enlargement, and lead to cardiac failure.

Celiac Sprue

Celiac sprue is a chronic disorder associated with a sensitivity to dietary gluten, a protein found in wheat and wheat products. When gluten is ingested, injury to the intestinal mucosa results. Malabsorption of other nutrients, such as vitamin B_{12} and folic acid, occurs be-

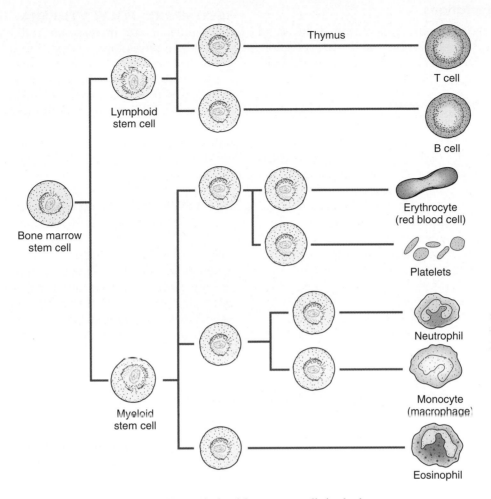

Figure 9-8 Blood cells are derived from stem cells in the bone marrow

cause of mucosal injury. As a result, anemia develops, as do the oral and clinical signs associated with it.

Clinical features and oral manifestations

Systemic symptoms include diarrhea, nervousness, and paresthesia of the extremities. Oral manifestations include a painful burning tongue (glossitis), atrophy of the papillae of the tongue, and ulceration of the oral mucosa.

Diagnosis and treatment

Patients should adhere to a gluten-free diet. Oral manifestations resolve when the systemic disease is under control.

Aplastic Anemia

In **aplastic anemia**, patients experience a dramatic decrease in all the circulating blood cells **(pancytopenia)** because of a severe depression of bone marrow activity. All the blood cells are produced in the marrow **(Figure 9-8)**. The cause of **primary aplastic anemia** is unknown. In **secondary aplastic anemia** the bone marrow failure is a result of a drug or chemical agent. Chemotherapy, radioactive isotopes, radium, or radiant energy have been associated with the development of aplastic anemia. Primary aplastic anemia occurs most frequently in young adults.

Oral manifestations

These are related to the generalized decrease in white blood cells and platelets and include infection, spontaneous bleeding, petechiae, and purpuric spots **(Figure 9-9).**

Diagnosis and treatment

In both forms of aplastic anemia, a generalized decrease of circulating blood cells occurs. In addition to anemia, **leukopenia** (a decrease in white blood cells) and **thrombocytopenia** (a decrease in platelets) occur. White blood cells are essential in the defense against infection (see Chapters 3 and 4), and platelets are essential in the clotting of blood. Primary aplastic anemia is usually progressive and fatal. Treatment of secondary aplastic anemia involves removing the cause.

Polycythemia

Polycythemia is characterized by an increase in the number of circulating red blood cells. This increase can be either an absolute or a relative increase. Normal red blood cell production is carefully regulated and involves both the precursor cells in the bone marrow and the hormone erythropoietin, which is produced by the kidney.

Types of polycythemia

The three forms of polycythemia are (1) polycythemia vera (primary polycythemia), (2) secondary polycythemia, and (3) relative polycythemia.

POLYCYTHEMIA VERA (PRIMARY POLYCYTHEMIA). In polycythemia vera, a neoplastic proliferation of bone marrow stem cells results in an abnormally high number of circulating red blood cells. The production of red blood cells is uncontrolled. The cause of this disorder is unknown. It is somewhat more common in men than in women, and the age of onset is usually between 40 and 60 years. It is generally seen in white individuals and is extremely rare in black individuals. The symptoms of polycythemia vera include headache, dizziness, and itching of the skin (pruritus). The increase in red blood cells leads to impaired blood flow, vascular stasis, and poor circulation. The formation of thrombi can cause a disruption of the blood supply to the brain, heart, or peripheral vessels. A decrease in platelets (thrombocytopenia) can occur because of the disruption of the marrow from which they are derived.

SECONDARY POLYCYTHEMIA. In secondary polycythemia, the increase in red blood cells is caused by a physiologic response to decreased oxygen. A decrease in oxygen in the blood triggers an increase in erythropoietin by the kidneys, which results in increased production of red blood cells. A number of factors can cause a decrease in oxygen, including pulmonary disease, heart disease, living at high altitudes, and an elevation in carbon monoxide. The increase in carbon monoxide has been associated with tobacco smoking.

RELATIVE POLYCYTHEMIA. This is caused by a decreased plasma volume and not an increase in red blood cells. In acute forms the cause is usually easily recognized. Causes of acute relative polycythemia include diuretic use, vomiting, diarrhea, or excessive sweating. A chronic form of relative polycythemia has been called stress polycythemia. Most patients with this type of polycythemia are middle-aged white men who are under physiologic stress, mildly overweight, hypertensive, and heavy smokers. The risk of cerebrovascular accidents (stroke) and myocardial infarction (heart attack) is increased in these patients.

Oral manifestations

The oral mucosa in patients with polycythemia may appear deep red to purple, and the gingiva may be edematous. The gingiva may bleed easily, and submucosal petechiae, ecchymosis, and hematoma formation can be present. There can be excessive bleeding after oral surgical procedures. Abnormalities of the oral mucosa result from an increase in circulating red blood cells, the impaired blood flow, and thrombocytopenia.

Figure 9-9 Aplastic anemia. Severe oral infection occurred after extraction of teeth in this patient with aplastic anemia. (Courtesy Dr. Harry Lumerman.)

Diagnosis and treatment

Diagnosis of the different forms of polycythemia involves laboratory testing and measurement of the hemoglobin content and the hematocrit. Treatment is related to the type of polycythemia and may include removal of causative factors, chemotherapy, and phlebotomy (blood-letting). Oral lesions generally do not require local treatment; however, patients tend to have increased bleeding after oral surgery.

DISORDERS OF WHITE BLOOD CELLS

Three groups of white blood cells are found in the circulation: granulocytes, lymphocytes, and monocytes. The three types of granulocytes are polymorphonuclear leukocytes (neutrophils), eosinophils, and basophils. The primary function of the neutrophils is to defend the body against foreign invaders, such as bacteria, viruses, and fungi (described in Chapter 4). These cells are produced primarily in the bone marrow and are released into the circulating blood (see Figure 9-8). The response of these cells to infection is known as the **inflammatory response** (see Chapter 2).

Agranulocytosis

In **agranulocytosis** a significant reduction in circulating neutrophils occurs, which has serious consequences. An abnormally low white blood cell count is called **leukopenia**. Any of the white blood cells can be involved, but leukopenia most commonly involves the neutrophils. A reduction in the number of circulating neutrophils is called **neutropenia;** it can be seen in a variety of circumstances and is usually temporary and of little significance.

Agranulocytosis can result from either a problem in the development of neutrophils or a problem in accelerated destruction of neutrophils. Primary and secondary forms of agranulocytosis have been described. The cause of the primary form is unknown and may be an immunologic disorder. The secondary form of agranulocytosis is most commonly produced by drugs and other chemicals. Secondary agranulocytosis is most commonly seen in women.

Clinical features and oral manifestations

Clinically, patients experience a sudden onset of high fever, chills, jaundice **(icterus)**, weakness, and sore throat. Orally, the most characteristic feature is the presence of infection. Necrotizing ulcerations, excessive bleeding from the gingiva, and rapid destruction of the supporting tissue of the teeth have been described. Regional lymphadenopathy can accompany the oral problems.

Diagnosis and treatment

The diagnosis is made by laboratory testing. The white blood cell count, which is normally 5000 to 10,000 cells/mm^3, is dramatically reduced to less than 1000 cells/mm^3. Treatment includes transfusions, antibiotics to control infection, and, in the secondary form, removal of the causative agent. Infections can become overwhelming and cause death. All surgical procedures, including dental hygiene procedures, are contraindicated.

Cyclic Neutropenia

Cyclic neutropenia is a form of agranulocytosis. A severe depression of granulocytes (neutrophils) occurs at periodic intervals. Cyclic neutropenia is described in detail in Chapter 6.

Leukemia

Leukemias are malignant neoplasms of the hematopoietic (blood-forming) stem cells. They are disorders that primarily originate in the bone marrow. However, the most dramatic feature of leukemias is the excessive number of abnormal white blood cells in the circulating blood. The pathogenesis is unknown. However, current investigations are focusing on oncogenic viruses (see Chapter 7). Many different types of leukemias exist. Leukemias are classified by the cell type involved and the maturity of the neoplastic cells **(Table 9-2)**. Leukemias are de-

Table 9-2 Classification of Leukemias

Acute Leukemias	Chronic Leukemias
Acute lymphoblastic leukemia (lymphocytes)	Chronic lymphocytic leukemia
Acute nonlymphoblastic leukemia (granulocytes, monocytes, erythrocytes)	Chronic granulocytic (myeloid) leukemia

scribed in this chapter with other abnormalities of blood. They also have been included in Chapter 7, in which other neoplasms are described. Many different types of leukemias are known, and this text gives only an overview of them to discuss the oral manifestations. The student is encouraged to use other texts for a more complete description of leukemias. The two general categories of leukemias, acute and chronic, are described in this text. Oral lesions are most common in acute leukemias but may also occur in chronic forms of leukemia.

Acute leukemias

Acute leukemias are characterized by the presence of very immature cells (blast cells) and by a rapidly fatal course if not treated. Acute leukemias can involve immature lymphocytes (**acute lymphoblastic leukemia**) or immature granulocytes (**acute myeloblastic leukemia**). Acute lymphoblastic leukemia primarily affects children and young adults and has a good prognosis. Acute myeloblastic leukemia involves adolescents and young adults (age range, 15 to 39 years), and the prognosis is not as good. The onset of acute leukemia is sudden and dramatic.

CLINICAL FEATURES. Clinically, patients experience weakness, fever, enlargement of lymph nodes, and bleeding. The lymph node enlargement can include cervical lymphadenopathy (enlargement of the lymph nodes in the neck). A general loss of cells produced by the bone marrow occurs. The fatigue mainly results from anemia, the fever from infection, and the bleeding from a decrease in platelets (**throm-**

Figure 9-10 Generalized gingival hyperplasia in a patient with leukemia. (Courtesy Dr. Edward V. Zegarelli.)

bocytopenia). In advanced disease, enlargement of the spleen (**splenomegaly**) and liver (**hepatomegaly**) occurs when those organs are infiltrated by the leukemic cells.

ORAL MANIFESTATIONS. Oral manifestations can include gingival enlargement (which can be severe) caused by infiltration of leukemic cells (**Figure 9-10**) and oral infections (including acute necrotizing ulcerative gingivitis [ANUG]) because white blood cells are not functioning. In addition, if a decrease in platelets occurs, bleeding gums, petechiae, and ecchymoses may be present. Toothache as the result of invasion of the pulp by leukemic cells has been reported.

DIAGNOSIS AND TREATMENT. In acute leukemia, laboratory findings include an elevated white blood cell count with the presence of many immature cells, anemia, and a low platelet count. In young children with acute lymphocytic leukemia, the prognosis with treatment is very good. In adolescents and adults with acute myelocytic leukemia, the prognosis is poor. Remissions occur with chemotherapy, and then relapses occur. Bone marrow transplantation is a treatment for this form of leukemia.

Chronic leukemias

In addition, several different types of chronic leukemias exist. They are all characterized by a slow onset, and they all primarily affect adults. The disease can be present for months before a diagnosis is made, and occasionally the diagnosis is made during a routine physical examination based on laboratory testing. One of the forms of chronic leukemia, **chronic myeloid leukemia**, is associated with a distinctive chromosomal abnormality, the Philadelphia chromosome. Another form of chronic leukemia, **chronic lymphocytic leukemia**, is the most common form and accounts for about one quarter of the total cases of leukemia. It may be asymptomatic for a long time. About half the patients with this type of leukemia have abnormal karyotypes; however, the abnormality is different from the Philadelphia chromosome.

CLINICAL FEATURES AND ORAL MANIFESTATIONS. The clinical onset is slow. The symptoms are nonspecific and include easy fatigability, weakness, weight loss, and anorexia. Oral manifestations include pallor of the lips and gingiva, gingival enlargement, petechiae and ecchymosis, gingival bleeding, and atypical periodontal disease. Cervical lymphadenopathy may be an early manifestation of chronic leukemia.

DIAGNOSIS AND TREATMENT. The white blood cell count can increase to 500,000/mm^3, and most of the total cells can be leukemia cells. Remissions occur with chemotherapy; however, they are of short duration, and the long-term prognosis is poor. Bone marrow transplantation is used to treat both chronic and acute leukemia.

BLEEDING DISORDERS

Hemostasis

Patients with bleeding disorders can have one of a number of different defects.

Hemostasis (the cessation of bleeding) is a complex process that involves a number of events **(Figure 9-11).** When a blood vessel is damaged, marked constriction of the vessel (vasoconstriction) occurs in an attempt to stop the flow of blood. Platelets (thrombocytes) that are produced by the bone marrow and are circulating in blood adhere to the damaged surface and aggregate to form a tem-

Table 9-3 Factors Involved in Coagulation*	
Factor	**Name**
I	Fibrinogen
II	Prothrombin
III	Tissue factor
IV	Calcium ions
V	Proaccelerin
VII	Proconvertin
VIII	Antihemophilic factor
IX	Plasma thromboplastin
X	Stuart factor
XI	Plasma thromboplastin antecedent
XII	Hageman factor
XIII	Fibrin-stabilizing factor

*Factors are numbered in the order in which they were discovered and not in the order in which they function. (No factor VI is included.)

Figure 9-11 Hemostasis.

Figure 9-12 Coagulation cascade. Coagulation factors remain inactive until needed. As each coagulation factor becomes activated (a), it is responsible for the activation of another factor until all have been activated and the final clot is formed. The two pathways by which this cascade is activated are the intrinsic and extrinsic pathways.

Table 9-4 Laboratory Tests for Hemostasis

Test	Normal Values
Platelet count (number of platelets)	150,000–400,000/mm³
Bleeding time (platelet function)	1–6 minutes*
Prothrombin time (PT) (fibrin clot formation—extrinsic pathway)	11–16 seconds*
Partial thromboplastin time (PTT) (fibrin clot formation—intrinsic pathway)	25–40 seconds*

Normal values may differ according to the specific test used and the individual laboratory.

porary clot. To stop the bleeding permanently, it is necessary for fibrin to be produced. Fibrin tightly binds the aggregating platelets to form a clot. A cascade of circulating plasma proteins that are made almost exclusively in the liver and called **clotting factors** or **coagulation factors** is necessary to convert the precursor fibrinogen to fibrin **(Table 9-3; Figure 9-12).**

Finally, anticlotting mechanisms are activated to prevent the spread of more clots and to allow the clot to dissolve so that the damaged vessel can be repaired. This complexity is necessary to prevent inappropriate clotting. Successful hemostasis is dependent on the walls of the blood vessels, adequate numbers of functioning platelets, and adequate levels of properly functioning clotting factors.

Defects in hemostasis are caused by abnormalities of either platelets or coagulation factors. These defects can be diagnosed with a few laboratory tests **(Table 9-4).** Normal values may differ according to the specific test used and the individual laboratory.

Platelet count

The **platelet count,** which is usually requested with a CBC, provides a quantitative or numeric evaluation of platelets. A normal platelet count should be 150,000 to 400,000/mm³. A platelet count less than 100,000/mm³ is considered thrombocytopenia. Spontaneous gingival bleeding can occur when a patient's platelet count is less than 20,000/mm³. In addition, a physician can request specific clotting factor assays, which can also be performed in patients with suspected or known clotting factor deficiencies. Nearly all bleeding disorders are caused by abnormalities of either platelets or clotting factors. Rarely, bleeding disorders result from capillary fragility or weakness of the blood vessel walls.

Bleeding time

The **bleeding time** provides an assessment of the adequacy of platelet function, not platelet number. The test measures how long it takes a standardized skin incision to stop bleeding by the formation of a temporary hemostatic plug or clot. The normal range of bleeding time is dependent on the way the test is performed but is usually between 1 and 6 minutes. The bleeding time is prolonged, or greater than 5 to 10 minutes, in patients with platelet abnormalities.

Prothrombin time

The **prothrombin time (PT)** measures the patient's ability to form a clot. It is performed by measuring the time it takes for a clot to form when calcium and a tissue factor are added to the patient's plasma. A normal PT is usually between 11 and 16 seconds. The value is usually compared with a normal control, which is generated daily by the laboratory using standardized plasma. A prolonged or greater than normal PT can be associated with postoperative bleeding because of abnormal clot formation. A prolonged PT is usually not associated with bleeding unless it is longer than 1.5 times the control. Most often physicians use PT to monitor anticoagulant therapy (as in coumarin or warfarin sodium) for preventing myocardial infarction. A more accurate determination of PT is the INR, an expression of the ratio of PT to thromboplastin activity. The INR is more accurate because it is standardized from laboratory to laboratory. Values less than 3.0 are considered within normal range. Patients on anticoagulants, like warfarin, may have INR values of 4 to 5.

Partial thromboplastin time

The **partial thromboplastin time (PTT)** also measures the effectiveness of clot formation. Two different pathways exist by which clot formation occurs. PT measures one of these, and PTT measures the other. The test is performed by measuring the time it takes for a clot to form after the addition of kaolin, a surface-activating factor, and cephalin, a substitute platelet factor, to the patient's plasma. A normal PTT is usually 25 to 40 seconds. Prolongation of the PTT to 45 to 50 seconds can be associated with mild bleeding problems.

With further prolongation (more than 50 seconds), severe bleeding can occur. PTT is also used by physicians to monitor heparin therapy, which is commonly used for kidney hemodialysis in patients with renal failure.

Purpura

Purpura is a reddish-blue or purplish discoloration of the skin or mucosa that results from spontaneous extravasation of blood. It can be caused by a defect or deficiency in blood platelets or an increase in capillary fragility. A significant oral clinical finding is the oozing of blood at the gingival margins in several sites without the presence of gingivitis or inflammation. Petechiae, ecchymoses, and hemorrhagic blisters can also be present.

Thrombocytopenic purpura

Thrombocytopenic purpura is a bleeding disorder that results from a severe reduction in circulating platelets. The normal platelet level is 150,000 to 400,000/mm³ of blood. Spontaneous bleeding occurs when platelet levels fall to less than 20,000/mm³. When the cause is unknown, the condition is called **idiopathic thrombocytopenic purpura.** An autoimmune type of process has been identified for thrombocytopenia, and therefore it is sometimes called **immune thrombocytopenia.** The condition can also be secondary to an existing disease or condition. **Secondary thrombocytopenic purpura** is often associated with drugs, including those used for cancer chemotherapy. The idiopathic or primary form is usually seen in young patients, with the greatest incidence occurring before the age of 10 years. No age predilection for the secondary type and no sex predilection for either type is seen.

CLINICAL AND ORAL MANIFESTATIONS. Clinically, spontaneous purpuric or hemorrhagic lesions of the skin develop that can vary in size and severity. Additionally these patients bruise easily, can have blood in the urine (hematuria), and have frequent nosebleeds (epistaxis). Oral manifestations include spontaneous gingival bleeding and clusters of petechiae or purpuric spots.

DIAGNOSIS AND TREATMENT. Laboratory tests show a significant decrease in platelets. Bleeding time can be prolonged to an hour or more, and the capillary fragility test result is positive. Treatment depends on the cause and includes transfusions, corticosteroids, and splenectomy. Any dental surgical procedure, including scaling, is contraindicated until laboratory test results confirm sufficient improvement in the patient's bleeding problem.

Nonthrombocytopenic purpura

Nonthrombocytopenic purpuras are bleeding disorders that can result from either a defect in the capillary walls or disorders of platelet function. Vascular wall alterations occur in vitamin C deficiency and infections and can also result from chemicals and allergy. Many factors can cause disorders of platelet function, including drugs, allergy, and autoimmune disease. By far the most common reason for a prolonged bleeding time is the ingestion of drugs that affect platelet function. Ingestion of small doses of aspirin (0.3 to 1.5 g) produces an impairment of platelet function for 7 to 10 days. The nonsteroidal antiinflammatory drugs (e.g., ibuprofen, naproxen, indomethacin) can also adversely affect platelet function. Patients with kidney failure and those with leukemia can have impaired platelet function. **von Willebrand disease** is an autosomal dominantly inherited disorder of platelet function. Both men and women may be affected with this disorder.

ORAL MANIFESTATIONS. The oral manifestations in nonthrombocytopenic purpura are the same as those that occur in thrombocytopenic purpura and include spontaneous gingival bleeding, petechiae, ecchymoses, and hemorrhagic blisters.

DIAGNOSIS AND TREATMENT. The platelet count is normal in nonthrombocytopenic purpura. The bleeding time is prolonged. Treatment includes systemic corticosteroids, splenectomy, and permanent or temporary discontinuation of the causative agent.

Hemophilia

Hemophilia is a disorder of blood coagulation that results in severely prolonged clotting time. The problem results from a deficiency of one of the plasma proteins involved in the coagulation cascade that is necessary for the conversion of fibrinogen to fibrin (see Figure 9-12).

Types of hemophilia

The two most common types of hemophilia are type A and type B. These types of hemophilia are inherited as X-linked diseases and are therefore transmitted through an unaffected carrier daughter to a son. The carrier mother may have a mildly prolonged coagulation time. (Inheritance patterns including sex-linked inheritance, are described in Chapter 6.)

Type A hemophilia is the classic and most common type and is caused by a deficiency of the clotting factor called plasma thromboplastinogen or Factor VIII. This deficiency is characterized by severe hemorrhage after even mild to moderate injury or surgery. Type B, or Christmas disease, is less common. The clotting defect is in **plasma thromboplastin** or **Factor IX.**

Oral manifestations

The oral manifestations of hemophilia are spontaneous gingival bleeding, petechiae, and ecchymoses. Patients have a risk of hemorrhage after oral surgery procedures and scaling.

Diagnosis and treatment

The bleeding time and PT in hemophilia are normal, and the PTT is prolonged. Diagnosis involves identifying the missing factor, and treatment involves replacing it.

Immunodeficiency

Immunity is described in Chapter 3. Immunodeficiency can involve the different parts of the immune system either alone or together. Immunodeficiency can involve the cell-mediated (T cell) response or the humoral (B cell or antibody) response. Deficiencies in phagocytosis can also be considered deficiencies in immunity. Immunodeficiency diseases are divided into primary and secondary immunodeficiencies. Primary immunodeficiencies are those of genetic origin, and secondary immunodeficiencies result from some other underlying disorder. The signs and symptoms that occur in a person with immunodeficiency depend on the degree of the deficiency and the type of immune response involved. The most common complications arising in persons with either primary or secondary immunodeficiency is infection. The type of infection is related to the type of immunodeficiency. Individuals with deficiency in humoral immunity are more likely to develop bacterial infections; those with deficiency in cell-mediated immunity are more likely to develop viral infections, fungal infections, and infections by intracellular bacteria such as tuberculosis. Autoimmune diseases and neoplasm may also be associated with certain immune deficiencies.

PRIMARY IMMUNODEFICIENCIES

Primary immunodeficiencies are immunodeficiencies of genetic origin and can involve B cells, T cells, or both. These primary immunodeficiencies have provided much information about the functions of the different immunologic responses and are extremely rare.

Three examples are included here. The first is **Bruton disease**, also called **X-linked congenital agammaglobulinemia** (lack of immunoglobulins), which is a disorder in which B cells do not mature. Plasma cells are deficient throughout the body; T cells are normal. Autoimmune diseases are common in these patients.

The second example is **DiGeorge syndrome**, which is also called **thymic hypoplasia**. It is a disorder in which the thymus is deficient or lacking, and therefore T lymphocytes do not mature. Infants and children with this syndrome are extremely susceptible to fungal, viral, and those bacterial infections that require T- and B-cell cooperation. B lymphocytes and immunoglobulins are not affected.

The third example is **severe combined immunodeficiency**. Most infants with this type of immunodeficiency die within the first year of life and are vulnerable to all forms of viral, fungal, and bacterial infections.

SECONDARY IMMUNODEFICIENCIES

Secondary immunodeficiencies are those that occur as a result of an underlying disorder. They are much more common than the primary immunodeficiency disorders. Disorders that can have accompanying immunodeficiency include malnutrition, which can lead to inadequate synthesis of antibodies; viral infection; cancer; renal diseases in which antibodies are excreted abnormally; and Hodgkin's disease. They can also occur with the use of immunosuppressive drugs, including corticosteroids; drugs that are used, along with radiation, to suppress the immune system in organ and bone marrow transplantation and to treat autoimmune diseases; and drugs used for cancer chemotherapy. **Table 9-5** lists some of the most common drugs that can cause immunodeficiency and the reasons they are generally used. Acquired immunodeficiency syndrome (AIDS), which occurs as a result of infection with the human immunodeficiency virus (HIV), is an example of a secondary immunodeficiency. HIV infection is described in detail in Chapter 4.

Oral Manifestations of Therapy for Oral Cancer

Oral cancer can be treated by surgery, radiation therapy, or chemotherapy, or any combination of the three. Radiation therapy and chemotherapy can result in the development of several different oral manifestations.

RADIATION THERAPY

During radiation therapy the patient often experiences mucositis (**Figure 9-13**, *A–C*), which begins about the second week of therapy and subsides a few weeks after its completion. The mucositis is painful and appears as erythematous and ulcerated mucosa. Difficulty in eating, pain on swallowing, and loss of taste can occur as a result of the mucositis. If the

Table 9-5 Examples of Drugs That Can Cause Immunosuppression

Name	Use
Azathioprine	Prevention of rejection of renal transplants
	Treatment of rheumatoid arthritis
Cyclosporine	Prevention of rejection of renal transplants
Cyclophosphamide	Cancer chemotherapy
Methotrexate	Cancer chemotherapy
Prednisone	Treatment of autoimmune diseases (such as rheumatoid arthritis, pemphigus vulgaris, Behçet's syndrome, lupus erythematosus)

radiation affects the major salivary glands, irreversible salivary gland destruction can occur, resulting in severe xerostomia. As a result, the mucosal tissues are easily irritated and the patient is prone to the development of rampant caries **(Figure 9-14)** and oral candidiasis. Pilocarpine hydrochloride taken during the course of radiation treatment decreases the severity of radiation-induced xerostomia. A patient who has received radiation therapy for oral cancer is also at risk for the development of **osteoradionecrosis** (necrosis of bone from radiation therapy) because of the decreased blood supply to the bone after radiation therapy. Osteoradionecrosis develops in the mandible more frequently than in the maxilla, and the risk for its development does not decrease with time.

Patients for whom head and neck radiation is planned should have an oral evaluation before the initiation of radiation therapy. Potential sources of oral infection should be eliminated and teeth for which the prognosis is questionable should be removed. The role of the dental hygienist in the management of patients receiving head and neck radiation treatment expected to result in xerostomia involves fluoride application both by the dental hygienist and the patient, patient education in oral hygiene care, and frequent follow-up appointments to ensure patient compliance.

Saliva substitutes can be used by the patient for symptomatic relief of xerostomia.

Figure 9-13 **A** and **B,** Radiation mucositis. **C,** Post-radiation xerostomia.

Figure 9-14 Clinical appearance of radiation caries. (Courtesy Dr. Jonathan A. Ship.)

CHEMOTHERAPY

The complications of cancer chemotherapy are predictable and differ for the various types of chemotherapy used. Mucositis and oral ulceration are frequent complications because drugs used for cancer chemotherapy affect rapidly dividing cells and therefore affect the basal cells of the epithelium. The epithelium becomes atrophic and ulcerated with minor irritation. Cells of the bone marrow are also affected, and therefore a decrease in all blood cells (red blood cells, white blood cells, and platelets) can result. The patient can experience anemia because of a decrease in red blood cells, is at increased risk for opportunistic infections (e.g., candidiasis) because of a decrease in white blood cells, and is at increased risk for bleeding problems because of a decrease in the number of platelets.

Before the initiation of cancer chemotherapy, the patient should receive an oral evaluation to identify and eliminate any source of oral infection that may exacerbate during the course of chemotherapy.

Effects of Drugs on the Oral Cavity

Many drugs can cause changes in the oral tissues. Xerostomia can be caused by drugs used to control blood pressure. Antianxiety medications, antipsychotic medications, and antihistamines can also cause xerostomia **(Figure 9-15)**. Drugs such as prednisone that suppress the immune system can increase the risk of candidiasis and other oral infections **(Figure 9-16)**. Antibiotics can also increase the risk of candidiasis. Tetracycline taken when teeth are forming can cause tooth discoloration **(Figure 9-17)**. Phenytoin (Dilantin) and nifedipine (Procardia) can cause gingival enlargement **(Figure 9-18**, *A* to *C*). Cyclosporine, an immunosuppressant drug used to prevent rejection of transplanted organs, can also cause gingival enlargement.

The complete medical history should include a listing of the medications taken by a patient and is useful in establishing the diagnosis of drug-induced oral lesions.

Figure 9-15 Xerostomia caused by chlorpromazine (Thorazine) administration.

Figure 9-16 Candidiasis in a patient taking prednisone for rheumatoid arthritis.

Figure 9-17 Discoloration of teeth caused by tetracycline ingestion.

Figure 9-18 Drug-induced gingival hyperplasia. **A,** Gingival enlargement caused by phenytoin (Dilantin). **B** and **C,** Gingival hyperplasia caused by nifedipine (Procardia). (**A** courtesy Dr. Edward V. Zegarelli; **B** and **C** courtesy Dr. Victor M. Sternberg.)

Selected References

Books

Little JW, Falace DA: *Dental management of the medically compromised patient,* ed 6, St Louis, 2002, Mosby.

Neville BW et al: *Oral and maxillofacial pathology,* ed 2, Philadelphia, 2002, WB Saunders.

Regezi JA, Sciubba JJ: *Oral pathology. Clinical-pathologic correlations,* ed 4, Philadelphia, 2003, WB Saunders.

Sonis ST, Fazio RC, Fang LST: *Oral medicine secrets,* Philadelphia, 2003, Hanley & Belfus.

Journal Articles

Avcu N et al: The relationship between gastric-oral *Helicobacter pylori* and oral hygiene in patients with vitamin B$_{12}$-deficiency anemia, *Oral Surg Oral Med Oral Pathol Oral Radiol Endod* 92:166, 2001.

Centers for Disease Control and Prevention: Iron deficiency—United States, 1999-2000, *Morb Mortal Wkly Rep* 51:89, 2002.

Chavez EM et al: A longitudinal analysis of salivary flow in control subjects and older adults with type 2 diabetes, *Oral Surg Oral Med Oral Pathol Oral Radiol Endod* 91:166, 2001.

Collin H et al: Oral symptoms and signs in elderly patients with type 2 diabetes mellitus, *Oral Surg Oral Med Oral Pathol Oral Radiol Endod* 90:299, 2000.

Fletcher PD, Scopp IV, Hersh RA: Oral manifestations of secondary hyperparathyroidism related to long-term hemodialysis therapy, *Oral Surg Oral Med Oral Pathol* 43:218, 1977.

Garg AK, Malo M: Manifestations and treatment of xerostomia and associated oral effects secondary to head and neck radiation therapy, *J Am Dent Assoc* 128:1128, 1997.

Genco R et al: Molecular factors influencing neutrophil defects in periodontal disease, *J Dent Res* 65:1379, 1986.

Guggenheimer J et al: Insulin-dependent diabetes mellitus and oral soft tissue pathologies. I. Prevalence and characteristics of non-candidal lesions, *Oral Surg Oral Med Oral Pathol Oral Radiol Endod* 89:564, 2000.

Guggenheimer J et al: Insulin-dependent diabetes mellitus and oral soft tissue pathologies. II. Prevalence and characteristics of *Candida* and candidal lesions, *Oral Surg Oral Med Oral Pathol Oral Radiol Endod* 89:570, 2000.

Inokuchi T, Sano K, Kamingo M: Osteoradionecrosis of the sphenoid and temporal bones in a patient with maxillary sinus carcinoma: a case report, *Oral Surg Oral Med Oral Pathol* 70:278, 1990.

Johnson WT, Leary JM: Management of dental patients with bleeding disorders: review and update, *Oral Surg Oral Med Oral Pathol* 66:297, 1988.

Khocht A, Schneider LC: Periodontal management of gingival overgrowth in the heart transplant patient: a case report, *J Periodontol* 68:1140, 1997.

McDonough RJ, Nelson CL: Clinical implications of factor XII deficiency, *Oral Surg Oral Med Oral Pathol* 68:264, 1989.

Miranda J et al: Prevalence and risk of gingival enlargement in patients treated with nifedipine, *J Periodontol* 72:605, 2001.

Moore PA et al: Type 1 diabetes mellitus and oral health: assessment of periodontal disease, *J Periodontol* 70:409, 1999.

Moore PA et al: Type 1 diabetes mellitus and oral health: assessment of coronal and root caries, *Community Dent Oral Epidemiol* 29:183, 2001.

Moore PA et al: Type 1 diabetes mellitus, xerostomia and salivary flow rates, *Oral Surg Oral Med Oral Pathol Oral Radiol Endod* 92:281, 2001.

Ohishi M et al: Acute gingival necrosis caused by drug-induced agranulocytosis, *Oral Surg Oral Med Oral Pathol* 66:194, 1988.

Park JB, Park N-H: Effect of chlorhexidine on the in vitro and in vivo herpes simplex virus infection, *Oral Surg Oral Med Oral Pathol* 67:149, 1989.

Redding SW, Luce EB, Boren MW: Oral herpes simplex virus infection in patients receiving head and neck radiation, *Oral Surg Oral Med Oral Pathol* 69:578, 1990.

Sreebny LM, Valdini A, Yu A: Xerostomia. II. Relationship to nonoral symptoms, drugs and diseases, *Oral Surg Oral Med Oral Pathol* 68:419, 1989.

Vernillo AT: Diabetes mellitus. Relevance to dental treatment, *Oral Surg Oral Med Oral Pathol Oral Radiol Endod* 91:263, 2001.

Wahlin YB: Effects of chlorhexidine mouth rinse on oral health in patients with acute leukemia, *Oral Surg Oral Med Oral Pathol* 68:279, 1989.

Wu J, Fantasia JE, Kaplan R: Oral manifestations of acute myelomonocytic leukemia: a case report and review of the classification of leukemias, *J Periodontol* 73:664, 2002.

Review Questions

1. Hyperpituitarism results from an excessive production of growth hormone. Which of the following most often causes it?
   A. Pituitary adenoma
   B. Pituitary sarcoma
   C. Carcinoma in situ
   D. Ameloblastoma
   E. Pleomorphic adenoma

2. Hyperthyroidism in children can lead to:
   A. Partial anodontia
   B. Amelogenesis imperfecta
   C. Ankylosis
   D. Early exfoliation of the deciduous dentition and early eruption of the permanent teeth
   E. Hypercementosis

3. Hypercalcemia, hypophosphatemia, and abnormal bone metabolism are characteristic of which of the following conditions?
   A. Hyperthyroidism
   B. Hypothyroidism
   C. Hyperparathyroidism
   D. Hyperpituitarism
   E. Cherubism

4. All of the following are chronic complications of diabetes mellitus *except*:
   A. Eye damage
   B. Nerve damage
   C. Atherosclerosis
   D. Kidney failure
   E. Ketoacidosis

5. Polydipsia, polyuria, and polyphagia are all characteristic of which of the following?
   A. Fibrous dysplasia
   B. Hyperthyroidism
   C. Type 1 diabetes mellitus
   D. Type 2 diabetes mellitus
   E. Hypothyroidism

6. Which of the following is *not* a feature of type 2 diabetes mellitus?
   A. Those with it have increased insulin resistance.
   B. It occurs at 40 years of age or older.
   C. Autoimmunity is the key to its development.
   D. Glucose control can be achieved without daily insulin injections in many cases.
   E. Onset is usually gradual.

7. Which of the following oral complications is *not* associated with diabetes mellitus?
   A. Candidiasis
   B. Xerostomia
   C. Excessive periodontal bone loss
   D. Mucormycosis
   E. Purpura

8. Which one of the following is *false* concerning Addison disease?
   A. It is also known as primary adrenal cortical insufficiency.
   B. It is characterized by an insufficient production of adrenal steroids.
   C. It may be caused by malignant tumor that destroys the adrenal gland.
   D. It is a disease in which the pituitary gland increases production of ACTH.
   E. It is a condition in which the pituitary adenoma destroys the adrenal gland.

9. Which of the following statements is *false* regarding diabetes mellitus?
   A. Candidiasis may be indicative of compromised immunity in a diabetic patient.
   B. Insulin pump therapy may lead to more predictable control of blood sugar.
   C. Hypoglycemic agents are more commonly used in the treatment of type 2 diabetes than in type 1 diabetes.
   D. Diabetes mellitus is not appropriately considered a syndrome.
   E. Autoimmunity appears to play a role in the cause of type 1 diabetes.

10. Which of the following statements is *false*?
    A. Primary immunodeficiencies are less common than are secondary immunodeficiencies.
    B. Persons with T-lymphocyte deficiencies are susceptible to viral and fungal infections.
    C. All primary immunodeficiencies are combined B-lymphocyte and T-lymphocyte deficiencies.
    D. Secondary immunodeficiency can result from corticosteroid medication.
    E. HIV infection is an example of a secondary immunodeficiency.

11. Iron-deficiency anemia can be caused by:
    A. Chronic blood loss
    B. A deficiency of iron intake
    C. An increased requirement for iron
    D. All of the above
    E. Both A and B

12. Thalassemia major is:
    A. Caused by a nutritional deficiency
    B. The same as celiac sprue
    C. An inherited disease
    D. Associated with a severe hemolytic anemia
    E. Both C and D

13. Achlorhydria, failure to absorb vitamin B_{12}, and megaloblastic anemia are characteristic features of which of the following?
    A. Pernicious anemia
    B. Thalassemia
    C. Sickle cell anemia
    D. Thrombocytopenic purpura
    E. Celiac sprue

14. Which of the following are characteristic of sickle cell anemia?
    A. It is an inherited blood disorder found predominantly in blacks.
    B. It occurs as a result of an abnormal type of hemoglobin and decreased oxygen in the red blood cells.
    C. The individual with sickle cell anemia can experience weakness, fatigue, and joint pain.
    D. Red blood cells are crescent shaped.
    E. All of the above are correct.

15. Which of the following is characterized by a decrease in platelets?
    A. Celiac sprue
    B. Thrombocytopenia
    C. Thalassemia
    D. Plummer-Vinson syndrome
    E. Polycythemia

16. Secondary aplastic anemia can be caused by:
    A. Chemotherapy
    B. Dental radiographs
    C. A genetic disorder
    D. An autoimmune factor
    E. An unknown factor

17. Which of the following is characterized by an abnormal increase in the circulating red blood cells?
    A. Leukopenia
    B. Polydipsia
    C. Thrombocytopenia
    D. Polycythemia
    E. Leukemia

18. Leukopenia most often involves which cell type?
    A. Eosinophils
    B. Neutrophils
    C. Basophils
    D. Erythrocytes
    E. Mast cells

19. If a patient's white blood cell count is 1000/mm^3, the patient has:
    A. Leukopenia
    B. Thrombocytopenia
    C. Hemophilia
    D. Cyclic neutropenia
    E. Anemia

20. Excessive numbers of abnormal white blood cells are characteristic of:
    A. Agranulocytosis
    B. Leukopenia
    C. Cyclic neutropenia
    D. Leukemia
    E. Polycythemia

21. Normal bleeding time is usually between:
    A. 1 and 6 minutes
    B. 2 and 3 minutes
    C. 15 and 45 seconds
    D. 10 and 15 minutes
    E. 15 and 30 minutes

22. The normal PT is:
    A. 2 to 5 minutes
    B. 11 to 16 seconds
    C. 10 to 15 minutes
    D. 1 to 6 seconds
    E. 45 seconds to 1 minute

23. The INR is:
    A. An expression of the ratio of PT to thromboplastin activity
    B. More accurate than the PT because it is standardized from laboratory to laboratory
    C. Within normal range when the value is less than 3.0
    D. Used to determine the patient's ability to form a clot
    E. All of the above

24. Symptoms of leukemia can be similar to those found in:
    A. Hepatitis
    B. Amelogenesis imperfecta
    C. Nonthrombocytopenic purpura
    D. Mononucleosis
    E. Pernicious anemia

25. Which of the following is not characteristic of primary hyperparathyroidism?
    A. Osteoclastic resorption
    B. Excessive production of parathyroid hormone
    C. Cotton-wool radiographic appearance
    D. Increased serum calcium
    E. Giant cell lesions in bone

Chapter 9 Synopsis

Condition/ Disease	Cause	Age/Race/Sex	Location
Hyperpituitarism	Excess growth hormone produced by the pituitary gland	Children: gigantism	Generalized bone involvement
	Most commonly caused by a pituitary adenoma	Adults (most common fourth decade): acromegaly	Affects only certain bones
Hyperthyroidism (Graves Disease)	Excessive production of thyroid hormone	Children and adults	Systemic disease
Hypothyroidism	Decreased production of thyroid hormone	Children: cretinism	Systemic disease
Hyperpara-thyroidism	Excessive secretion of parathyroid hormone	Usually adults	Systemic disease
	Primary: may be caused by hyperplasia or tumor of parathyroid glands		
	Secondary causes include renal disease and vitamin D deficiency		

*Not covered in text.

Clinical Features	Radiographic Features	Microscopic Features	Treatment	Diagnostic Process
Excessive growth of the skeleton overall	*	N/A	May involve pituitary gland surgery	Laboratory
Enlargement of the hands and feet, increase in rib size Enlargement of the mandible, maxilla, and maxillary sinus Separation of teeth with malocclusion Frontal bossing and enlargement of the nasal bones	*	N/A		
Rosy complexion, erythema of the palms, excessive sweating, fine hair and softened nails, exophthalmus Anxiety, weakness, restlessness, cardiac problems Children: premature exfoliation of deciduous and premature eruption of permanent teeth Adults: osteoporosis Dental caries and periodontal disease appear to progress rapidly	*	*	Suppression of thyroid activity May involve surgery, medication, radioactive iodine	Laboratory
Children: thickened lips, enlarged tongue, delayed eruption of teeth Adults: enlarged tongue	Delayed eruption pattern may be observed	*	*	*
Joint pain or stiffness, lethargy Loosening of teeth	Well-circumscribed bone lesions, changes in trabeculation, partial loss of lamina dura	Bone lesions—indistinguishable from central giant cell lesion	Dependent on cause	Laboratory

Continued

Chapter 9 Synopsis—cont'd

Condition/ Disease	Cause	Age/Race/Sex	Location
Diabetes Mellitus	Abnormally high blood glucose levels resulting from the lack of the hormone insulin	Type I (IDDM) peak age of onset, 20 yrs Type 2 (NIDDM) 40 years or older	Systemic disease
Addison Disease	Insufficient production of adrenal steroids caused by: Autoimmune disease Malignant tumor of adrenal gland Tuberculosis Cause may be undetermined	*	Systemic disease
Iron Deficiency Anemia	Nutritional deficiency of iron intake Chronic blood loss Poor iron absorption Increased requirement of iron	May occur at any age	Systemic disease

*Not covered in text.

Clinical Features	Radiographic Features	Microscopic Features	Treatment	Diagnostic Process
Accelerated atherosclerosis resulting in impaired circulation of blood. Increased risk of ulceration, gangrene of the feet, high blood pressure, kidney failure, and stroke Eye damage and blindness Neurologic complaints Decreased resistance to infection including oral candidiasis Slow wound healing Bilateral salivary gland enlargement Xerostomia (usually with uncontrolled diabetes) Accentuated response to dental plaque	Increased severity of periodontal bone loss	N/A	Control of blood glucose with insulin injections, oral hypoglycemic agents, and diet	Laboratory
Brown pigmentation of the skin and oral melanotic macules	N/A	*	Steroid replacement therapy	*
Often asymptomatic Weakness, fatigue, skin pallor. Oral: angular cheilitis pallor, erythematous and depapillated tongue Plummer-Vinson syndrome: long-term iron deficiency, dysphagia, atrophy of upper alimentary tract, increased risk of oral and esophageal cancer	N/A	Microcytic and hypochromic red blood cells	Increase in dietary iron intake	Laboratory

Continued

Chapter 9 Synopsis—cont'd

Condition/Disease	Cause	Age/Race/Sex	Location
Pernicious Anemia	Deficiency of intrinsic factor (produced by parietal cells of the stomach) Autoimmune mechanism most likely	Usually adults	Systemic disease
Folic Acid and Vitamin B$_{12}$ Deficiencies	Malnutrition Increased metabolic requirements		Systemic disease

Thalassemia
Thalassemia Major (Homozygous)
Thalassemia Minor (Heterozygous)
	Inherited disorder (autosomal dominant)	Begins in early childhood	Systemic disease
			  Thalassemia major—severe symptoms
			  Thalassemia minor—asymptomatic or mildly symptomatic

Sickle Cell Anemia Sickle Cell Trait (Heterozygous)	Inherited disorder (autosomal dominant pattern) Abnormal hemoglobin in red blood cells	Before age 30 Most in black individuals and those of Mediterranean origin Women > Men	Systemic disease
Celiac Sprue	Sensitivity to dietary gluten resulting in injury to the intestinal mucosa and subsequent anemia	N/A	Systemic disease

*Not covered in text.

Clinical Features	Radiographic Features	Microscopic Features	Treatment	Diagnostic Process
Weakness, fatigue, skin pallor, nausea, dizziness, diarrhea, abdominal pain, loss of appetite, weight loss Oral: angular cheilitis, pallor, painful, erythematous and depapillated tongue, mucosal ulceration	N/A	Abnormally large red blood cells (megaloblastic anemia)	Vitamin B_{12} by injection	Laboratory
Weakness, fatigue, skin pallor, nausea dizziness, diarrhea, abdominal pain, loss of appetite, weight loss Oral: angular cheilitis, pallor, painful, erythematous and depapillated tongue, oral ulcers	N/A	Abnormally large red blood cells (megaloblastic)	Dietary supplements	Laboratory
Yellowish skin pallor, fever, malaise, weakness, enlarged liver and spleen Facies: prominent cheekbones, depression of the bridge of the nose, prominent premaxilla, protrusion or flaring of the maxillary anterior teeth	Atypical trabecular pattern ("salt and pepper effect") Thinning of the lamina dura Circular radiolucencies in the alveolar bone also described	*	Experimental	Clinical Laboratory
Weakness, shortness of breath, fatigue, joint pain, nausea	Loss of trabeculation with large, irregular marrow spaces	Sickle-shaped red blood cells on blood smear	Symptomatic and supportive Oxygen, intravenous and oral fluids	Laboratory
Same clinical features as anemias	N/A	*	Adherence to a gluten-free diet	*

Continued

Chapter 9   Synopsis—cont'd

Condition/ Disease	Cause	Age/Race/Sex	Location
Aplastic Anemia	Decrease in all circulating blood cells because of a severe depression of bone marrow activity Primary—cause unknown Secondary—because of drug or chemical agent	Primary—young adults Secondary—any age	Systemic disease
Polycythemia	Abnormal increase in circulating red blood cells	Usually adults	Systemic disease
Polycythemia Vera (Primary polycythemia)	Neoplastic		
Secondary Polycythemia	Physiologic response to decreased oxygen		
Relative Polycythemia	Decreased plasma volume, not an increase in red blood cells		
Agranulocytosis	Marked reduction in circulating neutrophils (neutropenia) Primary—may be immunologic Secondary—drugs and other chemicals	N/A	Systemic disease
Cyclic Neutropenia	See Chapter 6		
Leukemia	Neoplastic Oncogenic viruses suggested	Children (acute lymphoblastic) Adolescents and young adults (acute myoblastic)	Systemic disease

*Not covered in text.

Clinical Features	Radiographic Features	Microscopic Features	Treatment	Diagnostic Process
Infection, spontaneous bleeding, petechiae and purpuric spots	N/A	N/A	Primary— experimental, poor prognosis Secondary—removal of cause	Laboratory
Oral mucosa may appear deep red to purple Gingiva may be edematous and bleed easily	N/A	N/A	*	*
Petechiae, ecchymosis and hematoma formation can be present	N/A	N/A	*	*
Sudden onset of high fever, chills, jaundice, weakness, and sore throat Oral infection with rapid periodontal destruction Gingival bleeding	N/A	N/A	Transfusions Antibiotics to control infection Removal of causative agent if identified	Laboratory
Weakness, fever, lymph node enlargement, bleeding, enlarged liver, and spleen Gingival enlargement because of infiltration of leukemic cells, oral infections, spontaneous gingival bleeding, petechia, and eccymoses	N/A	Enlarged gingiva— infiltration of tissue by leukemic cells	Chemotherapy Bone marrow transplantation	Laboratory

Continued

Chapter 9 Synopsis—cont'd

Condition/ Disease	Cause	Age/Race/Sex	Location
Leukemia—cont'd		Adults (chronic leukemias)	Systemic disease
Thrombocytopenic Purpura	Severe reduction in circulating platelets		Systemic disease
Idiopathic Type (Primary Type)	Cause unknown	Primary and immune types	
Immune Type	Autoimmune disease	Usually children and young adults	
Secondary Type	Drugs—often chemotherapeutic agents	No age predilection for secondary type	
Hemophelia A and B	Inherited (X-linked)	Identified in childhood Affects boys	Systemic disease

Clinical Features	Radiographic Features	Microscopic Features	Treatment	Diagnostic Process
Slow onset of symptoms Easy fatigability, weakness, weight loss, anorexia Pallor of the lips and gingiva, gingival enlargement, petechiae, ecchymosis, gingival bleeding, and atypical periodontal disease	N/A	Enlarged gingiva—infiltration of tissue by leukemic cells	Chemotherapy Bone marrow transplantation	Laboratory
Spontaneous hemorrhagic lesions of the skin and/or mucosa Gingival bleeding Frequent nose bleeds Blood in urine (hematuria)	N/A	N/A	Systemic corticosteroids, splenectomy Discontinuation of causative agent	Laboratory
Spontaneous bleeding, petechiae, ecchymoses Risk of hemorrhage after oral surgery and dental hygiene procedures	N/A	N/A	Replacement of missing clotting factor	Laboratory

Chapter 10

Diseases Affecting the Temporomandibular Joint

Kenneth E. Fleisher
Anthony J. Casino

Objectives

After studying this chapter, the student will be able to:

1. Label the following on a diagram of the temporomandibular joint: glenoid fossa of the temporal bone, articular disk, mandibular condyle, joint capsule, and superior belly of the lateral pterygoid muscle.

2. State the function of the muscles of mastication.

3. State three factors that have been implicated in the cause of temporomandibular disorders (TMDs), and three questions that would be appropriate to ask of a patient suspected of having a TMD.

4. List at least two symptoms that are suggestive of temporomandibular dysfunction.

5. State the function of radiographs in the evaluation of a patient with symptoms suggestive of temporomandibular dysfunction.

6. List five types of TMDs.

7. List and describe the two main categories of treatment of TMDs.

8. State the names of one benign and one malignant tumor that may affect the temporomandibular joint area.

Vocabulary

Arthrocentesis (ahr″thro-sen-te′sis) Surgical puncture of a joint usually for the withdrawal of fluid.

Arthrography (ahr-throg′rah-fē) Radiography of a joint after injection of opaque contrast material.

Arthroscopy (ahr-thros′cah-pē) Method for evaluating and manipulating a joint via the insertion of a camera and instruments.

Articulation (ar-tik-ū-lā′shin) Joint.

Auscultation (aws-kul-tā′shin) Listening to sounds within the body using a stethoscope.

Crepitus (krep′i-tus) Dry, crackling sound.

Iatrogenic (i-at″ro-jen′ik) Induced inadvertently by a medical or dental care provider or by medical treatment or a diagnostic procedure.

Magnetic resonance imaging (MRI) Noninvasive diagnostic technique that uses radio waves to produce computerized images of internal body tissues.

Palpation (pal-pa′shĕn) Physical examination using pressure of the hand or fingers.

Sign (sīn) Objective evidence of disease that can be observed by a health care provider rather than by the patient.

Symptom (simp′tĕm) Subjective evidence of disease or a physical disorder that is observed by the patient.

Trismus (triz′mĕs) Spasm of the muscles of mastication.

Knowledge of the anatomy and function of the temporomandibular joint enables the dental hygienist to understand the diseases that affect the joint. Disorders of the temporomandibular joint include myofascial pain and dysfunction (MPD), internal derangements syndrome, osteoarthritis, and rheumatoid arthritis. Benign and malignant tumors can also affect the temporomandibular joint.

Anatomy of the Temporomandibular Joint

The temporomandibular joint is the **articulation** between the condyle of the mandible and the glenoid fossa of the temporal bone **(Figure 10-1)**. It is a highly specialized joint that differs from other joints because of the fibrocartilage that covers the bony articulating surfaces, its **ginglymoarthrodial** (rotational and translational) movement, its function and overall health being dictated by jaw movement, and its dependence on the contralateral joint. An **articular disk** is interposed in the space between the temporal bone and the mandible. This disk divides the space into an upper (superior joint space) and a lower compartment (inferior joint space) (see Figure 10-1).

Translational movements occur in the upper compartment, whereas the lower compartment functions primarily as the hinge or rotational component. The superior and inferior spaces contain **synovial fluid,** which is produced by the **synovial membrane** that lines the joint. The synovial fluid provides nourishment and lubrication of the avascular structures.

The articular disk is attached to the lateral and medial aspects of the condyle, to the superior belly of the lateral pterygoid muscle, and to the joint capsule (see Figure 10-1). The disk and the bony surfaces are avascular (they do not contain blood vessels). The joint is further surrounded and protected by the fibrous connective tissue joint capsule.

Understanding the location and action of the **muscles of mastication** is important in the evaluation of disorders affecting the temporomandibular joint. **Palpation** of these muscles during a clinical evaluation is used to determine whether muscle spasm or dysfunctional muscle activity is occurring. The muscles of mastication comprise major muscles about the facial region that govern the movement of

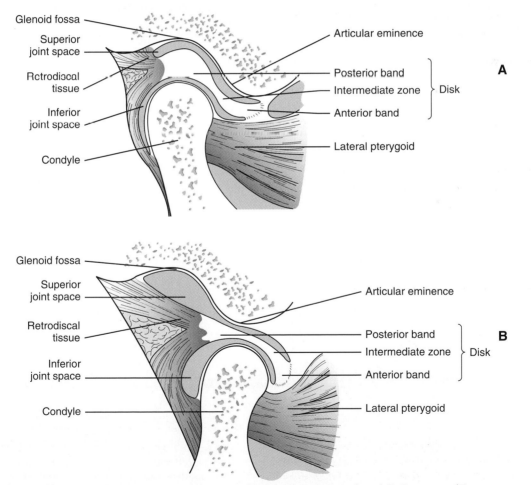

Figure 10-1 Lateral views of the temporomandibular joint. **A,** Jaw closed. **B,** Jaw open. (From Kaplan AS, Assael LA: *Temporomandibular disorders,* Philadelphia, 1991, WB Saunders.)

the mandible. These muscles include the masseter, temporalis, medial pterygoid, lateral pterygoid, anterior digastric, and mylohyoid (suprahyoids) **(Figures 10-2, 10-3, and 10-4).** The function of these muscles is to create the mandibular envelope of motion. Three of these muscles, the masseter, medial pterygoid, and temporalis, are elevator muscles that, when activated, close the mandible. The opening, or depressor, function is accomplished mainly by the lateral pterygoid muscle with some help from the anterior digastric muscle. Studies have shown that the two components of the lateral pterygoid muscle are active at different times in the functioning of the mandible (see Figure 10-4). The superior portion of the muscle seats the articular disk on the eminence of the articulating surface. The inferior belly is attached to the mandibular condyle and functions during mouth opening.

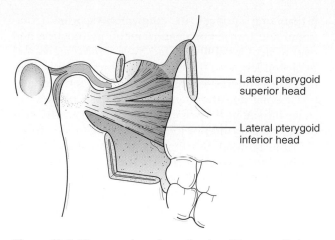

Figure 10-3 The muscles of mastication. The two distinct heads of the lateral pterygoid muscle are illustrated. (From Kaplan AS, Assael LA: *Temporomandibular disorders,* Philadelphia, 1991, WB Saunders.)

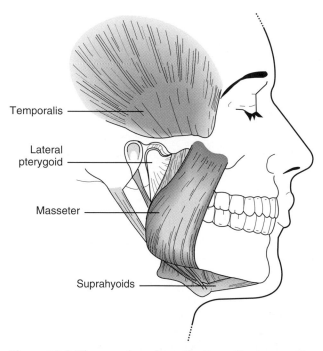

Figure 10-2 The muscles of mastication: the temporalis, lateral pterygoid, masseter, and suprahyoid muscles. (From Kaplan, AS, Assael LA: *Temporomandibular disorders,* Philadelphia, 1991, WB Saunders.)

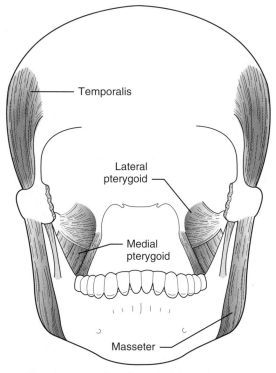

Figure 10-4 The muscles of mastication. Illustrated are the four paired muscles of mastication: the masseter, temporalis, medial pterygoid, and lateral pterygoid muscles. (From Kaplan AS, Assael LA: *Temporomandibular disorders,* Philadelphia, 1991, WB Saunders.)

Normal Joint Function

The harmonious function of the temporomandibular joint depends on various factors. The anatomic relationship of the condyle-disk complex governs the smooth functioning of the mandible. This articulation, along with the muscles of mastication, provides the movement of the mandible. Whereas the muscles of mastication are the machinery that powers mandibular movement, the anatomic joint structures, such as the condyle, articular eminence, and disk, act as the gears or bearings of the jaw.

In **normal joint function** the jaw begins at a rest position of maximum occlusal contact. In this position the mandibular condyle rests within the glenoid fossa, with the articular disk situated between the condyle, roof of the glenoid fossa, and articular eminence (see Figure 10-1, *A* and *B*). The first phase of opening is characterized by rotational (hinge) movement of the condyle followed by anterior translation (sliding movement) to approximately the anterior peak of the articular eminence. During translation the disk assumes a more posterior position in relation to the condyle. The inferior and superior joint spaces assume different configurations during each of these movements.

Temporomandibular Disorders

Temporomandibular disorders (TMDs) are caused by abnormalities in the functioning of the temporomandibular joint or associated structures and these have been a clinical and diagnostic challenge in dentistry for many years. Hippocrates documented jaw dysfunction problems as early as the fifth century BC. However, it was not until 1934 that a syndrome of temporomandibular joint diseases was described. Dentists and oral and maxillofacial surgeons began to study the TMJ and related structures in an attempt to accurately describe the pathophysiology of disorders of this joint and establish the most effective treatment. Most studies suggest that clinically significant TMD-related jaw pain, dysfunction, or both affects about 5% of the general population. Significantly more frequent and more severe TMD signs and symptoms are seen in women and older adults.

PATHOPHYSIOLOGY OF TEMPORO-MANDIBULAR JOINT DISORDERS

The cause of TMDs remains controversial, and many factors have been implicated. Trauma has been suggested as the most likely cause. Trauma affecting the temporomandibular joint is classified as *direct* (assault), *indirect* (whiplash injury), or secondary to *parafunctional habits* (clenching, bruxism). Other contributing factors include dentofacial deformities and psychosocial factors. Numerous studies continue to dispute the significance of occlusal relationships. TMJ abnormalities are also associated with a number of different systemic diseases. Rheumatoid arthritis and osteoarthritis are the most common and are described later in this chapter. Temporomandibular joint disorders may also be the result of disorders in growth and development as seen in condylar hyperplasia or hypoplasia. Iatrogenic causes (resulting from the action of a health care provider) of TMDs include the indiscriminate use of corticosteroid injection into the joint.

PATIENT EVALUATION

Temporomandibular dysfunction can be caused by disorders of the muscles of mastication or internal derangements of the components of the joint. Evaluation involves a comprehensive history and a thorough clinical examination. An understanding of the procedures used in the evaluation of temporomandibular joint disorders is important to the dental hygienist. The dental hygienist does not generally perform a comprehensive examination of the temporomandibular joint area but may participate in diagnostic procedures related to the joint.

History

A history of aberrant growth, previous injuries, illnesses, musculoskeletal complaints, and possible emotional disturbances are important considerations in the evaluation of patients with TMDs. The patient history specific to TMDs includes questions regarding the following:

- Joint symptoms (clicking, popping)
- Pain
- Problems with mastication

- Trismus
- Malocclusion
- Parafunctional habits (bruxing, clenching)
- Dental symptoms
- Extensive dental or orthodontic treatment
- History of surgical treatment of the jaws
- Progression of symptoms (sudden, gradual)
- Precipitating events (mastication, spontaneous, yawning)

Examination

A comprehensive examination of a patient related to temporomandibular joint disorders includes an examination of the joint, muscles of mastication, oral cavity, and cervical spine. Joint examination involves **auscultation** (using a stethoscope) and palpation. The clinician relates joint noises such as clicking, crepitus (crackling), or popping to the mandibular movement cycle. The muscles of mastication are palpated to determine tenderness. In addition to a thorough oral examination, the patient is asked to move the mandible in a normal rotation (hinge) and translatory (forward slide) cycle. Interincisal opening is measured along with any obvious deviation of motion to the right or left side. The patient's ability to manipulate the mandible into right and left lateral excursions is noted. The patient is asked to protrude the mandible in order to determine whether any deviations or disk interferences exist within the joint. Finally, the patient's occlusion is evaluated to determine gross abnormalities and whether the occlusal abnormalities are related to the patient's temporomandibular problem.

Imaging

Radiographic studies may be helpful in determining the cause of the patient's pain or dysfunction. Several different types of radiographs and views are obtained to determine the shape of the condyle and whether evidence of degenerative joint disease exists **(Figures 10-5** and **10-6).** Radiographic evaluation of patients with TMDs typically includes panoramic or transcranial imaging. These radiographs are limited to identifying gross changes in bone. Several specialized diagnostic studies that are useful in the diagnosis of TMDs have become available over the past several years. Tomography may provide greater accuracy in assessing condylar position and range of mobility.

Computerized tomography (CT) is the most accurate for identifying bone abnormalities, and MRI is mandatory for examining disk position, function, form, and the presence of joint effusions (inflammatory changes) **(Figure 10-7).** Arthrography may be useful when MRI is not tolerated and information regarding the position and morphology of the disk is required.

TYPES OF TEMPOROMANDIBULAR DISORDERS

Myofascial Pain and Dysfunction

MPD comprises at least 50% of all TMDs. It is characterized as a dysfunctional muscle hyperactivity with regional pain, tenderness of the affected muscles, and variable amounts of reduced opening and complaints of malocclusion.

Figure 10-5 Panoramic radiograph of a patient with temporomandibular dysfunction and normal anatomy of the mandibular condyles.

Internal Derangements

Internal derangements are divided into disk (meniscal) displacements, ankylosis, and hypermobility disorders.

Disk displacement

Disk displacements are problems in which the disk (meniscus) is displaced. In some cases the disk is displaced anteriorly and returns to normal position upon opening the mouth or movement away from the affected side (disk displacement with reduction). In another form of disk displacement, the displaced disk acts as an obstacle to the sliding condyle. In this type of displacement, patients complain of problems such as intermittent locking of the jaw; a sudden onset of limited mouth opening, usually associated with cessation of joint sounds; deflection of the mandible, with a midline correction upon opening; and restricted lateral excursive movements away from the affected side (disk displacement without reduction).

Ankylosis

Ankylosis of the TMJ is defined as immobility of the condyle because of fibrous or bony union between the articulating structures of the joint. Ankylosis can be classified by tissue type (fibrous, bony), location (intraarticular, extraarticular) and extent of fusion

Figure 10-6 Panoramic radiograph shows resorption of both the right and the left condyles. In this patient, degenerative arthritis followed bilateral surgery of the temporomandibular joint. The left coronoid process was removed during surgery.

Figure 10-7 A, Magnetic resonance imaging (MRI) scan of the right temporomandibular joint shows the normal position of the disk. Arrows point to the disk. **B,** MRI scan of the left temporomandibular joint in the same patient shows displacement of the disk. *C,* Condyle.

(complete, incomplete). Joint infection, usually after trauma, accounts for 50% of all TMJ ankylosis cases, but 30% result from trauma without infection. Fibrotic intraarticular ankylosis is the most common type seen in the TMJ. Trauma-induced hemorrhage (hemarthrosis) is a common cause of this type of ankylosis. Children are more prone to ankylosis because of greater osteogenic potential and less development of the joint meniscus.

Hypermobility disorders

Hypermobility disorders include **dislocation** and **subluxation**. Dislocation occurs when one or both of the condyles translates anterior to the articular eminence, resulting in an open lock that the patient cannot reduce. Subluxation refers to hypermobility in which the patient is able to relocate the mandible back into the glenoid fossa.

Arthritis

Arthritis is defined as inflammation of a joint and is classified as either **osteoarthritis** or **rheumatoid arthritis**. Osteoarthritis, also referred to as degenerative joint disease, is the most common disease affecting the TMJ. It is characterized by degenerative changes of the articular cartilage with associated remodeling. Patients may have pain symptoms that are worse in the evening, as well as limited opening, muscle splinting, and crepitus of the TMJ. Rheumatoid arthritis is an inflammatory, immunologic disorder of the joints. Approximately 50% to 75% of patients with rheumatoid arthritis have involvement of the TMJ during the course of the disease. In rheumatoid arthritis, patients may complain of pain that is worse in the morning, limited opening, occlusal changes, and preauricular edema and tenderness.

TREATMENT OF TEMPORO-MANDIBULAR JOINT DISORDERS

Nonsurgical Treatment

Treatment goals for TMDs involve improving function (range of motion) and reducing pain. Treatment typically begins with nonsurgical modalities. The first phase of nonsurgical treatment includes pharmacologic therapy, moist heat, physical therapy, soft mechanical diet, jaw stretching, and coordination exercises. This type of treatment is indicated for internal derangements, MPD, and the arthritides. Medications are used to control pain and inflammation. Muscle relaxants and antianxiety agents can be used to reduce muscle hypertonicity. Certain patients may also benefit from occlusal adjustment or orthodontic therapy to correct uneven tooth contacts or malocclusions respectively.

If a patient fails to improve or worsens after approximately 1 to 2 months of conservative nonsurgical management, the second phase may be initiated. The second phase involves the use of occlusal appliances. Depending on the type used, these function by relaxing muscles, protecting the dentition, stabilizing and protecting the joint, providing biofeedback by making patients aware of bruxing habits, or by relieving the load on the disk to allow repair of damaged retrodiscal tissues. Recently, botulism toxin (Botox®) has been used to treat severe bruxism by providing muscle relaxation and thereby reducing inflammation of the masseter muscle and TMJ capsule.

Surgical Treatment

Patients with TMDs other than MPD may be considered for surgical treatment if they do not respond to nonsurgical therapy and continue to suffer from pain and functional impairment because of interferences in TMJ function. Various surgical techniques are used to treat TMDs. **Arthrocentesis** involves lavaging the joint through a needle. **Arthroscopy** allows direct visualization and manipulation of the

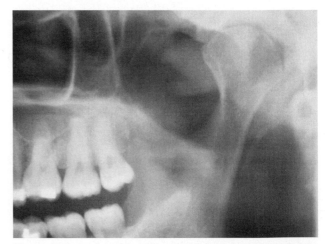

Figure 10-8 Panoramic radiograph of an osteochondroma of the mandibular condyle. (Courtesy Dr. David L. Hirsch.)

joint. Condylotomy involves surgical repositioning of the condyle. **Open joint surgery** is used to perform disk repositioning, replacement or excision, and total joint reconstruction using a prosthetic device or autogenous graft.

Multidisciplinary Management

Additional considerations for patients with oral, facial, and head and neck pain may necessitate referral to other specialists, such as a neurologist or otolaryngologist.

Tumors of the Temporomandibular Joint

Tumors arising in the temporomandibular joint are rare. The most common benign tumors that arise in the condyle include the osteochondroma **(Figure 10-8)**, osteoblastoma, chondroblastoma, and osteoma. Synovial chondromatosis is the most common benign neoplasm of the synovium and is characterized by the development of metaplastic, highly cellular cartilaginous foci in the synovial membrane that results in degenerative changes consistent with osteoarthritis. It is characterized by swelling, pain, and limitation of movement. Radiographic findings are variable and may include loose radiopaque bodies in the TMJ, degenerative changes of the articular surfaces, and variable widening or loss of joint space. Osteosarcoma (see Chapter 7) is one of the most frequently occurring malignant bone tumors. Approximately 6% to 8% of all osteosarcomas occur in the jaws. Osteosarcoma of the temporomandibular joint has been reported.

Selected References

Books

Kaplan AS, Assael LA: *Temporomandibular disorders,* Philadelphia, 1991, WB Saunders.

Lynch MA, Brightman VJ, Greenberg MS: *Burket's oral medicine,* ed 9, Philadelphia, 1997, JB Lippincott.

Neville BW et al: *Oral and maxillofacial pathology,* ed 2, Philadelphia, 2002, WB Saunders.

Regezi JA, Sciubba JJ: *Oral pathology: clinical-pathologic correlations,* ed 4, Philadelphia, 2003, WB Saunders.

Journal Articles

Akerman S et al: Relationship between clinical and radiologic findings of the temporomandibular joint in rheumatoid arthritis, *Oral Surg Oral Med Oral Pathol* 66:639, 1988.

Carlsson GE: Epidemiology and treatment need for temporomandibular disorders, *J Orofac Pain* 13:232, 1999.

Clark GT, Kim YJ: A logical approach to the treatment of temporomandibular disorders, *Oral Maxillofac Surg Clin North Am* 7:149, 1995.

De Bont LGM, Kijkgraaf LC, Stegenga B: Epidemiology and natural progression of articular temporomandibular disorders, *Oral Surg Oral Med Oral Path Oral Radiol Endod* 83:72, 1997.

Dworkin SF et al: Epidemiology of signs and symptoms in temporomandibular disorders: clinical signs in cases and controls, *J Am Dent Assoc* 120:273, 1990.

Epstein JB, Caldwell J, Black G: The utility of panoramic imaging of the temporomandibular joint in patients with temporomandibular disorders, *Oral Surg Oral Med Oral Pathol Oral Radiol Endod* 92:236, 2001.

Kuttila M et al: TMD treatment need in relation to age, gender, stress, and diagnostic subgroup, *J Orofac Pain* 12:67, 1998.

McNeill C et al: Temporomandibular disorders: diagnosis, management, education, and research, *J Am Dent Assoc* 120:253, 1990.

Parker MW, Holmes EK, Terezhalmy GT: Personality characteristics of patients with temporomandibular disorders: diagnostic and therapeutic implications, *J Orofac Pain* 7:337, 1993.

Stohler CS: Muscle-related temporomandibular disorders, *J Orofac Pain* 13:273, 1999.

Takehana dos Santos D, Cavalcanti MGP: Osteosarcoma of the temporomandibular joint: report of 2 cases, *Oral Surg Oral Med Oral Pathol Oral Radiol Endod* 94:641, 2002.

Tan E, Janovic J: Treating severe bruxism with botulism toxin, *J Am Dent Assoc* 131:211, 2000.

Trieger N, Hoffman H, Rodriguez E: The effect of arthrocentesis of the temporomandibular joint in patients with rheumatoid arthritis, *J Oral Maxillofac Surg* 57:537, 1999.

Review Questions

1. Disorders of the articulation between the mandible and maxilla are called:
   A. Synovial hyperplasias
   B. Mandibulomaxillary dysfunction
   C. Temporomandibular disorders
   D. Mandibular dysfunction
   E. Craniofacial disorders

2. Using a stethoscope to listen to abnormal noises in the temporomandibular joint is called:
   A. Audiology
   B. Auscultation
   C. Palpation
   D. Arthrography
   E. Crepitus

3. Which of the following is the most important aspect of the management of TMDs?
   A. Palpation of the muscles of mastication
   B. Using a nonsurgical approach
   C. Adjusting the occlusion
   D. Arthroscopy
   E. Establishing an accurate diagnosis

4. Translational movements of the temporomandibular movements are:
   A. Hinge movements
   B. Sliding movements
   C. Rotational movements
   D. Only used for diagnosis
   E. Only used as treatment exercises

5. Which of the following is considered a parafunctional habit?
   A. Palpation
   B. Mastication
   C. Bruxing
   D. Trauma
   E. Biofeedback

6. Which of the following is a symptom of a temporomandibular disorder?
   A. Pain
   B. Malocclusion
   C. A history of surgical treatment of the jaws
   D. Occlusal adjustment
   E. Orthodontic treatment

7. Which of the following comprises at least 50% of all temporomandibular disorders?
   A. Ankylosis
   B. Hypermobility
   C. Myofascial pain and dysfunction
   D. Internal disk derangements
   E. Osteoarthritis

8. Immobility of the temporomandibular joint because of fibrous or bony union between the articulating structures of the joint is called:
   A. Rheumatoid arthritis
   B. Hypermobility
   C. Ankylosis
   D. Disk displacement
   E. Osteoarthritis

9. Which of the following is **not** a form of *surgical* treatment used for temporomandibular joint disorders?
   A. Arthroscopy
   B. Arthrocentesis
   C. Condylotomy
   D. Joint reconstruction
   E. Occlusal appliance

10. Which of the following is the most common benign tumor of the synovium of the temporomandibular joint?
    A. Osteoblastoma
    B. Osteochondroma
    C. Chondroblastoma
    D. Synovial chondromatosis
    E. Osteoma

Glossary

A

Acantholysis Dissolution of the intercellular bridges of the prickle cell layer of the epithelium.

Acute Of short duration or of short and relatively severe course.

Agranulocytosis A marked decrease in the number of granulocytes, particularly neutrophils.

Alleles Genes that are located at the same level or locus in the two chromosomes of a pair and that determine the same functions or characteristics.

Allergy A hypersensitive state acquired through exposure to a particular allergen. Re-exposure to the same allergen elicits an exaggerated reaction.

Amenorrhea Abnormal temporary or permanent cessation of menstrual cycles.

Amino acid An organic compound containing the amino group NH_2. Amino acids are the main component of proteins.

Anaphylaxis A type of hypersensitivity or allergic reaction in which the exaggerated immunologic reaction results from the release of vasoactive substances such as histamine. The reaction occurs on re-exposure to a foreign protein or other substance after sensitization.

Anaplastic Characterized by a loss of differentiation of cells and their orientation to one another; a characteristic of malignant tumor tissue.

Anemia Reduction to less than normal of the number of red blood cells, quantity of hemoglobin, or the volume of packed red blood cells in the blood.

Ankyloglossia Extensive adhesion of the tongue to the floor of the mouth or the lingual aspect of the anterior portion of the mandible, caused by a short lingual frenum.

Ankylosed teeth Teeth that are fused to the alveolar bone; a condition especially common with retained deciduous teeth.

Anodontia Complete or almost complete congenital lack of teeth.

Anomaly Marked deviation from normal, especially as a result of congenital or hereditary defects.

Antibody A protein molecule, also called an immunoglobulin, that is produced by plasma cells and reacts with a specific antigen.

Antigen Any substance that is able to induce a specific immune response.

Aplasia (adjective, aplastic) Lack of development.

Arthralgia Severe pain in a joint.

Arthrocentesis Surgical puncture of a joint usually for the withdrawal of fluid.

Arthrography Radiography of a joint after injection of opaque contrast material.

Arthroscopy A method for evaluating and manipulating a joint by the insertion of a camera and instruments.

Articular disk A pad of fibrocartilage or dense fibrous tissue present in some synovial joints; for example, the temporomandibular joint.

Articulation (noun) A joint.

Atrophy The decrease in size and function of a cell, tissue, organ, or whole body.

Auscultation The act of listening to sounds within the body.

Autoantibody An antibody that reacts against an antigenic constituent of the person's own tissues.

Autoimmune disease A disease characterized by tissue injury caused by a humoral or cell-mediated immune response against constituents of the body's own tissues.

Autoimmunity Immune-mediated destruction of the body's own cells and tissues; immunity against self.

Autosomes (adjective, autosomal) The nonsex chromosomes that are identical for men and women.

B

B lymphocyte A lymphocyte, also called a B cell, that matures without passing through the thymus and later can develop into a plasma cell that produces antibodies.

Barr body Condensed chromatin of the inactivated X chromosome, which is found at the periphery of the nucleus of cells in women.

Benign Not malignant; favorable for recovery.

Benign fibro-osseous lesion A benign lesion of bone characterized histologically by cellular fibrous connective tissue admixed with irregularly shaped bone trabeculae or cementoid material.

365

Brachydactyly Short fingers or toes, or both.

Bulla (adjective, bullous; plural, bullae) A circumscribed, elevated, fluid-filled lesion that is larger than 5 mm in diameter and usually contains serous fluid.

C

Calcitonin A polypeptide secreted by the C cells of the thyroid gland.

Carcinoma A malignant tumor of epithelial tissue.

Carrier In genetics, a heterozygous individual who is clinically normal but who can transmit a recessive trait or characteristic; also, a person who is homozygous for an autosomal dominant condition with low penetrance.

Cell-mediated immunity Immunity in which the predominant role is played by T lymphocytes.

Centimeter (cm) One hundredth of a meter. Equivalent to a little less than ½ inch (0.393 of an inch).

Central In oral pathology, a lesion occurring within the maxilla or mandible.

Centromere The constricted portion of the chromosome that divides the short arms from the long arms.

Chemotaxis The directed movement of white blood cells to the area of injury by chemical mediators.

Chiasmata The intercrossing of chromatids of the same or homologous chromosomes that takes place at metaphase of first meiosis for the purpose of genetic recombination.

Chromatid Either of the two vertical halves of a chromosome that are joined at the centromere.

Chromatin A general term used to refer to the material (DNA) that forms the chromosomes.

Chronic Persisting over a long time.

Coagulation Formation of a clot.

Coalescence The process by which parts of a whole join together, or fuse, to make one.

Codominance The full expression in a heterozygote of both alleles of a pair of chromosomes, with neither influenced by the other. A good example is the AB blood group.

Codon The vertical sequence of three bases in DNA that codes for an amino acid.

Coloboma A cleft generally seen on the iris or the eyelids.

Commissure The site of union of corresponding parts; for example, the corners of the lips.

Concrescence A condition in dentistry in which two adjacent teeth are united by cementum.

Congenital Present at and existing from the time of birth.

Consanguinity Blood relationship. In genetics, the term is generally used to describe matings or marriages among close relatives.

Corrugated Having a surface that appears wrinkled.

Crepitus A dry, crackling sound.

Crossing over The exchange of segments between chromatids of the same or homologous chromosomes that takes place at metaphase of first meiosis. Crossing over is the result of chiasmata.

Cyst An abnormal pathologic sac or cavity that is lined with epithelium and is enclosed in a connective tissue capsule.

D

Deletion In genetics, the loss of part of a chromosome.

Dens in dente "A tooth within a tooth"; a malformed tooth caused by an invagination of the crown before it is calcified.

Dentinogenesis The formation of dentin.

Deoxyribonucleic acid (DNA) A substance composed of a double chain of polynucleotides; both chains coiled around a central axis form a double helix. DNA is the basic genetic code or template for amino acid formation.

Differentiation The distinguishing of one thing from another.

Diffuse In the description of a lesion, the borders of the lesion are not well defined, and it is not possible to detect the exact parameters of the lesion.

Dilaceration An abnormal bend or curve, as in the root of a tooth.

Diploid Having two sets of chromosomes; the normal constitution of somatic cells.

Dominant In genetics, a trait or characteristic that is manifested when it is carried by only one of a pair of homologous chromosomes.

Dysplasia Disordered growth. In epithelial tissue, alteration in size shape and organization of adult cells.

E

Ecchymosis A small, flat, hemorrhagic patch, larger than a petechia, on the skin or mucous membrane.

Emigration The passage of white blood cells through the endothelium and wall of the microcirculation into the injured tissue.

Encapsulated Surrounded by a capsule of fibrous connective tissue.

Erythema Redness of the skin or mucosa.

Expressivity In genetics, the degree of clinical manifestation of a trait or characteristic.

Exudate Inflammatory fluid formed as a reaction to injury of tissues and blood vessels.

F

Facies The appearance of the face.

Fever An elevation of body temperature to greater than the normal of 98.6° F (37° C).

Fibrin An insoluble protein that is essential to the clotting of blood.

Fissure A cleft or groove, normal or otherwise, showing prominent depth.

Fissured Having surface clefting or grooves.

Flare Redness of the skin or mucosa around an area of an irritant.

Fusion The union of two adjoining tooth germs.

G

Gamete Spermatozoon or ovum.

Gemination In dentistry, a single tooth germ splits completely or partially, forming separate crowns. The tooth usually has a single root and root canal; also called twinning.

Genetic heterogeneity Having more than one inheritance pattern.

Granuloma A tumor-like mass of inflammatory tissue consisting of a central collection of macrophages, often with multinucleated giant cells, surrounded by lymphocytes.

Granulomatous disease A disease characterized by the formation of granulomas.

H

Haploid A cell with a single set of chromosomes. A gamete is haploid.

Hematocrit The volume percentage of red blood cells in whole blood.

Hemolysis The release of hemoglobin from red blood cells by destruction of the cells.

Hemostasis The stoppage or cessation of bleeding.

Hepatomegaly Enlargement of the liver.

Heterozygote (adjective, heterozygous) An individual with two different genes at the allele loci.

Homozygote (adjective, homozygous) An individual having identical genes at the allele loci.

Hormone A chemical substance produced in the body that has a specific regulatory effect on certain cells or a certain organ or organs.

Humoral immunity Immunity in which antibodies play the predominant role.

Hypercalcemia An excess of calcium in the blood.

Hyperchromatic Staining more intensely than normal.

Hyperemia An excess of blood in a part of the body.

Hyperglycemia An excess of glucose in the blood.

Hyperplasia An enlargement of a tissue or organ resulting from an increase in the number of normal cells.

Hypersensitivity A state of altered reactivity in which the body reacts to a foreign agent with an exaggerated immune response.

Hypertelorism Abnormally increased distance between two organs or parts. Orbital or ocular hypertelorism abnormally increased distance between the orbits.

Hyperthermia Increased body temperature.

Hypertrophy An enlargement of a tissue or organ caused by an increase in size but not in number of cells.

Hypochromic Stained less intensely than normal.

Hypodontia Partial anodontia. The lack of one or more teeth.

Hypohidrosis Abnormally diminished secretion of sweat.

Hypophosphatemia Deficiency of phosphates in the blood.

Hypotrichosis Presence of less than the normal amount of hair.

I

Iatrogenic Induced inadvertently by a medical/dental care provider or by medical treatment or a diagnostic procedure.

Immune complex A combination of antibody and antigen.

Immunodeficiency A deficiency of the immune response caused by hypoactivity or decreased numbers of lymphoid cells.

Immunoglobulin A protein, also called an antibody, synthesized by plasma cells in response to a specific antigen.

Impacted teeth Teeth that cannot erupt into the oral cavity because of a physical obstruction.

In situ Confined to the site of origin without invasion of neighboring tissues.

Insulin A peptide hormone produced in the pancreas by the beta cells in the islets of Langerhans. Insulin regulates glucose metabolism and is the major fuel-regulating hormone.

Invasion The infiltration and active destruction of surrounding tissues.

K

Karyotype A photomicrographic representation of a person's chromosomal constitution arranged according to the Denver classification.

Ketoacidosis An accumulation of acid in the body resulting from the accumulation of ketone bodies.

L

LE cell A cell that is a characteristic of lupus erythematosus and other autoimmune diseases. It is a mature neutrophil that has phagocytized a spherical inclusion derived from another neutrophil.

Leukocytosis A temporary increase in the number of white blood cells circulating in blood.

Leukoplakia A clinical term used to identify a white, plaque-like lesion of the oral mucosa that cannot be wiped off and cannot be diagnosed as any other disease.

Lobule (adjective, lobulated) A segment or lobe that is part of a whole. Lobules sometimes appear fused together.

Local Confined to a limited part, not general or systemic.

Locus In genetics, the position occupied by a gene on a chromosome.

Lymphadenopathy Any disease process that affects lymph nodes such that they become enlarged and palpable.

Lymphoid tissue Tissue composed of lymphocytes supported by a meshwork of connective tissue.

M

Macrodontia Abnormally large teeth.

Macrophage A large, mononuclear phagocyte derived from monocytes. Macrophages become mobile when stimulated by inflammation and interact with lymphocytes in an immune response.

Macule A flat area on the skin or mucosa, usually distinguished by color, that is different from the surrounding tissue.

Magnetic resonance imaging (MRI) A noninvasive diagnostic technique that uses radio waves to produce computerized images of internal body tissues.

Malaise A vague, indefinite feeling of discomfort, debilitation or lack of health.

Malignant Likely to cause the death of the host.

Malignant tumor Cancer; a tumor that is resistant to treatment and frequently causes death; a tumor that has the potential for uncontrolled growth and dissemination or recurrence, or both.

Margination A process during inflammation in which white blood cells tend to move to the blood walls.

Meiosis The two-step cellular division of the original germ cells, which reduces the chromosomes from 4nDNA to 1nDNA.

Metaphase The phase of cellular division in which the chromosomes are lined up evenly along the equatorial plane of the cell and in which the chromosomes are most visible.

Metastasis (plural, metastases) The transport of neoplastic cells to parts of the body remote from the primary tumor and the establishment of new tumors in those sites.

Metastatic tumor A tumor formed by cells that have been transported from the primary tumor to a site not connected to the primary tumor.

Microcirculation Small blood vessels, including arterioles, capillaries, and venules.

Microcyte A red blood cell that is smaller than normal.

Microdontia Abnormally small teeth.

Millimeter (mm) One thousandth of a meter (a meter is equivalent to 39.3 inches). The periodontal probe is of great assistance in documenting the size or diameter of a lesion that can be measured in millimeters.

Mitochondria Cytoplasmic organelles having their own DNA in a circular chromosome.

Mitosis The way in which somatic cells divide so that the two daughter cells receive the same number of identical chromosomes.

Mitotic figures Dividing cells caught in the process of mitosis.

Mucositis Mucosal inflammation.

Multifactorial conditions Those conditions in which the phenotype results from a combination of genetic factors and environmental influences.

Multilocular A term used to describe a radiographic appearance of multiple, rounded compartments or locules. These can appear "soap bubble like" or "honeycomb-like."

Mutation A permanent change in the arrangement of genetic material.

Myalgia Muscle pain.

N

Natural killer cell (NK cell) A lymphocyte that is part of the body's initial inate immunity, which by unknown mechanisms is able to destroy cells recognized as foreign.

Necrosis The pathologic death of one or more cells or a portion of tissue or organ, resulting from irreversible damage.

Neoplasia The process of the formation of tumors by the uncontrolled proliferation of cells.

Neoplasm Tumor; a new growth of tissue in which the growth of tissue is uncontrolled and progressive.

Neoplastic Pertaining to the formation of tumors by the uncontrolled proliferation of cells.

Neutropenia A diminished number of neutrophils in the blood.

Nevus (plural, nevi) A benign, localized overgrowth of melanocytes; also, a birthmark.

Nikolsky's sign Seen in some bullous diseases, such as pemphigus vulgaris and bullous pemphigoid; the superficial epithelium separates easily from the basal layer on exertion of firm sliding manual pressure.

Nodule A palpable, solid lesion in soft tissue that is up to 1 cm in diameter and may be above, level with, or beneath the skin or mucosal surface.

Nondysjunction The result of chromosomes that were crossing over and did not separate; therefore, both migrate to the same cell.

Nucleotide A hydrolytic product of nucleic acid formed by a nitrogen-containing base, a five-carbon sugar (deoxyribose), and a phosphate.

O

Odontogenic Tooth forming.

Oncology The study of tumors or neoplasms.

Oogenesis The process of formation of female germ cells (ova).

Opportunistic infection A disease caused by a microorganism that does not ordinarily cause disease but becomes pathogenic under certain circumstances.

Osteoporosis A hereditary disease marked by abnormally dense bone.

Ovulum Ovum, the mature female germ cell.

P

Pallor Paleness.

Palpation The act of feeling with the hand.

Papillary Describing a small nipple-shaped projection or elevation usually found in clusters.

Papule A small circumscribed lesion usually less than 1 cm in diameter that protrudes above the surface of normal surrounding tissue.

Parathormone Parathyroid hormone.

Parenteral Administered by injection.

Paresthesia An abnormal sensation such as prickling or tingling.

Pathogenic microorganism A microorganism that causes disease.

Pavementing Adherence of white blood cells to the walls of a blood vessel during inflammation.

Pedunculated Attached by a stem-like or stalk-like base.

Penetrance The prevalence of individuals with a given genotype that manifest clinically the phenotype associated with that trait.

Peripheral Located away from the center; indicates that the location of a lesion is in the soft tissue surrounding a bone.

Petechia A minute red spot on the skin or mucous membranes resulting from escape of a small amount of blood.

Phagocytosis A process of ingestion and digestion by cells.

Phenotype The physical and clinical visible characteristics of an individual. Genotype is the genetic composition. Phenotype is its observable appearance.

Platelet A disk-shaped structure, also called a thrombocyte, found in the blood, which plays an important role in blood coagulation.

Pleomorphic Occurs in various forms.

Polycythemia An increase in the total red blood cell mass in the blood.

Polydactyly The presence of extra fingers or toes, or both.

Polydipsia Excessive thirst.

Predilection A disposition in favor of something; preference.

Primary tumor The original tumor; the source of metastasis.

Pruritis Itching.

Purpura A group of disorders characterized by purplish or brownish-red discolorations caused by bleeding into the skin or tissues.

Purulent Containing or forming pus.

Pustule Varying-sized circumscribed, pus-filled, elevated lesions.

R

Radiolucent The black or dark areas in a radiograph that result from the ability of radiant energy to pass through the structure. Less dense structures (e.g., the pulp) are radiolucent.

Radiopaque The white or clear appearance in a radiograph that results from the inability of radiant energy to pass through a structure. The more dense the structure (i.e., amalgam restorations), the whiter it appears in the radiograph.

Receptor A cell surface protein to which a specific hormone can bind; such binding leads to biochemical events.

Recessive In genetics, a trait or characteristic manifested clinically with a double gene dose in autosomic chromosomes or with a single dose in males if the trait is X-linked.

Regeneration The process by which injured tissue is replaced with tissue identical to that present before the injury.

Repair The restoration of damaged or diseased tissues.

Rheumatoid factor A protein, an immunoglobulin M (IgM), found in serum and detectable on laboratory tests. It is associated with rheumatoid arthritis and other autoimmune diseases.

Ribonucleic acid (RNA) Single strands of polynucleotides found in all cells; different types of RNA have different functions in the production of proteins by the cell.

Ribosome The cytoplasmic organelles in which proteins are formed based on the genetic code provided by RNA.

Root resorption Observed radiographically when the apex of the tooth appears shortened or blunted and irregularly shaped. It occurs as a response to stimuli, which can result from a cyst, tumor, or trauma.

S

Sarcoma A malignant tumor of connective tissue.

Scoliosis Lateral curvature of the spine.

Serous A substance having a watery consistency; relating to serum.

Sessile Broad based.

Sign Objective evidence of disease that can be observed by a healthcare provider rather than by the patient.

Somatic cells All the cells of the human body with the exception of the primitive germ cells (oogonia and spermatogonia).

Spermatogenesis The process of formation of spermatozoa (sperm).

Spermatozoon The mature masculine germ cell.

Spina bifida A defect in the spine caused by a lack of the vertebral arches through which the spinal cord protrudes.

Spina bifida occulta Similar to spina bifida, but with little or no protrusion.

Splenomegaly Enlargement of the spleen.

Stomodeum The embryonic structure that becomes the oral cavity.

Subclinical infection An infectious disease not detectable by the usual clinical signs.

Supernumerary In excess of the normal or regular number, as in teeth.

Symptom Subjective evidence of disease or a physical disorder that is observed by the patient.

Syndactyly Soft tissue or bone fusion, or both, of fingers and toes.

Syndrome A set of signs or symptoms, or both, occurring together.

Synovial The transparent, viscous fluid that is secreted by the synovial membrane and found in joint cavities.

Synovial membrane Tissue that forms a portion of the lining of some joints; for example, the temporomandibular joint.

Systemic Pertaining to or affecting the body as a whole.

T

T lymphocyte A lymphocyte that passes through the thymus before migrating to tissues. The T lymphocyte, also called a T cell, is responsible for cell mediated immunity and may modulate the humoral immune response.

Thrombocyte A platelet.

Thrombocytopenia Decrease in the number of platelets in circulating blood.

Thymus A lymphoid organ that is situated in the chest. It reaches maximal development at about puberty and then undergoes gradual involution.

Translocation A portion of a chromosome attached to another chromosome.

Trismus Spasm of the muscles of mastication.

Trisomy A pair of chromosomes with an identical extra chromosome.

Tumor A neoplasm; also, a swelling or enlargement.

U

Undifferentiated Absence of normal differentiation; a characteristic of tumor tissue.

Unilocular A term used to describe a radiographic appearance of a single, rounded compartment or locule.

V

Vesicle A small, elevated, fluid-filled lesion that is less than 1 cm in diameter.

W

Well circumscribed The borders of the lesion are specifically defined, and one can clearly see the exact margins and extent of the lesion.

Wheal A localized swelling of tissue due to edema during inflammation often accompanied by severe itching.

Whitlow An infection involving the distal phalanx of a finger.

X

Xerophthalmia Abnormal dryness of the eyes.

Xerostomia Dryness of the mouth caused by a decrease in salivary flow.

Answers

Chapter 1

1. C	13. E
2. D	14. B
3. E	15. E
4. B	16. A
5. E	17. D
6. A	18. A
7. E	19. C
8. E	20. E
9. A	21. A
10. C	22. E
11. A	23. B
12. B	24. E

27. D	39. C
28. A	40. B
29. C	41. B
30. E	42. A
31. E	43. C
32. A	44. B
33. D	45. E
34. B	46. E
35. A	47. D
36. D	48. E
37. C	49. E
38. B	50. B

Chapter 2

1. B	14. C
2. B	15. E
3. D	16. B
4. B	17. E
5. E	18. B
6. E	19. B
7. D	20. A
8. E	21. B
9. A	22. B
10. E	23. C
11. D	24. E
12. C	25. C
13. A	26. D

Chapter 3

1. C	14. C
2. B	15. B
3. D	16. A
4. A	17. C
5. E	18. D
6. C	19. A
7. D	20. D
8. A	21. B
9. B	22. C
10. E	23. E
11. A	24. B
12. C	25. E
13. B	26. D

27. C	29. E
28. E	30. D

Chapter 4

1. E	16. E
2. B	17. E
3. B	18. E
4. E	19. E
5. E	20. B
6. C	21. C
7. B	22. C
8. C	23. E
9. D	24. E
10. B	25. A
11. E	26. D
12. D	27. C
13. C	28. C
14. C	29. D
15. D	30. D

Chapter 5

1. C	8. E
2. A	9. D
3. D	10. C
4. E	11. A
5. E	12. B
6. E	13. A
7. B	14. B

15. D	31. B
16. C	32. A
17. E	33. D
18. E	34. A
19. C	35. B
20. A	36. D
21. B	37. C
22. B	38. E
23. C	39. A
24. D	40. B
25. E	41. D
26. A	42. C
27. D	43. E
28. A	44. C
29. E	45. D
30. B	

Chapter 6

1. C	11. A
2. A	12. D
3. B	13. C
4. D	14. C
5. B	15. B
6. A	16. A
7. B	17. A
8. D	18. E
9. E	19. C
10. D	20. E

Chapter 6—cont'd

21. B	25. E
22. D	26. A
23. A	27. E
24. B	

Chapter 7

1. D	11. C
2. D	12. C
3. C	13. D
4. C	14. C
5. A	15. D
6. E	16. B
7. C	17. A
8. D	18. A
9. B	19. C
10. E	20. A

21. D	31. C
22. A	32. A
23. C	33. C
24. A	34. B
25. A	35. C
26. C	36. E
27. B	37. B
28. C	38. E
29. D	39. B
30. B	40. C

Chapter 8

1. D	9. B
2. D	10. E
3. B	11. C
4. D	12. A
5. E	13. B
6. A	14. C
7. C	15. A
8. C	

Chapter 9

1. A	14. E
2. D	15. B
3. C	16. A
4. E	17. D
5. C	18. B
6. C	19. A
7. E	20. D
8. E	21. A
9. D	22. B
10. C	23. E
11. D	24. D
12. E	25. C
13. A	

Chapter 10

1. C	6. A
2. B	7. C
3. E	8. C
4. B	9. E
5. C	10. D

Index

Note: Page numbers in *italics* refer to illustrations; page numbers followed by t refer to tables.